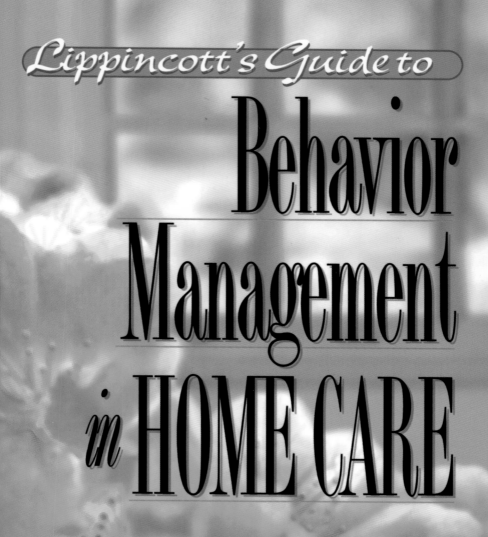

Lippincott's Guide to

Behavior Management in HOME CARE

Nina A. Klebanoff

Nina Maria Smith

Lippincott

Abbreviations and Acronyms

AA: Alcoholics Anonymous
ACHPR: Agency for Health Care Policy and Research
ADLs: activities of daily living
AIDS: acquired immunodeficiency syndrome
ARF: at risk for falls
AST: aspartate transaminase
B/P: blood pressure (lying, sitting, and standing)
CAD: coronary artery disease
CHF: congestive heart failure
CMD: cognitive mental disorder
CNS: central nervous system
CO$_2$: carbon dioxide
COPD: chronic obstructive pulmonary disease
CP: cardiopulmonary
CPR: cardiopulmonary resuscitation
CV: cardiovascular
d: day
DAT: dementia of the Alzheimer's type
DSM-IV: *Diagnostic and Statistical Manual of Mental Disorders, 4th ed.*
ECG: electrocardiogram
ECT: electroconvulsive therapy
EENT: eye, ears, nose, and throat
EPS: extrapyramidal syndrome
f/c: family/caregiver
FDA: Food and Drug Administration
GI: gastrointestinal
GU: genitourinary
HCl: hydrochloric
HIV: human immunodeficiency virus
IADLs: instrumental activities of daily living
LSD: lysergic acid diethylamine
MAOI: monoamine oxidase inhibitor
mEq/L: milliequivalent per liter
μg: microgram

mg: milligram
MI: myocardial infarction
MID: multi-infarct dementia
mL: milliliter
MSW: medical social worker
NA: Narcotics Anonymous
NIMH: National Institute of Mental Health
NMS: neuroleptic malignant syndrome
NSAID: nonsteroidal anti-inflammatory drug
OC: obsessive-compulsive
OCD: obsessive-compulsive disorder
OT: occupational therapist, therapy
p/c: patient/caregiver
PCA: patient-controlled analgesia
pcg: primary caregiver
pCO$_2$: carbon dioxide partial pressure or tension
PCP: phencyclidine
p/f/c: patient/family/caregiver
pH: hydrogen ion concentration
PMS: premenstrual syndrome
po: orally
PO$_2$: oxygen partial pressure or tension
prn: as needed
pt: patient
PT: physical therapist, therapy
PTSD: post-traumatic stress disorder
REM: rapid eye movement
s/s: signs and symptoms
SSRI: selective serotonin reuptake inhibitor
STDs: sexually or socially transmitted diseases
TENS: transcutaneous electrical nerve stimulation
THA: tetrahydroaminoacridine
VD: venereal disease

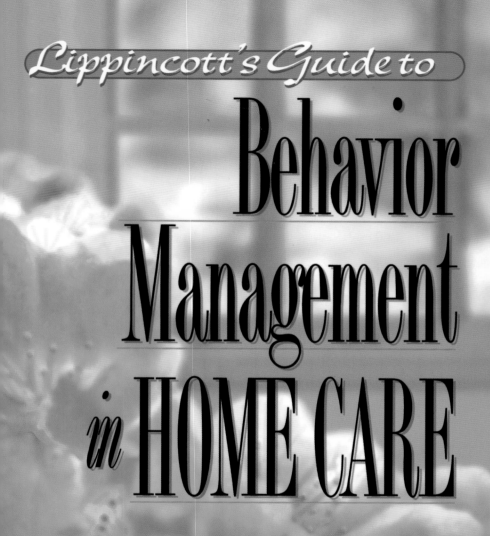

Lippincott's Guide to

Behavior Management *in* HOME CARE

Nina A. Klebanoff

Nina Maria Smith

Lippincott

Abbreviations and Acronyms

AA: Alcoholics Anonymous
ACHPR: Agency for Health Care Policy and Research
ADLs: activities of daily living
AIDS: acquired immunodeficiency syndrome
ARF: at risk for falls
AST: aspartate transaminase
B/P: blood pressure (lying, sitting, and standing)
CAD: coronary artery disease
CHF: congestive heart failure
CMD: cognitive mental disorder
CNS: central nervous system
CO_2: carbon dioxide
COPD: chronic obstructive pulmonary disease
CP: cardiopulmonary
CPR: cardiopulmonary resuscitation
CV: cardiovascular
d: day
DAT: dementia of the Alzheimer's type
DSM-IV: *Diagnostic and Statistical Manual of Mental Disorders, 4th ed.*
ECG: electrocardiogram
ECT: electroconvulsive therapy
EENT: eye, ears, nose, and throat
EPS: extrapyramidal syndrome
f/c: family/caregiver
FDA: Food and Drug Administration
GI: gastrointestinal
GU: genitourinary
HCl: hydrochloric
HIV: human immunodeficiency virus
IADLs: instrumental activities of daily living
LSD: lysergic acid diethylamine
MAOI: monoamine oxidase inhibitor
mEq/L: milliequivalent per liter
µg: microgram

mg: milligram
MI: myocardial infarction
MID: multi-infarct dementia
mL: milliliter
MSW: medical social worker
NA: Narcotics Anonymous
NIMH: National Institute of Mental Health
NMS: neuroleptic malignant syndrome
NSAID: nonsteroidal anti-inflammatory drug
OC: obsessive-compulsive
OCD: obsessive-compulsive disorder
OT: occupational therapist, therapy
p/c: patient/caregiver
PCA: patient-controlled analgesia
pcg: primary caregiver
pCO_2: carbon dioxide partial pressure or tension
PCP: phencyclidine
p/f/c: patient/family/caregiver
pH: hydrogen ion concentration
PMS: premenstrual syndrome
po: orally
PO_2: oxygen partial pressure or tension
prn: as needed
pt: patient
PT: physical therapist, therapy
PTSD: post-traumatic stress disorder
REM: rapid eye movement
s/s: signs and symptoms
SSRI: selective serotonin reuptake inhibitor
STDs: sexually or socially transmitted diseases
TENS: transcutaneous electrical nerve stimulation
THA: tetrahydroaminoacridine
VD: venereal disease

Lippincott's Guide to
Behavior Management
in HOME CARE

Lippincott's Guide to

Behavior Management

in HOME CARE

Nina A. Klebanoff, PhD, RN, CS, LPCC
Behavioral Health Consultant
Independent Practice
Carson, New Mexico

Nina Maria Smith, RNC, MEd
President
Integrated Behavioral Health Consultants
Consultant
National Behavioral Health Programs
Western Medical Services
Fort Collins, Colorado

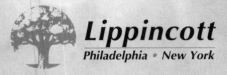

Lippincott
Philadelphia • New York

Acquisitions Editor: Margaret Zuccarini
Editorial Assistant: Emily Cotlier
Project Editor: Sandra Cherrey Scheinin
Production Manager: Helen Ewan
Production Coordinator: Kathryn Rule
Design Coordinator: Doug Smock
Indexer: Victoria Boyle

9   8   7   6   5   4   3   2   1

Library of Congress Cataloging in Publication Data

Klebanoff, Nina A.
    Lippincott's guide to behavior management in home care / by Nina
A. Klebanoff, Nina M. Smith. — 1st ed.
        p.   cm.
    Includes bibliographical references and index.
    ISBN 0-397-55432-X (alk. paper)
    1. Home nursing.   2. Behavior modification.   3. Nurse and patient.
I. Smith, Nina M. (Nina Marie)
    [DNLM: 1. Home Care Services—handbooks.   2. Behavior—handbooks.
3. Activities of Daily Living—handbooks.   4. Mental Disorders-
-nursing—handbooks.   WY 49 K63L 1997]
    RT120.H65K56   1997
    610.73—dc21
    DNLM/DLC
    for Library of Congress   96–53511
                                                                         CIP

Care has been taken to confirm the accuracy of the information presented and to describe generally accepted practices. However, the authors, editors, and publisher are not responsible for errors or omissions or for any consequences from application of the information in this book and make no warranty, express or implied, with respect to the contents of the publication.

The authors, editors and publisher have exerted every effort to ensure that drug selection and dosage set forth in this text are in accordance with current recommendations and practice at the time of publication. However, in view of ongoing research, changes in government regulations, and the constant flow of information relating to drug therapy and drug reactions, the reader is urged to check the package insert for each drug for any change in indications and dosage and for added warnings and precautions. This is particularly important when the recommended agent is a new or infrequently employed drug.

Some drugs and medical devices presented in this publication have Food and Drug Administration (FDA) clearance for limited use in restricted research settings. It is the responsibility of the health care provider to ascertain the FDA status of each drug or device planned for use in their clinical practice.

⊚This Paper Meets the Requirements of ANSI/NISO Z39.48-1992 (Permanence of Paper).

To my wonderful parents, Elizabeth Kasarda Klebanoff and M. Robert Klebanoff, to Mellis I. Schmidt for her unwavering support and love, and to Baby John.

—*Nina Klebanoff*

To my family—Bob, Cara, and Rachel—for their unending love, help, and belief in me; to Janet Erinakes for teaching me home care; to Linda Brown for being there during the crunch; and to Western Medical Services for its enthusiastic support for this project.

—*Nina Smith*

Preface

In this current environment of health care cost-cutting, shorter hospitalizations, and managed health care, it is increasingly likely that individuals will receive health care at home. An array of home health care professionals is necessary to care for them. It is the intent of *Lippincott's Guide to Behavior Management in Home Care* to aid the home care nurse and other health care professionals in sifting through the behavioral problems inherent in providing health care services to adults and older adults in the home care setting, and in providing guidance in identifying appropriate and effective interventions. This guide presents useful clinical approaches that are specifically geared for use in the home setting to provide comprehensive, holistic care.

We are using the phrase "in-home behavioral health care" instead of in-home mental health care, psychiatric home health care, or other variations. We feel that "in-home behavioral health care" focuses on the client and family or caregiver. The family or caregiver (abbreviated as "f/c") includes those persons affiliated, formally or informally, with the patient and who are directly or indirectly involved in the provision of home care. Behavioral health care encompasses ambulatory care and services for the following: the behavioral aspects of primary care; psychiatric, mental illness, and chemical dependency or substance abuse treatment; mental illness and substance abuse prevention; and health teaching, mental wellness, and health promotion.

TEXT CONTENT

This book is divided into two parts. Part I, **Essentials of Behavior Management in Home Care,** is an introduction to communication and caretaking from a behavior management perspective. This includes caretaker self-awareness and communication; safety and crisis intervention skills; defensive, protective, and coping mechanisms; family or caregiver dynamics and communication; and home management problems and solutions. Part I also includes content about mental status examinations and treatment planning in the home setting, documentation guidelines specifically for use in home behavioral health care, and an outcome measurement system.

Part II, **Common Problems Encountered in Home Care,** delineates problems commonly encountered in the home care arena. The format for each behavioral problem includes:

- Problem Description
- Problem Identification, including Characteristics and Observable Behaviors and Factors Related to the Problem
- Problem List
- Problem Management
- Nursing Interventions, and Rationale for the following areas: Behavioral, Emotional, Cognitive, Physical, Social, and Spiritual
- Nursing Goals
- Patient Goals
- Patient and Family/Caregiver Outcomes
- Resources and Information

Medication Management is included for all problems where it is a part of treatment.

The behavioral problems are in tabbed alphabetical order for easy retrieval, and are cross-referenced in order to guide you to related information. For ease of use, lists and tables condense information and problem characteristics. This concise, thorough presentation is easy to consult quickly.

The appendices contain the frequently used, standardized behavior assessment tools and instruments, as noted for each problem. All these assessment tools are appropriate for in-home behavioral health care. The tools are in alphabetical order; each is complete with description, source information, and complete administration and scoring information. A bibliography of background readings is also included in the appendices.

KEY FEATURES

The guide includes the following key features to assist the home health care provider:

- Compact size that can easily be carried for ready reference
- Overview of behavioral problems and interventions in the home care setting
- Tabbed and alphabetically ordered entries for easy retrieval
- Consistent, easy-to-consult format with lists and tables
- Icons that highlight the following areas of intervention: Behavioral, Emotional, Cognitive, Physical, Social, and Spiritual
- Cross-referencing for additional information
- Practical resources of support groups and information for many common problems
- Appendix with multiple Assessment Tools

The creation of the first edition has been an incredible opportunity for us to share our experience in and research about an important topic in the changing health care system. We are proud of this work and trust that you will find the guide useful in enhancing the therapeutic process in the home health care milieu. Beyond that, we want to inspire and encourage providers to care holistically for patients and their families or caregivers in the least restrictive, most natural, and productive environment—the home.

Nina A. Klebanoff, PhD, RN, CS, LPCC

Nina M. Smith, RNC, MEd

Contents

Part 2
Common Problems Encountered in Home Care   *49*

Abbreviations and Acronyms   *50*

A

B

C

D

E

F

G

H

I

L

M

N

O

P

R

S

T

Toileting Problems *(See Activities of Daily Living Problems)*

V

Violence, Directed at Self, Other(s), or Property *(See Abusive Behaviors, Aggressive Behaviors, Self-Mutilation, and Suicidal and Homicidal Behaviors)*

W

Part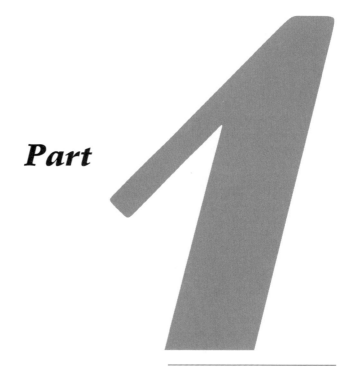

ESSENTIALS OF BEHAVIOR MANAGEMENT IN HOME CARE

Introduction to Behavior Problems in Home Health Care

HOME MANAGEMENT PROBLEMS AND SOLUTIONS

The pt's and f/c's need to manage and function in the home is the premise on which home care is based. A safe, hygienic, growth-promoting environment provides support to assist the pt in maintaining functional independence. Home management provides resources to meet self-care needs, safety, coping, decision-making skills, and relationship management and formation.

The pt needing assistance to manage at home is lacking:

1. Skills to function independently
2. Confidence
3. Interdependence with others
4. A perception of self as capable
5. Structure and assistance in maintaining a clean environment
6. The knowledge to correct these limitations

The f/c request assistance when the burden becomes overwhelming because they lack the ability to assist the pt or they are unable to provide the level of care required.

Factors related to the inability of the pt to maintain home management include:

1. Inadequate support systems
2. Inadequate financial resources
3. Impaired cognitive or emotional functioning
4. Disorganized or dysfunctional living environment
5. Disease or injury
6. Lack of role modeling
7. Unfamiliarity with resources available

Assessment: Identifying the Problem

The provider assesses the pt's:

1. Ability to function independently
2. Previous level of highest functioning
3. Home environment
4. The f/c situation and relationship
5. Continuum of care needs
6. Secondary gains from being ill
7. Support systems
8. Financial resources
9. Spiritual and cultural needs
10. Knowledge base of disease and medications
11. Coping skills
12. Self-care
13. Deficits in communication
14. Decision-making skills
15. Health and safety hazards
16. Motivation to maintain self in a functionally independent situation

Intervention: Determining the Solutions

The provider then gives the assistance necessary to allow the pt and f/c to:

1. Plan for care
2. Meet emotional needs through significant relationships and social activities
3. Deal with stress
4. Maintain as much independence as possible
5. Develop and practice daily living skills
6. Make decisions regarding care
7. Adopt behaviors reflecting life-style changes to create and sustain a healthy, growth-promoting environment

Community resources are effectively used and optimal health and f/c functioning is improved through effective communication and healthy coping skills. Understanding home management provides the premise for assisting the pt and f/c to understand the disease concept, medications necessary, and intervention techniques and skills that will maintain the pt successfully in his or her own home.

Diagnosis/Problem, Medication, and Symptom Education Checklists

Patient/Family Caregiver Knowledge Checklist

Teach the pt and f/c the following diagnosis-related information:

_____   Psychiatric diagnosis of the pt's disorder.
_____   S/s of the pt's psychiatric disorder.

_____   The disease- and illness-imposed requirements for the management of the pt's psychiatric disorder.

_____   Medical diagnosis of the pt's condition.

_____   S/s of the pt's medical condition.

_____   Disease- and illness-imposed requirements for the management of the pt's medical condition.

_____   Specific home health care problems and outcomes associated with the pt's psychiatric and medical disorders.

Management of Medication Teaching Checklist

Teach the pt and f/c the following medication-related information:

_____   The therapeutic effects of the medication(s).

_____   How the medication(s) is to work.

_____   Length of time it will take the medication(s) to achieve the desired effects.

_____   Key signs that indicate the medication(s) is working.

_____   The side effects of the medication(s).

_____   The adverse effects of the medication(s).

_____   Foods, drugs, and other substances to avoid while taking the medication(s) that the pt is taking.

_____   The possible consequences of not taking the medication(s) as directed by the prescriber.

_____   Tests, medical examinations, or other procedures that might be necessary to monitor the medication(s).

Symptoms Management Checklist

Use this checklist as a guide to teach the pt and f/c the following symptoms-management information:

_____   The need for monitoring the symptoms of the pt's disease and illness.

_____   General health, environmental surroundings, attitude, and behavioral variables may positively influence to the restoration, maintenance, and achievement of an optimal level of independent functioning and wellness and have identified individual indicators that relate to the pt's recovery and healing.

_____   General health, environmental surroundings, attitude, and behavioral variables may trigger a relapse and have identified the pt's individual symptoms that relate to relapse.

_____   The need to establish effective symptom management techniques.

_____   An emergency plan to implement if the symptoms become severe and the pt's current coping skills are not sufficient.

SELF-AWARENESS AND COMMUNICATION

Self-Awareness

Self-awareness is important for home care nurses, especially those engaged in behavioral or psychiatric care. It is necessary to know yourself and your preferred communication style before you try to help another person. Some needs to consider are your own awareness and need to love and be loved, control and be controlled, and take care of and be taken care of. Self-awareness helps the nurse maintain boundaries, adapt communication style to the specific situation, and focus on the pt and f/c.

Self-awareness also helps the nurse develop empathy and understanding for pt's and f/c's perspectives. Different people have different expectations of themselves and others, different strengths and limitations, and different reactions to the same stimulus. An appreciation of the varying behavioral styles of the pt, f/c, and providers makes for clearer, more effective communication, in addition to reduced conflict and a healthier home care climate.

Table 1-1 presents different styles of communication. Most people are a blend of these styles. Considering the styles of all the involved parties is productive. Instead of anticipating a stressful, adversarial interaction you can learn to grow and be creative, rather than avoid, deny, or fight out the conflict.

Communication

Communication uses verbal and nonverbal interactions to convey ideas and meanings to another person. Tone of voice, choice of words, facial expression, and gestures communicate ideas and feelings in addition to the actual words used. There are several kinds of communication. Directive communication assigns duties, gives definite information, or demonstrates how to perform a procedure. Creative communication assists another to determine what should be done and how to do it. Therapeutic communication is empathic and perceptive. When communication is therapeutic, the pt is the focus of communication. From initial contact throughout delivery of home care, the provider must assess the pt's grasp of the communication. Through therapeutic techniques, the provider can help the pt to express thoughts and feelings so that needs can be identified.

Table 1-2 outlines health provider interactions that enhance human dignity; Table 1-3 lists health provider interactions that dehumanize the pt. Table 1-4 presents blocks to therapeutic communication, which are to be avoided, along with measures to counter the blocks.

Physical and Cultural Blocks to Communication

When you deal with pts and f/c who have physical reasons why they cannot communicate fully or who are of different cultures than yourself, additional considerations are needed to foster clear communication. Strategies to deal with more obvious physical and cultural blocks to communication are:

- Assess and understand the background and experience of each pt, including whether or not the person is in pain, fatigued, nervous, weak, or ill.
- Find out if you are speaking the same language; if not, use an interpreter to translate the words and the message.
- Avoid indiscriminate use of nursing, medical, or home health care terminology and abbreviations.
- If communication seems difficult, ask if there is something you can do to enable the person to better understand you.
- Face the person directly and at the same level (especially if pt is in a wheelchair), or lower if the pt might feel powerless.

Text continues on p. 11.

Table 1-1
Four Behavioral Styles and Their Differences

	Senser (Doer)	Intuitor (Imaginer)	Thinker (Concentrator)	Feeler (Meditator)
Description	Understands world by senses; results matter	Understands world by ideas; long-range planner	Understands world by analysis; details matter	Understands world by emotions; systems oriented
Pace	Dead run and then collapse	Fast-paced glide	Moderate to slow, steady march	Moderately paced glide to trot
Best way to approach	Be brief; get right to point; emphasize results and urgency; be on time; give direct answers	Relate to general, big picture; speak in terms of future; show interest in creative ideas; use imaginative approach; plan unhurried meeting; play with ideas; avoid saying "it can't be done"	Have all facts, data, and options; be professional, conservative, low-key; emphasize specific, sound, reliable statistics; ask for data-type feedback; talk clearly and slowly; provide rational appraisal	Be warm, personal, and enthusiastic; use firsthand testimonials and personal stories; be helpful and supportive; use eye contact and make emotional connection

continued

Table 1-1
Four Behavioral Styles and Their Differences Continued

Senser (Doer)	Intuitor (Imaginer)	Thinker (Concentrator)	Feeler (Meditator)
Strengths			
Turns ideas into action; driving force on the team; moves ahead with determination; will take risks	Original, creative, visionary problem solver; sees new patterns and long-term effects; has new and exciting methods; willing to move ahead	Consistently produces; cool and calm under pressure; objective stabilizing member of team	Skilled in communication; is warm and nurtures team; reads between lines
Limitations			
Fails to see long-term effects of actions; low tolerance for different pace of others; fears losing control, being bored, or looking weak	Unrealistic ideas; in "ivory tower"; wonderful ideas, but would take too much time; fears blame and humiliation	Plays it too safe; likely to say "no" if pressured; lacks enthusiasm; fears confusion, lack of clarity, confrontation, and feelings	Overreacts; relies on gut feelings not facts; too concerned about others' feelings; impulsive; fears criticism, not being liked, conflict, and alarming messages
Can be more effective by			
Being patient; giving more information; participating in the team	Being objective; managing time; paying attention to detail and organization	Adjusting better to change; varying routines; stating feelings	Being less emotionally reactive and more businesslike

Adapted from Keys (1985); Siegel (1992).

Table 1-2
Health Provider's Interactions that Enhance the Human Dignity of the Patient

Health Provider Interactions	Patient Reaction
1. Calling/referring to the pt by proper name and title (expression of warmth and respect)	1. Pt feels that he or she has a separate identity and is special
2. Recognizing the pt's presence (respectful care)	2. Pts feel that they count
3. Listening to what the pt has to say (respectful care)	3. Pt feels that what he or she has to say is important
4. Allowing the pt to *own* the problem (self-empowering care)	4. Pt feels that he or she has some control over the problem and can make decisions
5. Being consistent in the care that is given (continuity of care)	5. Pt develops a sense of direction and security and knows he or she can depend on certain consequences of certain behaviors
6. Relating to pt as an adult, regardless of age (respectful care)	6. Pt receives clear directions and does not feel put-down
7. Setting limits for the pt's benefit and not the provider's convenience (respectful care)	7. Pt receives positive, fair directions without a threat, which eliminates the need to test the limits
8. Focusing on the strengths of the pt, giving credit for positive behavior (respectful care)	8. Pt feels useful, significant, and receives the message that he or she can make decisions
9. Allowing the pt to do as much as possible for the self, depending on fluctuations in the pt's condition (respectful care)	9. Pt feels a sense of improvement and that he or she can be more independent
10. Trusting the pt's desire to find more positive behaviors than currently have (respectful care)	10. Pt feels that the provider has trust in him or her; pt receives a sense of hope
11. Promising only what can be realistically and reasonably done (complete information)	11. Pt feels that he or she can depend on the provider
12. Holding the pt responsible for behavior (knowledge of agency policies and procedures and expectations)	12. Pt develops a sense of responsibility and learns to view limits set as a consequence of, instead of punishment for behavior

Table 1-3
Health Provider's Interactions that Dehumanize the Patient

Health Provider Interactions	Patient Reaction
1. Talking about pts in their presence	1. Pt feels like an object
2. Reminding pts that they will not do something	2. Sets the pt up to act out (see Box 1-1) by reinforcing negative behavior
3. Threatening pts or otherwise showing them who the "boss" is	3. Pt complies through fear
4. Conversing with another home health team member or family member or caregiver instead of pt while caring for pt	4. Pt feels like he does not exist and that he is a nobody
5. Referring to pt by diagnosis	5. Pt feels like a nonperson
6. Disregarding the pt's plan of care and doing your "own thing"	6. Pt is confused as to what is expected and becomes more insecure if the plan changes
7. Repeating what the pt says in a mimicky way	7. Pts feel like they do not have anything of worth to say or become afraid to express their thoughts and feelings
8. Not listening to the pt	8. Pt feels that no one understands or cares
9. Demeaning, discounting, or belittling the pt	9. Pt feels hopeless and helpless and a sense of being trapped
10. Teasing the pt	10. Pt feels put down
11. Treating the pt as a child	11. Pt feels as though they no longer have control over their own life and that they have lost their "power base"
12. Provoking guilt in a pt	12. Pt feels depressed and can become outwardly angry
13. Ridiculing a pt	13. Pts feel that they have failed and that they cannot possibly succeed
14. Exploiting a pt	14. Pt feels used
15. Flirting with a pt	15. If pts perceive the behavior as genuine they will be confused by the home health provider's response
16. Displacing (see Table 1-5) your angry feelings on a pt	16. Pt becomes fearful of expressing needs because of the danger of retaliation
17. Clowning around in the presence of a pt who is confused or disoriented, or otherwise expressing humor that is not relevant to the home care situation	17. Pt becomes more confused by the environmental stimulation, which can trigger aggressive outbursts
18. Expressing favoritism about another pt	18. Pt becomes jealous and may begin to act out (see Box 1-1)

Table 1-4
Blocks With Counters to Therapeutic Communication

Block	Counter
1. Using reassuring clichés	1. Ask for more information
2. Giving advice	2. Help pts explore their thoughts so that they can arrive at their own solutions; supply pertinent information that may give them a better basis for decision-making
3. Giving approval	3. Focus on the pt's values and feelings
4. Requesting an explanation	4. Encourage pt to describe feelings
5. Agreeing with the pt	5. Accept pt's statements and encourage elaboration through use of general leads or reflection
6. Expressing disapproval	6. Accept the pt's own values
7. Listening only for words	7. Listen for how words are said—the content, meaning, intention, and the feeling—to determine the message

- If the individual has had several losses, such as hearing as well as vision, reduce background noises (turn off the television or radio, close the door, or move to a quieter place).
- Knowing that a person who is legally blind may not be totally blind, increase the light, read information, or describe the location of items, if that will help the pt to "see" better.
- Check with the person who is hearing impaired if one ear is better than the other and make sure that, if a person is wearing a hearing aid, it is clean and supplied with a good battery; speak in a slow, calm, and clear voice at a lower frequency, but do not drop your volume at the end of your sentences.
- Move slowly.

Promoting Effective Communication

Five "Rs" and four "Cs" of communication can help to promote effective and empathic communication.

The five "Rs" of communication are to:

1. Reassess
2. Reconsider
3. Rechannel
4. Redirect
5. Reinforce

The four "Cs" of communication are:

1. Calmness
2. Caring
3. Clarity
4. Consistency

Guidelines for Moving Communication Conflict From Problem to Positive Change

When conflict occurs, the following guidelines can assist in creating positive change.

1. Breathe and let go of viewing it as a problem.
2. Listen using empathy for signals that bring a new solution.
3. "See" the situation as resolved.
4. Take responsibility for your part in the event.
5. Determine what you want to say and how you can simply say it.
6. Ask open-ended questions.
7. Wait to hear the answers without interruption.
8. Mean what you say by keeping your tone of voice, facial expression, and actions in harmony with the content of your message and adjusting them to the way you would like to be addressed.
9. Try to evaluate objectively all that you see and hear.
10. Ask how you can help.
11. Listen to the feedback.
12. Summarize and validate the information.
13. Check the impact of the communication.

SAFETY CONCERNS: ASSESSMENT AND INTERVENTIONS

The level of function, cognition, and emotional status; the social and health history; drugs and medications used; and sensory and neurologic deficits can all present risks for crises and accidents in the home setting for the pt, f/c, and providers. Falls, various behavior problems, suicide, and homicide are some of the accidents and crises that can result from these risks if providers do not intervene.

Fall Prevention

On admission, it is important to assess the pt for the risk of falling and institute a fall prevention program if the pt is deemed at risk for falls. (See the Appendix for an "At Risk for Falls and Falls Risk Factors Assessment" tool.)

Documentation of planned interventions should be included in the plan of care. Pts may be taken off the fall prevention program after their condition improves or their environment is manipulated to prevent falls.

The assessment for potential falls includes asking and observing:

1. Are handrails or grab bars placed in the pt's area, stairs and hallways, and bathroom?
2. Are there scatter rugs that are not taped down or removed to prevent slipping and tripping?
3. Is lighting adequate and proper and are pathways clear in all stairways, hallways, and other areas?
4. Is the air temperature in the home not too low to prevent a drop in body temperature, which leads to dizziness and falls?

5. Is the air temperature in the home not too high to prevent restlessness, which leads to falls?
6. Is the hot water temperature on a low setting (no more than 120°F) and are ground fault interrupters in the bathroom and kitchen outlets to prevent falling in response to accidental scalding or shock?
7. Is the pt oriented?
8. If the pt is in a hospital bed, are there side rails?
9. Can the pt easily obtain assistance?
10. Does the pt need assistance to ambulate or to transfer?
11. Does the pt take narcotics or sedatives?
12. Does the pt exercise regularly?
13. Does the pt wear proper footwear?
14. Are there other hazards in the home, such as step stools without rails, open landings, unfastened electrical cords, malfunctioning assistive devices, or slippery surfaces in the home environment?

Provider Home Visit Safety

The safety of providers is paramount, and certain precautions, if taken, will ensure a successful home visit. Currently there are no federal Occupational Safety and Health Administration rules for home health care. The following steps are recommended:

Plan Your Home Visit

Before the first visit to a pt, consider:

- Agency resources, program, and goals
- The community in which the pt lives (eg, community resources; socioeconomic, cultural, and environmental factors; and access to neighborhood and safety factors)
- Data from referral sources and reviewing referral information to make certain all necessary information is provided
- Knowledge of nursing and medical practices
- Your own strengths, values, and limitations
- Consultation with experienced staff
- Development of a specific plan to reduce your own anxiety
- Development of a specific plan that is pt and f/c centered, achievable in the allowable time, realistic, and appropriate
- Visitation by appointment; ALWAYS make arrangements to visit before you actually arrive at the pt's home
- Clear identification of yourself and the purpose of the home visit
- Self-defense and crisis prevention techniques

The Initial and Ongoing Home Visits

NEVER hesitate to take safety precautions, even if it means a missed or delayed home visit, and take the following home visit precautions:

- Do not act hesitant or apologetic.
- Never walk into a home uninvited or force your way into a home because the pt and f/c have a right to refuse service.

- Know exactly where you are going (use a map and get precise directions to the home).
- Carry and wear identification, a functional and well maintained cellular telephone, and telephone numbers of the agency, police and fire departments, and the pt who you will be visiting (if it is in an apartment building, get the manager's telephone number and apartment number).
- Be sure that your car is in good working order and that you have sufficient gasoline as well as provisions, such as a snack and water and a blanket in the winter.
- Do not carry excessive amounts of money with you, but do have enough for emergency transportation and telephone calls.
- Avoid carrying a purse or bag, and keep your money and identification in a pocket.
- Park as close to and in view of the pt's home as possible, and lock your car doors and place all valuables in a locked trunk.
- When walking, avoid groups of people.
- Carry your car keys in your hand with a personal safety alarm or emergency response device attached.
- Wear clothing and shoes that fit comfortably and well so that you can move safely and quickly, if necessary.
- Never knock on unmarked doors or on doors of homes other than those of the pt's whom you are visiting.
- Be alert at all times, trust your intuition or instincts, and if you have any doubts about the safety of entering a home or apartment building, do not do so, and notify your supervisor immediately.
- If during a home visit you have fears or doubts about safety, remain calm, speak softly, and leave the home as quickly as possible.
- If a person in the home appears intoxicated, reschedule the home visit and leave.
- If any weapons are present, either ask that they be secured or, if they are not removed or you are afraid to ask for their removal, quietly leave.
- If a pet is excessively obnoxious or is hostile to you, ask that it be put in another room or leave in a composed manner.
- Do not engage in lengthy conversation (not related to the pt's care) with the f/c or neighbors of the pt outside of the home.
- Note all possible exits from the house and sit so that you have easy access to these exits should an emergency arise.
- If you carry an equipment bag, keep it where you can see it, and keep it closed when you are not using it.
- If a serious verbal argument occurs in the home, simply leave.
- If someone in the home or a pt's neighborhood becomes a safety problem, make a joint visit with another provider, arrange for an escort (eg, from a neighborhood police station), or make the home visit when the person is gone.

CRISIS INTERVENTION SKILLS

A crisis, or a sudden change, event, or turning point usually lasts from 4 to 6 weeks. A crisis can include physical, emotional, financial, and interpersonal aspects. In a crisis the pt or f/c is highly stressed or overwhelmed and may not be able to use the usual problem-solving and coping skills. Effective crisis intervention reduces the severity, duration, and incidence of mental problems and disorders (Chandler, 1993).

General Guidelines for Crisis Intervention

1. Determine if anyone involved is a safety risk to the self or others, and initiate precautions if necessary.
2. Assist the pt and f/c to confront reality and identify the facets of the crisis.
3. Encourage the people involved to express their emotions nondestructively and assist with and allow catharsis (emotional ventilation), but discourage the pt and f/c from blaming others or self.
4. Encourage the pt and f/c not to focus on all of the implications of the crisis at once.
5. Avoid giving false reassurances.
6. Identify the effectiveness of past and current coping mechanisms, strengths and assets, and other resources.
7. Assist in the development of new coping mechanisms, strengths, and resources to deal with the current crisis, if indicated.
8. Clarify any fantasies with facts and identify misinformation and misperceptions.
9. Assist those involved to identify alternative courses of action, evaluate the possible courses, to decide on a course of action with a stated time frame, and evaluate if the crisis was resolved by the chosen course of action.
10. Encourage those affected by the crisis to seek help and provide referrals that you can endorse.
11. Assist the pt and f/c to identify and mobilize resources to help with the day-to-day tasks of living and home management until they are able to resume their roles.
12. Anticipate with those involved what coping skills, strengths, and resources can be used in the future (Carpenito, 1992; Chandler, 1993).

Telephone Crisis Intervention

Often, a care provider learns through a telephone call that a pt or f/c member is distressed enough to be considering suicide. Prompt, practical, and caring responses are vital for successful intervention. These telephone crisis interventions should be followed.

1. Ask the pt:
   - What the telephone number is
   - Where he or she currently is
   - If pt is alone or with someone (and if with someone, ask who)
   - If pt has taken any medication(s), and if so, which medication and how many were taken
   - If pt has any other plans to harm the self, and if so, what the plans are, what will be used to harm the self, and if the means are available now
2. If pt is alone, has taken an overdose of medications, or has a plan or another means to harm the self:
   - Make a contract with the pt that he or she will answer the telephone because you are going to hang-up, but will call right back.

- Hang up and call 911, or other means of summoning emergency assistance.
- Report the incident, providing the pt's name, address, your name, company or agency, and relationship with the pt.
- Call the pt back and stay on the telephone until the emergency responders (eg, the police and paramedics) arrive; if the pt does not answer the telephone, call the emergency responder system back to report that the pt is not answering the telephone and they might need to break into the home.
- Provide any further information requested by the emergency responders (eg, the pt's physician(s) and telephone number and the names and numbers of pertinent family members).
- Call the pt's physician and your supervisor to report the incident in detail.
- Document the incident completely and file an incident report.

In-Home Emergency Crisis Prevention and Intervention

Violent situations, drug or alcohol abuse, and pt ideation involving self-harm or harm to others may be present when the nurse is at the home care site. The following steps should be implemented, and the safety precautions detailed previously should also be considered.

- Immediately contact your clinical supervisor if there is suspected substance abuse or violent activity in the home.
- If drug or alcohol usage is within view during your home visit, ask those present to wait until the visit is completed, and if this is not done, notify the pt and f/c that you are leaving, and will reschedule the home visit for a later date.
- Any pt who verbalizes ideation involving thoughts of self-harm or harm to others (See Section 2) will be considered for inpatient assessment, placed on suicide evaluation, or 24-hour watch depending on the intensity of the suicidal or homicidal thoughts and feelings.
- Establish and reassess a 24-hour on-call policy and procedure (Burgess, 1983; Klebanoff, 1996).

DEFENSIVE, PROTECTIVE, AND COPING MECHANISMS

A defense or protective mechanism is used, usually unconsciously, to protect the self from internal impulses, thoughts, and feelings of conflict and anxiety. Using a defense or protective mechanism can be one's internal response to an external event, such as a death of a family member, or an internal circumstance like fatigue and illness, or emotional stress and personality problems. Defense or protective mechanisms are how a person deals with internal experiences.

Coping is the conscious or unconscious ways a person successfully adjusts and adapts to external, environmental demands. Coping mechanisms are how a person deals with the external environment; they are learned and varied. When coping mechanisms are used effectively, they protect the person. When a person overuses or does not use coping mechanisms effectively, the person does not adapt well and the quality of life suffers.

The assessment of the pt's and f/c's thinking processes, feelings, and behavioral responses will assist you to determine whether the pt and f/c are effectively or ineffectively using defense, protective, and coping mechanisms. Box 1-1 lists and briefly describes the frequently used defense and protective mechanisms. Box 1-2 describes some common coping mechanisms.

BOX 1-1. **Defense and Protective Mechanisms**

Acting out: outwardly manifesting inner need in an impulsive way

Altruism: connecting desire to satisfy one's own needs with desire to satisfy needs of others in a constructive and rewarding manner

Anticipation: acknowledging both intellectually and emotionally an upcoming situation that is thought to cause anxiety

Avoidance: unconsciously avoiding any situation, object, or behavior because it would produce too much anxiety

Compensation: exaggeration of one trait to make up for feelings of inferiority or inadequacy in another parameter

Conversion: when unable to express feelings, person reacts with body symptoms

Denial: external reality is not consciously recognized because it is too frightening or threatening to tolerate and would produce anxiety if acknowledged

Displacement: emotional aspect of an unacceptable idea of object is transferred to more acceptable one

Dissociation: mental or behavioral processes are compartmentalized from rest of person's awareness

Distortion: reshaping of external reality to suit internal needs

Fantasy: using nonrational mental activity to escape from responsibilities

Humor: when difficult situation cannot be fully acknowledged, humor is used to deal with anxiety without expense to self or others

Identification: patterning of self after another person to extent that self is altered

Intellectualization: reasoning or logic is used to try and avoid a confrontation with an impulse that would cause discomfort

Introjection: symbolic internalization of a hated or loved external object

Isolation: separation of idea or memory from feeling of idea or memory

Passive aggression: passively or inactively involves expression of indirect aggression or covert noncompliance to external demands

Projection: attributing to another (usually unconscious) undesirable, unacceptable ideas, feelings, thoughts, and impulses in the self

Rationalization: irrational or unacceptable feelings, motives, and behavior are logically justified or made tolerable by plausible means

Reaction formation: when an impulse or feeling is unacceptable, exact opposite of that which is unacceptable results

---

continued

BOX 1-1. Defense and Protective Mechanisms Continued

Regression: partial or total return to earlier patterns of adaptation

Repression: unconsciously unacceptable mental information is kept out of consciousness

Splitting: seeing situations and people as either all good or all bad

Sublimation: diversion of unacceptable energy connected with unacceptable impulses to socially and personally acceptable areas

Substitution: replacement of an unacceptable emotion, desire, impulse, or goal with an acceptable one

Suppression: consciously controlling and inhibiting unacceptable impulses, feelings, or thoughts

Symbolization: one idea or object comes to represent another because they are somehow similar

Transference: related to projection, this is unconscious linking of attitudes, feelings, and desires associated with an important person from one's earlier life onto another or others

Undoing: symbolically act out in reverse something unacceptable that has already been done, sometimes in a repetitive fashion

Adapted from Barry (1996); Kaplan & Sadock (1988)

BOX 1-2. Common Coping Mechanisms

1. Talking problems out with a trusted other person
2. Seeking input from others on how to cope, reduce tension, negotiate, confront, and compromise
3. Crying, laughing, yelling, or otherwise expressing emotion in an intense but safe way
4. Seeking comfort from other persons, leisure and recreational activities, treasured objects and places, sleeping, and journal writing
5. Exercising, physically moving, or otherwise manually working off tension safely
6. Using a step-by-step approach to solve problems
7. Gathering information about and becoming involved in health-related activities
8. Reframing a threat or problem as neutral or potentially beneficial
9. Engaging in stress-management practices, such as relaxation therapies, imagery, music therapy, assertiveness education, praying, painting, and energy work

Adapted from Barry (1996); Gorman, Sultan, & Luna-Raines (1989); Kaplan & Sadock (1988)

FAMILY OR CAREGIVER DYNAMICS AND COMMUNICATION

A family or caregiving network is a system of interrelated "parts" that is greater than the sum of its whole. When even one internal or external factor in the family or caregiving system changes (eg, one member becomes sick or loses a job), then all members in the system will respond to these changes. A crisis or change in one family member or caregiver will affect all members of the system until the roles, life-style, patterns, and routines can be redefined. Healthy systems adapt well to these changes. Family and interpersonal dynamics can greatly interfere with the overall effectiveness of home health care, from preadmission to discharge and continuing care planning. Even though the identified pt may be viewed as the provider's primary responsibility, the f/c greatly influences the course of care and may add extra demands. It is important to first assess the patterns of communication between or among the pt and f/c.

Key Assessment Questions

To assess if communication patterns in the family or caregiving system are healthy or not:

1. Are feelings freely expressed?
2. What decision-making processes are used?
3. Who makes decisions?
4. How do the parties interact with each other?
5. Whom does the pt talk about?
6. Who in the system is close by and likely to be involved in the course of home care?
7. What are the pt's and the f/c's criteria for deciding if a f/c is "involved" in the home care situation?
8. Do the members really listen to each other?
9. Who is the spokesperson?
10. Who presents issues and problems?
11. Before referral to the home care service did the f/c participate in the care of the pt?
12. What are the unique factors present in this system that affect the communication patterns?

Dysfunctional Patient and Family or Caregiver Interactions

Often dysfunctional interaction patterns exist in the home care situation. These can either be long-standing or can develop in response to the pt's illness and disease. These patterns negatively affect the f/c's work of keeping, getting, and performing on the job, the maintenance and nourishing of relationships, keeping one's identity, and running of the home. The most common dynamics, which are particularly prevalent in dysfunctional families, that affect the delivery of home care services and providers are:

1. *Triangulation*—an emotional process occurs when there is difficulty (eg, too much stress or intensity) between two people in a relationship (a dyad). Bringing in a third person, object, issue, or group forms a "triangle" and this is an attempt to re-

duce the tension in the dyadic relationship. This stabilizes the system by reducing the anxiety and intensity through avoidance of direct communication.

2. *Covert roles*—Covert roles are taken on by family members in a subconscious attempt to improve the dysfunctional family situation; unfortunately, as these roles are reinforced, they maintain dysfunction instead. The most common covert roles are: the mascot, who smooths over conflicts with humor; the "family hero," who is visibly successful and provides self-worth to the family; the scapegoat, whose problems or negative behavior provide a distraction and focus to the family system; and the lost child, who gets little attention and remains in the background, providing relief to the system.

3. *Unwritten rules*—certain, particular rules that guide thoughts, feelings, and behavior in a f/c system. All f/c systems have unwritten, covert rules. Some common examples of unwritten, covert rules are: "Ask Mom first for what you want and she'll talk Dad into it"; "Don't talk about Dad's drinking"; and "It's not OK to get angry."

Table 1-5 outlines problematic f/c system dynamics and therapeutic ways to counter the problems.

Table 1-5
Problematic Family or Caregiver Dynamics and Ways to Counter the Problems

Problem	Counter
1. Differing visions of course of illness or its management among f/c	1. Provide opportunities for family or caregivers to express feelings and identify sources of conflict, exact nature of the problem, and search for course that is shared and fair
2. The p/f/c feel overwhelmed	2. Assist them to come up with shared goals and actions; review progress made toward achieving goals
3. Expressions of disharmony (eg, manipulating, demeaning, or withholding)	3. Arrange for opportunities to express feelings openly; make referrals to other home health care professionals or community resources
4. F/c is angry, frustrated, overburdened, or worn out	4. Simplify, if possible, home care management and regimen; remain accessible and reinforce home health care team availability
5. Person, including the home health care provider, is in uncomfortable triangulated position in family system or caregiving system	5. Educate regarding concept of triangulation and identify dynamic; encourage key persons in triangle to identify their emotional "buttons" to take control of and change their part in dynamic; maintain enough emotional distance to observe process, including covert roles and unwritten rules, while maintaining emotional contact with other members; seek consultation

Functional Family or Caregiver Interactions

Functional f/c systems adapt to changes and are not bound by rigid roles and expectations. A functional f/c situation is characterized by:

1. Not keeping score or justifying one's behavior based on the past behavior of another
2. Accepting personal responsibility, not assigning blame, and actively trying to solve problems
3. Talking from the heart instead of lecturing
4. Being nonjudgmental about the perceptions and feelings of others
5. Being rigorously honest
6. Keeping behavior and being separate
7. Being persistent
8. Regarding others with positive esteem
9. Interacting within the f/c unit and with the community

RESOURCES AND INFORMATION FOR HOME SAFETY AND EMERGENCIES

1. U.S. Consumer Product Safety Commission (request "Safety for Older Consumers")
   4330 East West Highway
   Bethesda, MD 20814
   501-504-0580
2. Alzheimer's Association
   919 North Michigan Avenue
   Chicago, IL 60611
   1-800-272-3900
   312-335-8700
3. Injury Prevention for the Elderly Education Modules. Each module contains a book, video, and teaching materials for the following home safety practices:
   a. Preventing Falls (ISBN 0-8342-0823-7, #20823)
   b. Preventing Burns and Scalds (ISBN 0-8342-0826-1, #20826)
   c. Preventing Hyperthermia, Hypothermia, and Drowning (ISBN 0-342-0833-4, #20833)
   Available from Aspen Publishers, Inc.
   PO Box 990
   Frederick, MD 21705
   1-800-638-8437
   Fax: 301-417-7650
   http://www.aspen.pub.com

Section 2

Mental Status Examinations in the Home Setting

Meeting the complex needs of the home health care pt and f/c depends on accurately assessing the emotional and mental health care needs of the pt so that appropriate interventions, outcomes, and goals can be identified. Information about the pt is gathered from the referral source, the pt's history, physical examination, laboratory or diagnostic tests, and the mental status examination. These sources provide valuable data for use in developing the overall comprehensive and individualized care or treatment plan.

Aspects of the pt's functioning and quality of life that must be considered to address all facets of a pt's life are:

1. Behavioral
2. Emotional
3. Cognitive and psychological
4. Physical and biologic
5. Social and cultural
6. Spiritual

With in-home behavioral health care, a pt's primary, specific problem may be medical or physiologic in nature. The pt may have concurrent medical and psychiatric disorders or a blend of any combination of problems that are behavioral, medical, psychiatric, cognitive and psychological, social and cultural, and spiritual in nature. An integrated, complete, holistic assessment must be performed to adequately address problems, develop interventions, and evaluate the care given. For example, a pt with a cardiac condition will often need to be assessed for depression or suicidal thoughts.

MENTAL STATUS EXAMINATION

The mental status examination is the basic, essential component of all behavioral assessments. The mental status examination is a method of organizing the assessment of a pt's current psychological functioning, through observation and direct questioning.

The categories of the mental status examination include:

1. Appearance, grooming, dress, and physical characteristics
2. Eye contact and facial expressions

3. Posture and motor behavior
4. Speech and communication
5. Thought processes and content
6. Perceptions, thoughts, and beliefs
7. Mood or affect (feeling state) and emotions
8. Orientation and level of awareness
9. Memory (recent, intermediate, and remote) and recall
10. Level and fund of knowledge
11. Concentration
12. Abstract thinking and judgment
13. Insight
14. Potential for harm to self or others
15. Attitude and style of relating to others
16. Strengths

Using valid, reliable, standardized tools, the provider obtains baseline data, assesses for changes in mental status, communicates with other health care professionals, and obtains data that can be used in quality management activities. From the data obtained, problem statements and diagnoses can be defined, the pt's strengths and limitations can be identified, and appropriate interventions and teaching activities can be designed. The data are also used to establish goals and subsequent evaluations and to plan discharge and continuing care.

CHANGES IN THE MENTAL STATUS EXAMINATION

Because changes in mental status can reflect both medical and psychiatric disorders, the tool used must provide objective data and detect changes caused by physiologic or psychological factors, which are often reversible if detected and treated early. It is important to obtain information about a pt's mental status at various milestones—before admission to a home care agency or service, on admission to home care, during the course of home care, and at discharge.

Section 3

Treatment Planning in the Home Setting

The assessment process begins before a pt is admitted to a home care service or program. Based on the informal and formal assessments, most home health situations will have behavioral health aspects. Home health care providers should be able to function and use resources effectively in the home health care milieu; possess the necessary interpersonal and psychomotor skills to perform interventions; and know the scientific rationale for the interventions (Bulechek & McCloskey, 1992).

The following basic content applies to home health care or treatment plans with behavioral health aspects. Modify the content as appropriate to the pt's age and other factors that will affect the provision of care.

COMMON PROBLEMS LIST

- Adjustment, Impaired
- Anxiety
- Defensive Coping
- Denial, Ineffective
- Energy Field Disturbance
- Family Coping: Compromised, Ineffective
- Family Coping: Disabling, Ineffective
- Family Coping: Potential for Growth
- Family Processes, Altered
- Fear
- Health Maintenance, Altered
- Health Seeking Behaviors (Specify)
- Home Maintenance Management, Impaired
- Ineffective Individual Coping
- Injury, Risk for
- Knowledge Deficit (Specify)
- Loneliness, Risk for
- Role Performance, Altered
- Self Esteem, Chronic Low
- Self Esteem Disturbance

- Self Esteem, Situational Low
- Spiritual Well Being, Potential for Enhanced
- Therapeutic Regimen: Individual, Ineffective Management of

PROBLEM MANAGEMENT

Common Prevention, Maintenance, and Restorative Interventions and Rationales

- Provide emergency measures as necessary and obtain a consultation for inpatient evaluation *to preserve life.*
- Provide routine and emergency interventions, as indicated, *to maintain life and function.*
- Continually monitor the pt for subtle and overt changes in mental and physical status, and if detected notify members of the in-home team and the physician(s) *to intervene early, prevent complications, and reverse disease processes.*
- Continually assess treatment and possible causes of symptoms, as indicated, *to individualize home care and improve the pt's overall health and well-being.*
- Correct any reversible abnormality found during the mental status examination, physical examination, laboratory studies, home environment, or other assessment(s) *to prevent complications and permanent damage.*
- Remove any potentially harmful objects in the pt's immediate environment *to prevent falls, injuries, or harm.*
- Make sure that the if the pt wears eyeglasses or a hearing aid, or uses a walker or other assistive device, that the pt uses them *to enhance vision, hearing, ambulation, and self-esteem.*
- Provide for assistance with personal hygiene and activities of daily living (ADLs) *to meet the pt's basic needs.*
- Accept the pt and f/c at their current level of function *to establish a trusting relationship, design effective treatment, establish realistic goals and outcomes, and promote the dignity of the pt and the f/c.*
- Assist the pt and f/c *to maintain the pt's health status and make plans in anticipation of changes.*
- Assist the pt and f/c *to compensate for lost functions.*
- Assess for and treat any discomfort or painful condition (eg, arthritis, constipation, or denture problems), especially if the pt is unable to adequately express him or herself, *to relieve pain and discomfort.*
- Teach the pt and f/c to use individualized distraction techniques (eg, music, television, breathing, etc) alone or with other modalities *to focus attention from unpleasant sensations, such as pain.*
- Effectively design, provide, and evaluate interventions *to promote wellness and recovery, or maximize rehabilitation.*
- Teach the pt to make positive self-statements, use direct eye contact, identify own strengths, and list previous accomplishments *to increase self-esteem and self-worth.*
- Initiate referrals to other providers, services, and for equipment and supplies, as indicated, *to provide integrated, comprehensive, holistic home care.*

- Try to understand the underlying feelings communicated by others *to avoid threatening the pt and f/c.*
- Communicate your calmness, caring, and competency and listen with empathy, for feelings and impulses *to respond in a nonanxious, noncritical manner to establish and maintain a professional, therapeutic relationship with the pt and f/c.*
- Center yourself (take a moment, focus on your breathing, and slowly, deeply breathe while letting go of present tensions and concerns) before entering the home or speaking with a pt or f/c *to be fully present and available to the pt and f/c.*
- Promote a safe, stable, familiar environment for the pt *to facilitate health and healing.*
- Involve the pt and f/c in the plan of care *to obtain pt and f/c participation and satisfaction.*
- Teach stress reduction, relaxation, and other such techniques *to optimize health and alleviate problems.*
- Use verbal and nonverbal therapeutic communication skills *to effectively interact with the pt and f/c.*
- Focus on pt strengths and assets *to create constructive solutions to current and future problems.*
- Encourage the pt to develop new skills and formulate own opinions *to create a sense of competency to solve current and future problems.*
- Provide matter-of-fact, immediate responses and feedback *to minimize confusion and optimize pt and f/c participation in the plan of care.*
- Use a qualified translator, if needed, *to maintain confidentiality and ensure accuracy of information.*
- Assist the pt and f/c to develop a structured daily routine *to provide stability, security, and predictability.*
- Teach and allow for sufficient time for medication(s) to take effect *to optimize adherence with the treatment regimen.*
- Provide information about the pt's diagnosis or problem, causes of the disorder, medications, treatments, and measures *to prevent relapse.*
- Support the pt's and f/c's efforts to communicate with their health care providers *to encourage participation in and responsibility for health care.*
- Provide sources of support and resources *to organize a community support network for the pt and f/c.*
- Assist the pt only when necessary and provide positive reinforcement *to promote independent behavior.*
- Teach the f/c to assist the pt only when necessary and provide positive reinforcement *to promote independent behavior.*
- Take into account and keep of utmost concern the safety considerations of the pt, f/c, and provider *because if safety is not ensured, care will not be received.*
- Assess the pt and f/c for impulse control and signs of impending violent behavior with the assessment tools (see Aggressive Behaviors and Assaultive Behaviors) *to prevent harm, injury, or death.*
- Assess for suicidal or homicidal ideation with the standardized assessment tools (see Appendix), and every visit or contact thereafter, *to obtain a baseline measure of severity of symptoms and an ongoing assessment of the pt's status.*

- Instruct regarding suicide awareness, safety, and prevention *to prevent harm, injury, or death.*
- Obtain a verbal and written contract for the pt not to harm self, others, or property, if suicidal or homicidal ideation is expressed, *to prevent harm, injury, death; organize and institute a 24-hour pt watch, arrange for a consultation, or inpatient evaluation, if indicated.*
- Instruct the pt and f/c that feelings of anger may be appropriate in a situation but need to be expressed in an acceptable manner rather than being acted on in a destructive manner *for the preservation of life, health, and property.*
- Instruct the pt and f/c that verbal and nonverbal expression of emotions, such as anger, withdrawal, agitation, guilt, or self-blame *may indicate an avoidance of dealing with grief and loss, which will help in problem-solving.*
- Instruct the pt and f/c in the importance of setting realistic objectives and goals *to set ones that are applicable to the immediate situation.*
- Use an constructive, congruent, genuine, and positive approach to the pt and f/c *to enhance the pt's and f/c's self-esteem.*
- Provide and teach the f/c to give back rubs, foot massages, simple massage, touch, and so forth *to enhance the pt's self-worth, provide stimulation, and feeling of connection.*

NURSING MANAGEMENT

Nursing Interventions and Rationale

☆ Common Behavioral Interventions

- Understand your own feelings toward the pt and f/c *to prevent prejudices from interfering with treatment.*
- Maintain and model a calm, nonthreatening demeanor when working with the pt *because the pt will develop feelings of security in the presence of calm caregivers.*
- Assist with and institute activity therapy and limit setting as modes of intervention *to increase the range, frequency, or duration of the pt's activity and promote effective treatment and healing.*
- Role play, rehearse, and confront the pt and f/c *to clarify and augment specific role behaviors to improve relationships.*
- Identify and encourage actions *to support the f/c to positively enhance their involvement, clarify roles, and facilitate interventions.*
- Promote changes in life-style and habits slowly, beginning with one aspect at a time, *to allow time for the pt to adjust to a change and increase the chance that the change will be enduring.*
- Use standardized, accepted assessment tools and instruments *to assess the pt and f/c to validate the presence of the condition, obtain a baseline measure of the problem, evaluate the effectiveness of care, and make appropriate referrals.*
- Develop an individualized plan of care with the pt and f/c and a transdisciplinary team *to find and deliver the most effective treatment.*
- Teach and rehearse assertive communication *to help the pt and f/c learn new skills.*
- Observe and assess the pt and f/c on admission and each visit after for symptoms of _____ that are indicators of _____ *to minimize or prevent complications.*

- Observe and assess responses to the pt's symptoms *to assist in the modification of behaviors to guide further interventions.*
- Instruct the pt and f/c to identify symptoms of _____ that are indicators of _____ *to minimize or prevent complications.*
- Instruct the pt and f/c to identify situations that precipitate the onset of _____ *because often recognition is the first step in the elimination of maladaptive responses.*
- Instruct the pt and f/c in ways of reviewing past coping strategies and successes *because in seeking to create change, it is helpful to identify strengths and past responses that were effective and successful.*
- Instruct the pt and f/c in positive coping and relaxation skills (eg, deep breathing, muscle relaxation, imagery, meditation, warm baths, and diversional activities) *to minimize stress and forestall health problems.*
- Instruct the pt and f/c in the importance of setting realistic goals and assist and educate the pt regarding the setting of appropriate short-term and long-term goals that are applicable to the situation *so that there is success and progress rather than frustration and setback.*
- Instruct the pt and f/c how to modify behavior *so that health is enhanced and quality of life is improved.*
- Instruct the pt and f/c to participate in self-care and ADLs *to help the pt maintain activity tolerance, increase independence, and enhance self-worth.*
- Instruct the pt and f/c to discuss past experiences with crises and illnesses, inviting comparisons with the current situation, *to heighten awareness, identify previous coping mechanisms, increase self-confidence, facilitate resolution of past events, and decide which coping approaches to use at this time.*
- Monitor the pt's progress and report favorable and adverse responses to the other provider(s) *to maintain current communication, avoid misunderstandings, and revise the treatment plan.*
- Offer praise and remind the pt of what must be accomplished *to evaluate the pt's response to treatment and evaluate the course of care.*
- Explain any task in short, simple steps *because a task will be easier to accomplish for the pt if it is broken down into a series of smaller steps.*
- Repeat instructions as necessary and in different forms (eg, verbal and written) *because the pt and the f/c may not be able to remember all of the steps to the task at once.*
- Set clear limits and boundaries (ie, the parameters of accepted and desired behaviors), be direct in instructions, and offer win–win choices *to decrease the incidence and duration of undesirable behaviors, avoid behavioral acting out and control battles.*
- Provide reality orientation, if indicated, through a consistent approach; verbal and written orientation to person, place, time, and situation; labeling items in the pt's environment; using environmental cues (eg, clocks, calendars, etc), aids to increase sensory input, addressing by name, and other measures *to promote the pt's awareness of and personal identity, time, and home environment.*

⚕ Common Emotional Interventions

- Assist the pt to label and recognize feelings *to identify emotions that the pt is feeling and accurately reduce inaccurate interpretations of situations, events, and interactions that generate emotional arousal to provide reassurance, acceptance, and stress management guidance.*

- Explore emotional issues with the pt and f/c *because this can be an effective mode of intervention for current problem-solving through emotional resolution.*
- Observe and assess the pt and f/c on admission and each visit for functional and dysfunctional patterns of communication between and among the pt and f/c (see Section 1) *to intervene early if the home milieu changes and to identify areas for teaching.*
- Instruct the pt and f/c in the importance of verbalizing thoughts and feelings *to appropriately identify the relationship between feelings and events or stressors to more effectively deal with them.*
- Instruct the pt and f/c in the importance of expressing honest feelings as a more effective means of communication *so that change can occur.*
- Instruct the pt and f/c to safely express powerful feelings and to cry when needed *to help reduce bottled-up feelings.*
- Instruct the pt and f/c to use appropriate expressions of anger and promote discussions of ways *to identify and cope with underlying feelings to manage anger.*
- Assist the pt to identify feelings related to a positive self-appraisal *to arrive at constructive solutions to current and future problems.*
- Instruct the pt and f/c to counter feelings of inadequacy, worthlessness, fear of rejection, and incompetence *because they can contribute to poor self-esteem, anger, hostility, aggression, anxiety, and depression.*
- Instruct the pt and f/c to discuss feelings about the fears rather than the fears themselves *to focus on feelings and not the fear of physical or mental problems.*
- Instruct the pt and f/c to verbalize about realities without confrontation, *which begins resolutions and acceptance.*
- Instruct the pt and f/c to assertively express feelings *because it is self-enhancing and empowering.*
- Instruct the pt and f/c to talk about traumatic experiences of _____ in a non-threatening environment *to help the p/f/c identify and come to terms with unresolved issues to appropriately use defense, protective, and coping mechanisms for protection from feelings of inadequacy, incompetence, and worthlessness.*
- Instruct the pt and f/c to emotionally imagine increasing the difficulty of goals *to help gain confidence and independence.*
- Instruct the pt and f/c to verbalize thoughts and feelings related to illness and disability *to help with agreeing on the problem, problem-solving, and future planning.*
- Instruct the pt and f/c to explore feelings of lack of control over stress and life events *because they may have helpless and powerless feelings and not independently recognize them.*
- Arrange for the use animals or pets, if available and accepted, for the pt to hold, pet, stoke, watch, play with, exercise, feed, groom, and so forth *to provide feelings of love and affection, relaxation, diversion, and overall well-being.*
- Instruct the pt and f/c to nurture their emotional strength *to affect their ability to engage in self-care and other activities.*

△ **Common Cognitive Interventions**

- Teach and administer modes of intervention such as clarification, problem-solving, reality orientation, psychosocial education, reality testing, as well as imagery and visualization, which can be effective, *to promote mental health and prevent mental illness.*

- Provide or arrange for supportive psychotherapy *because it is an effective mode of therapy.*
- Monitor the pt's and f/c's ability to remember and interpret information *to gauge their awareness, comprehension, and ability to learn.*
- Encourage the f/c to make arrangements for informal or formal respite care *because the f/c needs to know that it is acceptable to take time off.*
- Assess and observe the mental status of the pt and f/c on admission and each visit using the assessment tools (see Appendix) *for subtle and overt changes in mental status and for s/s of depression, anxiety, mania, psychosis, and so forth to intervene early and prevent complications.*
- Test and provide reality orientation *to determine the pt's level or orientation and prevent complications.*
- Instruct the pt and f/c regarding reality-based thinking techniques *to regain, maintain, or promote congruent thinking.*
- Instruct the pt and f/c in the definition, description, process, and prevention of _____ *to help them gain control over their health status.*
- Instruct the pt and f/c to observe _____ behaviors *to see the relationship between thinking, feeling, and the corresponding _____ behavioral response because they may be unaware of the relationship between thoughts, emotions, and behaviors.*
- Instruct the pt and f/c regarding the _____ thoughts and ineffective coping behavior *because they may occur from the disease process.*
- Instruct the pt and f/c to keep a journal of events preceding, during, and after the _____ behavior occurs *to help them recognize themes, patterns, and events that may precipitate the _____ behavior to minimize or prevent it.*
- Instruct the pt and f/c to write down coping strategies *for use when needed for anticipated or potential areas of difficulty.*
- Instruct the pt and f/c in the importance of verbalization about thoughts and realities without confrontation *to help begin resolution and acceptance.*
- Instruct the pt and f/c to substitute positive thoughts for negative ones *to allow alternative ways of problem-solving and positive expectations to emerge.*
- Instruct the pt and f/c to set realistic goals to avoid setups for failure and to identify positive or neutral areas in life *to promote thoughts of power and independence.*
- Instruct the pt and f/c in the importance of thinking about a feared object or situation before it occurs to allow them *to view fears as more manageable and come up with a plan to gain control over them.*
- Encourage the continuation of therapy after discharge *to teach the pt and f/c so as to retain gains and prevent relapse.*
- Teach the pt and f/c about how cultural thoughts, beliefs, and practices affect how people express and accept the grieving process *to facilitate awareness and optimize the healing process.*
- Instruct the pt to identify activities that foster self-esteem *to draw on those activities that were successful in the past for elevating the pt's self-esteem now.*
- Instruct the pt in the differences between irrational, distorted thinking (eg, all or nothing and overgeneralization) and rational, logical thinking *to assist the pt to change dysfunctional thinking patterns and see the experience more realistically.*
- Assign homework and bibliotherapy exercises to the pt *to identify personal strengths and techniques for improving self-esteem, imparting insight, and to strengthen the pt's commitment to change.*

- Reinforce all teaching with educational materials, homework assignments, audiotapes, videotapes, and so forth *to meet the pt's and f/c's needs for information and counseling.*
- Instruct the pt to keep a journal *to help identify thoughts and feelings that are important.*
- Instruct the pt in a step-by-step approach to problem-solving (ie, identify the problem, explore alternatives, evaluate consequences of the alternatives, make a decision, and evaluate the course of action) *to give the pt awareness of a logical process for examining and resolving problems.*

⊓ Common Physical Interventions

- Make liquids and food available that require little effort to eat and drink to the pt at all times *to encourage the pt to eat and ingest fluids when interested in satisfying hunger or thirst.*
- Instruct the pt or f/c to make fortified shakes or high nutritional meals available *to provide maximum nutrition for the pt who does not ingest an adequate nutritional intake.*
- Prescribe activity therapy *because it is a mode of intervention that can enhance the pt's overall well-being.*
- Perform the prescribed treatment for the underlying disease or condition *to restore, maintain, or enhance the pt's status.*
- Teach awareness of the interrelatedness of the "bodymind" (a "state of integration that includes body, mind, and spirit") (Dossey, Keegan, Guzzetta, & Kolkmeier, 1995, p. 88) as evident in the psychophysiology of the endocrine, immune, and autonomic systems *to provide opportunities for affecting "bodymind" responses and promote healing.*
- Assess for physical conditions that mimic psychiatric disorders or concurrent problems and diagnoses *because it is important to consider the whole person to effectively design comprehensive interventions.*
- Teach the use of relaxation measures (eg, deep or progressive muscle relaxation, audiotapes, meditation, etc) *to activate the relaxation response that inhibits the activation of the flight-or-fight response of the autonomic nervous system.*
- Observe and assess the pt and f/c on admission and each visit for signs, symptoms, precipitants of abusive behavior and for neglect and exploitation (see Abusive Behavior and Neglect and Exploitation) *to prevent or minimize abusive, neglectful, or exploitative behavior.*
- Observe and assess the pt and f/c on admission and each visit for medication management and effectiveness *to determine medication compliance and efficacy.*
- Ensure nutritional balance; adequate oxygenation; sufficient fluids and fluid balance; adequate sleep, rest, and activity; and elimination patterns *to promote biologic integrity and wellness.*
- Observe and assess the pt for the status of vital signs and cardiovascular (CV) (including blood pressure lying, sitting, and standing) and cardiopulmonary (CP) function *to monitor systems status and minimize or prevent complications.*
- Observe and assess the pt for the status of nutritional and hydration state *to monitor and prevent weight loss and dehydration and to determine nutritional causes for _____ and to maintain healthy eating and elimination patterns.*
- Observe and assess the pt for the status of the gastrointestinal (GI) state *to prevent constipation and impaction.*

- Observe and assess the pt for the status of the genitourinary (GU) system *to prevent urinary tract infections, stress incontinence, urinary retention, or other problems.*
- Observe and assess the pt for the status of the neurologic state *to monitor and prevent problems with sleep, pain, gait, and other parameters.*
- Observe and assess the pt for the status of the musculoskeletal system *to monitor and prevent unsafe ambulation and prevent accidents and injury.*
- Observe and assess the pt for the status of the skin and tissue state *to monitor integrity and prevent complications.*
- Observe and assess the pt for the status of the immunologic, hormonal, and metabolic patterns and state *to monitor physical regulation and prevent compromise.*
- Observe and assess the pt for the status of the results of the history, laboratory tests, physical examination, and observations or behavior *to detect possible physiologic causes of mental symptoms.*
- Observe and assess the pt for the status of the effectiveness, side effects, adverse reactions and interactions, safety, contraindications, and overdose of medications for _____ *to ensure safety and facilitate cooperation with therapy.*
- Observe and assess the pt for the status of somatic complaints *because they are likely to be present.*
- Observe and assess the pt for the presence of physical symptoms of _____, _____, and _____ *because of the pt's actual or potential condition(s).*
- Observe and assess the pt and f/c for the status of physical strength *to accurately determine the ability to assume responsibility for self-care and engage in activities.*
- Observe and assess the f/c for the status of desire and capability to learn cardiopulmonary resuscitation (CPR) *to strengthen their self-confidence and support.*
- Observe and assess the pt and f/c for access to an emergency medical system *to decrease complications and strengthen the support system.*
- Observe and assess the pt for presence of a Medic Alert identification *to decrease complications and strengthen the support system.*
- Observe and assess for the availability of a thorough written medical history and do not resuscitate documents, if applicable, for easy access by emergency personnel *to decrease complications and strengthen the support system.*
- Instruct the pt and f/c about the relationship between stress and physical symptoms *to facilitate overall well-being.*
- Instruct the pt and f/c about the physical cues, body awareness, and relaxation *to develop a management plan to anticipate, recognize early, and prevent _____, as well as enhance the chance for new behaviors to be effective.*
- Instruct the pt and f/c to regularly exercise *to maintain physical integrity, assist with sleep and appetite, and for overall well-being.*
- Instruct the pt and f/c to eat nutritious food and ingest an adequate amount of fluids each day *to promote healing and digestion.*
- Instruct the pt and f/c to reduce or avoid alcohol, caffeine, drugs, and smoking *to minimize interactions with medication(s) and reduce anxiety.*
- Instruct the pt and f/c to develop a bedtime routine *to facilitate rest, sleep, and healing.*
- Instruct the pt and f/c about the effectiveness, side effects, adverse reactions and interactions, safety, contraindications, and overdose of medications for _____ *to ensure safety and facilitate cooperation with therapy.*
- Instruct the pt and f/c about bowel, GU, and bladder regimen; CV and CP management; and neurologic, sleep pattern, pain, musculoskeletal, and ambulation

management *to promote comfort, create regularity to the day, and minimize or prevent complications.*

- Instruct the pt and f/c that symptoms are real, even if there is no organic pathology, *to decrease physical and emotional discomfort.*
- Instruct the pt and f/c that the relationship between physical and emotional health as intertwined *to convey an appreciation of the "bodymind" (Dossey et al., 1995, p. 88) relationship.*
- Monitor the pt for health risks, skin integrity, tissue perfusion, infection, and bleeding tendencies *to detect subtle improvements or deterioration in the pt's condition for clinical decision-making.*

◯ Common Social Interventions

- Support the pt and f/c in altered role performance *to assist the healthy adjustment of the f/c system.*
- Assist the f/c to locate community resources or support groups and consider a medical social work referral *to help cope with the pt's condition, promote family cohesion and integrity, and assist the pt and f/c to locate food, clothing, transportation, and so forth.*
- Assist the f/c to organize a community support network and obtain a therapeutic companion *to help cope with the changed family organization and the pt's condition.*
- Act as a liaison and identify, refer (in written and verbal form), or consult with community resources and network *for continued contact and efficient, cost-effective use of existing resources.*
- Understand that the material resources and physical surroundings, the home, neighborhood, and community of the pt and f/c affect, positively or negatively, their ability and likelihood *to engage in activities that will promote wellness and recovery, or maximize rehabilitation.*
- Support socialization and provide emotional support as modes of intervention *to enhance the overall well-being of the pt and f/c.*
- Observe and assess the pt's and f/c's support system on admission and each visit *to facilitate the managing of daily living tasks.*
- Observe and assess the degree of the pt's and f/c's coping methods *to determine dysfunction and to make appropriate referrals.*
- Instruct the pt and f/c to seek assistance, such as community, self-help, advocacy, and support groups, from outside resources *to decrease strain, facilitate coping, and for continued information and referral services.*
- Instruct the pt and f/c that opportunities to interact with others *assists in maintaining a reality orientation and decreases social isolation.*
- Instruct the pt and f/c to discuss how they cope with illness *to help them to adjust to changes in roles and responsibilities.*
- Instruct the pt and f/c to identify role changes that have occurred as a result of sudden illness, recurrent hospitalizations, or other major life events *to improve communication, interventions, and expectations of treatment.*
- Instruct the pt and f/c to identify behaviors that are socially acceptable *to increase socialization and acceptance.*

- Instruct the pt and f/c in role playing and rehearsals concerning social contacts, adapting new behaviors, and giving positive reinforcement and feedback *to increase social skills.*
- Instruct the pt and f/c in the dangers of social isolation, contract for them to call one friend or family member a day, and encourage visits from others *to enhance social support and connection.*
- Instruct the pt and f/c to have social and family gatherings in the home *to encourage increased social contact and relieve social isolation.*
- Instruct the pt and f/c regarding social and cultural beliefs and practices *to show how they affect how people express and accept the grieving process.*

✦ Common Spiritual Interventions

- Clarify provider, pt, f/c, and agency values and beliefs regarding particular home care situations *to promote pt self-determination, spiritual well-being, and facilitate effective decision-making.*
- Establish a therapeutic and trusting relationship with the pt and f/c by actively listening and being nonjudgmental *to promote a safe, secure environment that will facilitate the pt and f/c to verbalize concerns about _____.*
- Offer and provide guidance on how to care for an ill, dependent, disabled, or older adult *because the f/c may lack the information to do so, coping the only way they know how, and feel out of control.*
- Coordinate activities and visits in the home *to promote the pt's and f/c's sense of self, feelings of belonging, and control.*
- Explain to the pt that you are concerned for the pt's safety and will help *to keep the pt as safe as possible to provide a sense of care and concern.*
- Involve the pt and f/c in the plan and scheduling of care *to convey a sense of control and involvement to the pt and f/c.*
- Encourage the pt and f/c to recognize and discuss thoughts, feelings, motivations, usual response patterns, life goals and priorities, strengths, and limitations *to explore and acknowledge that each person is unique.*
- Provide as many opportunities as possible for the pt and f/c to make decisions about care and the current home situation *to enhance coping, sense of self-control, and self-esteem.*
- Assist the pt and f/c to identify and list the positive and negative consequences of options for the future, and explore choices and desires *because the pt and f/c may feel powerless, with no perceived options, choices, or desires.*
- Provide information about services that are immediately available as well as other services in the community *because this information will help the pt feel more in control.*
- Provide or arrange for reminiscence, therapeutic or healing touch, and music therapy *because they are modes of intervention that can positively affect spiritual well-being.*
- Observe and assess the pt and f/c on admission and each visit for their perception of spiritual needs and the importance of establishing contact with an appropriate spiritual support system or representative *to assist in resolving the problem of _____ and for spiritual guidance and connection.*

- Observe and assess the pt and f/c on admission and each visit for referral to a spiritual support system or member of the clergy *to address spiritual needs, provide solace, and approach a resolution of spiritual concerns.*
- Instruct the pt and f/c on admission and each visit in the definition, description, process, and prevention of _____ *to help them gain control.*
- Instruct the pt and f/c on admission and each visit in the importance of establishing contact with their appropriate spiritual support system or representative *to assist in resolving the problem of* _____ *and for spiritual guidance.*
- Instruct the pt and f/c on admission and each visit to identify strengths and successes in fulfilling roles *to promote a sense of control over the current situation.*
- Instruct the pt and f/c on admission and each visit in the importance of positive planning and problem-solving for the future in order *to gain a sense of control over their life.*
- Instruct the pt and f/c on admission and each visit to set realistic goals, make achievable future plans, avoid setups for failure, and identify areas of life that are under control *to promote feelings of independence, power, and self-control.*
- Instruct the pt and f/c on admission and each visit to recognize and accept areas in life situations that are not within their ability to control *to aid in reality orientation regarding feelings of powerlessness and fear of failures.*
- Instruct the pt and f/c on admission and each visit to recognize areas of personal control (eg, taking medications on time, following treatment regimens, control with self-care, and choosing friends and foods) *to enhance self-mastery and self-control.*
- Instruct the pt and f/c on admission and each visit in the healing power of peer support and allowing friends and family to visit and communicate *to allow an opportunity to verbalize and share feelings.*
- Assist the pt and f/c to identify feelings of guilt or _____, the situations in which the feelings are aroused, and beliefs and behaviors generated *to cope with feelings and actual or potential feelings of responsibility.*
- Instruct the pt and f/c on admission and each visit to continue to hope for a cure, comfort measure, stronger medication, and so forth while remaining reality oriented, *to convey hope and serenity.*
- Instruct the pt and f/c on admission and each visit to regard self-worth with positive affirmations *to increase a positive view of the self and others.*
- Discuss and monitor with the pt their feelings, thoughts, and concerns regarding the assumption of responsibility for their present and future health status and self-care *to encourage the pt to assume more responsibility, encourage independence, communicate and clarify perceptions, identify areas where more responsibility can be assumed, and acquire support from others.*
- Provide spiritual counseling or a referral to a religious, spiritual, or cultural group for advocacy and continued monitoring, *to promote forgiveness of others and the self, as well as accountability to the pt, f/c, self, and community.*
- Instruct the pt and f/c on admission and each visit regarding information about services that are immediately available as well as other services in the community *because this information will help the pt feel more in control currently and for future use.*
- Help the pt to see humor in situations and laugh *to reduce despair and provide a different perspective.*

- Provide continuity of care throughout the length of stay *to foster trust and establish a therapeutic relationship.*
- Promote autonomy toward health-seeking behaviors *to encourage pt responsibility for own health and spiritual well-being.*

Common Nursing Goals

- Provide for the safety of the pt and f/c
- Treat reversible medical and psychiatric disorders as well as coexisting medical conditions
- Keep the pt as functional as possible
- Manage and treat behavioral problems
- Provide a safe, nurturing, and healing environment
- Help relieve or overcome their feelings of _____
- Assist the pt and f/c to recognize their strengths, limitations, capabilities, and liabilities
- Assist the pt to achieve functional independence
- Help the pt and f/c manage internal and external stressors
- Provide emotional support to the pt and f/c
- Help the pt and f/c develop appropriate coping mechanisms
- Promote self-confidence, self-worth, self-adequacy, and self-love
- Promote effective problem-solving techniques
- Promote effective stress reduction and coping strategies
- Facilitate verbal expression of feelings of _____
- Facilitate the identification of stress response to _____
- Help the pt and f/c identify life stresses or problems
- Help the pt and f/c develop alternative ways of dealing with stress and _____
- Organize a community network around the pt
- Promote a positive attitude of the f/c toward the pt
- Promote feelings of worth and uniqueness to the pt and f/c
- Help the pt to gain a sense of inner control and control of their own destiny
- Promote self-esteem
- Promote the identification and use of the pt's strengths and assets
- Provide a flexible, written plan of care
- Facilitate and support the individual goal-setting and functioning of the pt and the f/c
- Prevent hospitalization or rehospitalization
- Facilitate a transition to a more or less restrictive level of care
- Use resources and community referral judiciously

Common Patient Goals

- Be free of injury
- Be free of self-inflicted harm
- Have an improved ability to perform ADLs
- Live in the least restrictive environment possible
- Attain and maintain adequate levels or balance of nutritional, oxygenation, fluid, sleep, rest, activity, and elimination patterns

- Maintain health status
- Improve health status
- Maintain an adequate level of physical and diversional activity
- Be free of injury, not injure others, or destroy property
- Be free of harm inflicted by another
- Maintain adequate, balanced physiologic functioning
- Eat a balanced diet
- Obtain restful sleep
- Maintain a balance of activity and rest
- Identify life stresses
- Begin to develop an improved sense of self-esteem
- Modify life-style to prevent problems and minimize disability
- Become as functionally independent as possible
- Make decisions about treatment
- Report increased acceptance of change in health status
- Identify support systems outside of the home
- Identify the provider as a person to contact before or when problems arise
- Experience spiritual well-being
- Accept situation realistically
- Seek support from others
- Comply with the treatment regimen
- Assume responsibility for meeting own dependency needs
- Have an enhanced self-concept
- Establish a balance of rest, sleep, and activity
- Demonstrate weight _____
- Attain optimal level of independent functioning
- Cope adequately with threats to self-image
- Maintain a realistic self-perception
- Accept the self as a unique, valuable person
- Make positive self-statements and statements about others
- Alter negative coping mechanisms related to _____
- Become aware of negative thoughts and feelings about the self
- Assume responsibility for enhancing own self-concept
- Identify values and beliefs that create negative thoughts about self
- Feel competent
- Value own contributions
- Engage in constructive behaviors

Common Patient Outcomes

The patient will:

- Verbalize an absence of suicidality within _____ weeks
- Verbalize an absence of violent ideation within _____ weeks
- Verbalize _____ behaviors that are disruptive within _____ weeks
- State knowledge of when to call the physician, 911, or otherwise summon emergency assistance during crisis events within _____ weeks

- Verbalize acceptance of a therapeutic companion within _____ weeks
- Verbalize two management techniques of _____ disease within _____ weeks
- Verbalize two s/s of _____ illness within _____ weeks
- Report one precipitating event and demonstrate one coping skill to decrease _____ feelings and _____ thoughts within _____ weeks
- Exhibit goal-directed thoughts within _____ weeks as demonstrated by _____ by _____ (date)
- Exhibit conversation that exhibits a decrease in impaired _____ within _____ weeks as demonstrated by _____
- State to the provider that there is a decrease in _____ or _____ within _____ weeks
- Verbalize an understanding of uses and two side effects of all medications within _____ weeks
- Verbalize two techniques to assist with bowel or constipation management within _____ weeks
- Verbalize two techniques to assist with nutrition or hydration management within _____ weeks
- Verbalize two techniques to assist with CV impairments within _____ weeks
- Verbalize two techniques to assist with CP impairments within _____ weeks
- Sleep _____ hours per night within _____ weeks
- Verbalize and demonstrate the use of two coping skills within _____ weeks
- Demonstrate the use of stress reduction and relaxation techniques within _____ weeks
- Recognize events that precipitate _____ and intervene to minimize or prevent disabling behaviors by discharge
- Demonstrate two social skills within _____ weeks
- Make one social contact with one new person by _____ (date)
- Participate in _____ activity within _____ weeks
- Openly communicate with and verbally express feelings about _____ to the provider by _____ (date)
- Express feelings nonverbally in a safe manner regarding _____ by _____ (date)
- Identify their behavioral response to stress by _____ within _____ weeks
- Identify ways to deal with stress or other feelings of _____ by _____ (date)
- Demonstrate alternative ways to deal with stress by _____ as demonstrated by _____ by _____ (date)
- Demonstrate a decrease in physiologic, stress-related, or psychosomatic symptoms related to _____ as demonstrated by _____ by _____ (date)
- Discuss future plans, based on realistic self-assessment, as demonstrated by _____ within _____ weeks
- Learn about _____ illness and anticipate health status changes as demonstrated by _____ within _____ weeks
- Participate in the health care regimen as demonstrated by _____ by _____ (date)
- Participate in the plan of care as demonstrated by _____ within _____ weeks
- Choose and use distraction techniques, such as music, finger tapping, breathing, or _____ within _____ weeks
- Accept help with daily activity as demonstrated by _____ within _____ weeks

- Seek help from others and identify a support network as shown by contacting _____ within _____ weeks
- Assume responsibility for using social services and community resources as shown by contacting within _____ weeks
- Recognize problems related to _____ as demonstrated by _____ within _____ weeks
- Perform activities of daily living (specify: _____) as demonstrated by _____ within _____ weeks
- Verbalize an understanding of _____ and _____ medications as demonstrated by _____ within _____ weeks
- Verbalize importance of continued therapy or treatment for _____ as evidenced by _____ within _____ weeks

Common Family/Caregiver Outcomes

The family/caregiver will:

- Verbalize that they are receiving practical assistance and emotional support from the providers by _____ (date)
- Understand and implement the psychological, social, and environmental modifications (specify) that enhance the pt's functioning and safety by _____ (date)
- Verbalize concerns and fears regarding _____ within _____ weeks
- Communicate openly and honestly with the provider by _____ (date)
- Set realistic goals regarding _____ as evidenced by _____ by _____ (date)
- Develop and maintain a supportive and positive outlook as demonstrated by _____ by _____ (date)
- Recognize and accept the need for professional assistance as demonstrated by _____ by _____ (date)
- Discuss how the pt's _____ illness has altered established roles (specify: _____) and rules (specify: _____) within _____ weeks
- Participate in organizing a community network or obtaining a therapeutic companion for the pt by _____ (specify)
- Discuss the inequities in care responsibility (specify: _____) for the older, ill, dependent, or disabled pt as demonstrated by _____ within _____ weeks
- Revise caregiving and household responsibilities to correct inequities (specify: _____) as shown by _____ within _____ weeks
- Refrain from ineffective or dangerous coping methods, such as (specify) substance abuse, mistreatment of the pt, absences from work or school, withdrawal from or excessive involvement with the pt, or _____ as shown by _____ within _____ weeks
- Contact and attend support systems, such as (specify) extended family, community resources, self-help groups, respite service, religious organizations, or _____ for aid in the care and emotional support of the pt as shown by _____ contacts and the involvement of _____ by _____ (date)
- Report an increased ability to cope with the responsibilities of caring for an ill, dependent, disabled, or older adult as demonstrated by _____ within _____ weeks

- Discuss past experiences with change, crises, and illness within _____ weeks
- Discuss the perceived impact of _____ illness on f/c function (specify) as demonstrated by _____ within _____ weeks
- Establish _____ limits and _____ boundaries on the pt's _____ behavior and uphold them as demonstrated by _____ within _____ weeks
- Meet their own physical, emotional, social, spiritual, environmental, role, spiritual, and sexual needs and wants (specify) as demonstrated by _____ within _____ weeks
- Describe the cause, ss/s, usual course, and treatment of the pt's _____ disorder by _____ (date)

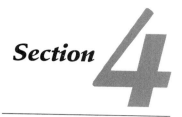

Documentation Guidelines and Tips for In-Home Behavioral Health Care

DOCUMENTATION GUIDELINES

1. Perform the assessments and complete the documents required by an agency.
2. Perform and document standard assessments for in-home care, including vital signs, CV, CP, GI, GU, skin, musculoskeletal, neurologic, functional, and pain status.
3. Assess and document:
   - History of frequent hospitalizations
   - Episodes or emotional crises with interventions
   - History of recurrent episodes of depression, mania, psychosis, or suicidal behavior
   - Impaired thought process
   - Multiple medical problems
   - Amount of personal care needed
   - Other skilled services needed
   - Behaviors or complications that cause a safety or high-risk concern
   - Nutritional or hydration problems
   - Multiple or restrictive functional limitations
   - Mental status impairment
4. In addition, perform and document the following assessments:
   - Mental status examination
   - Suicidal assessment
   - Age-appropriate depression tool
   - Psychiatric home safety
   - Spiritual well-being
   - Psychiatric emergency plan
   - Medication test
5. If indicated, perform and document:
   - Involuntary movements assessment

- Diagnosis or problem-specific assessments (eg, anxiety)
- Aggressive or assaultive behaviors assessment
- At risk for falls and falls risk factors assessment tool

6. Assess and document behaviors that require behavioral health intervention
   - Potential suicide attempts
   - Severe depression, feelings of doom, isolation, refusing to leave room or bed, or preoccupation with somatic complaints
   - Panic attacks with phobias, increased blood pressure, tachycardia, and tachypnea
   - Increased s/s of agitation, anxiety, and manic behaviors
   - Mismanagement and exacerbation of physical disease process related to emotional stability
   - Frequent falls secondary to an impaired state
   - Increased environmental or safety hazards secondary to impaired status or disease process
   - Anorexia with a weight loss of more than 10 pounds a month
   - Weight gain of more than 10 pounds a month
   - Mismanagement, noncompliance, or misunderstanding of medication regimen
   - Impaired and potential dangerous self-care and ADL care

IN-HOME BEHAVIORAL HEALTH DOCUMENTATION CHECKLIST

- Observe and assess mental status and psychosocial functioning for indications of impaired:
   - Mood and affect with _____ (specify related to what the pt said or did)
   - Thought process and content with _____ (specify related to what the pt said or did)
   - Perceptions with _____ (specify related to what the pt said or did)
   - Short-, intermediate-, and long-term memory as indicated by _____ (specify)
   - Self-care (appearance, appetite, sleep, and so forth) as indicated by _____ (specify)
   - Motivation related to _____ (specify) and indicated by _____ (specify)
   - Psychosocial functioning and behavior with _____ (specify)
   - Suicidal ideation with or without _____ (specify)

In-Home Behavioral Health Outcomes Measurement System

Outcome measurement systems provide feedback mechanisms that influence the quantity, quality, and type of treatments provided a patient in a particular service. Outcome measurements are based on the thesis that it is more efficient to match the patient to appropriate treatments and levels of service than it is to reduce benefits. This approach supports a partnership between payers and providers based on mutual acceptance of outcome standards.

PURPOSE OF BEHAVIORAL OUTCOMES

The purpose of an outcome measurement system is to:

1. Measure clinical effectiveness and outcomes
2. Measure patient satisfaction
3. Evaluate the level of satisfaction that the patient experiences with program elements
   a. Clinical staff and service delivery areas
4. Provide the patient with the most effective level of service
5. Assess history and course of illness
6. Evaluate viability of behavioral health home care
7. Assess level of functioning (ie, activities of daily living, work, social, family, etc)
8. Assess medical resources used
9. Demonstrate the effectiveness of clinical services to payers
10. Institute continuous quality improvement of clinical programs
11. Institute sound working relationships between provider organizations and payers, based on measurement of program effectiveness
12. Develop sound working relationships between providers and payers, based on accurate measures of program outcomes and on the delivery of the least restrictive most cost-effective treatment
13. Determine whether there are opportunities to improve staff performance
    a. Adjust patient expectations to be more realistic, thereby enhancing patient and f/c satisfaction with staff

Procedure

The outcome measurement system is designed to collect information from three separate sources: the participant, informant, and interviewer. The participant is the patient participating in the program. The informant is a f/c. The interviewer is the provider. With these sources of information, meaningful baseline data and outcomes can be reliably measured at specific points in time: intake, discharge, recertification, and follow-up. At intake, information is collected from all three sources. This validates the baseline information being gathered. At recertification information may be collected from the provider and the patient. On discharge, information may be obtained from the patient and the provider(s). Then at follow-up, information is collected from the patient and f/c.

Variables Measured

1. Baseline functioning
   - Mental health
   - Severity of depression
   - Physical health
   - Activities of daily living
   - Functional assessment of daily living
   - Medical resource use
2. Patient psychosocial characteristics
   - Diagnosis as outlined in *Diagnostic and Statistical Manual of Psychiatric Mental Disorders* (*DSM-IV*; American Psychiatric Association, 1994)
   - Age
   - Education
   - Treatment history
   - Service use
   - Living arrangement
   - Social resources
   - Economic resources
3. Treatment characteristics
   - Length of treatment
   - Number of visits
   - Reason treatment terminated
   - Continuing care recommended
   - Medications prescribed
4. Clinical outcomes
   - Mental health
   - Severity of depression
   - Physical health
   - Activities of daily living
   - Functional assessment of daily living
   - Medical resource use
5. Sampling

The outcome measurement system will sample (1) all patients with a primary or secondary psychiatric diagnosis being seen for skilled nursing in the home by a psychiatric nurse and (2) patients with behavioral or psychosocial problems being seen for skilled service in the home.

Assessment

Assessment tools are standardized measures of progress made during service and a means for measuring outcomes. A baseline level of functioning is collected on admission. The provider plans care to address the problems. At periodic intervals the provider reassesses the problem and analyzes the gains or setbacks and plans new strategies. An ongoing, structured outcome measurement system can be highly effective in creating a core of information that can be measured against individual organizations on a local or regional level. When integrated with larger information data bases, an organization's service can be measured against national norms.

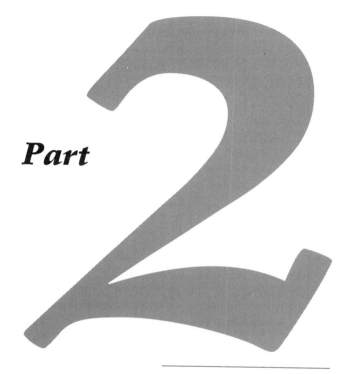

Part

COMMON PROBLEMS ENCOUNTERED IN HOME CARE

Abbreviations and Acronyms

AA: Alcoholics Anonymous
ACHPR: Agency for Health Care Policy and Research
ADLs: activities of daily living
AIDS: acquired immunodeficiency syndrome
ARF: at risk for falls
AST: aspartate transaminase
B/P: blood pressure (lying, sitting, and standing)
CAD: coronary artery disease
CHF: congestive heart failure
CMD: cognitive mental disorder
CNS: central nervous system
CO₂: carbon dioxide
COPD: chronic obstructive pulmonary disease
CP: cardiopulmonary
CPR: cardiopulmonary resuscitation
CV: cardiovascular
d: day
DAT: dementia of the Alzheimer's type
DSM-IV: *Diagnostic and Statistical Manual of Mental Disorders*, 4th ed.
ECG: electrocardiogram
ECT: electroconvulsive therapy
EENT: eye, ears, nose, and throat
EPS: extrapyramidal syndrome
f/c: family/caregiver
FDA: Food and Drug Administration
GI: gastrointestinal
GU: genitourinary
HCl: hydrochloric
HIV: human immunodeficiency virus
IADLs: instrumental activities of daily living
LSD: lysergic acid diethylamine
MAOI: monoamine oxidase inhibitor
mEq/L: milliequivalent per liter
μg: microgram

mg: milligram
MI: myocardial infarction
MID: multi-infarct dementia
mL: milliliter
MSW: medical social worker
NA: Narcotics Anonymous
NIMH: National Institute of Mental Health
NMS: neuroleptic malignant syndrome
NSAID: nonsteroidal anti-inflammatory drug
OC: obsessive-compulsive
OCD: obsessive-compulsive disorder
OT: occupational therapist, therapy
p/c: patient/caregiver
PCA: patient-controlled analgesia
pcg: primary caregiver
pCO₂: carbon dioxide partial pressure or tension
PCP: phencyclidine
p/f/c: patient/family/caregiver
pH: hydrogen ion concentration
PMS: premenstrual syndrome
po: orally
PO₂: oxygen partial pressure or tension
prn: as needed
pt: patient
PT: physical therapist, therapy
PTSD: post-traumatic stress disorder
REM: rapid eye movement
s/s: signs and symptoms
SSRI: selective serotonin reuptake inhibitor
STDs: sexually or socially transmitted diseases
TENS: transcutaneous electrical nerve stimulation
THA: tetrahydroaminoacridine
VD: venereal disease

A

Abusive Behaviors

PROBLEM DESCRIPTION

Abusive behaviors or abuse, also known as family or domestic violence; battering; incest; and marital rape, ranges from subtle and covert harm to life-threatening acts. Abuse is defined as a threat or behavior to coerce another to do what one wants in order to:

- Degrade or humiliate
- Gain or maintain a sense of control or power
- Act out inappropriate anger
- Cause pain or injury to another

The home care nurse may, in the course of providing care, observe that patients or the family/caregivers may be victims of abuse. Some forms of abuse, especially child abuse, are illegal, and must be reported to the authorities when detected. Other forms, such as emotional or spiritual abuse or elder abuse, create a negative, unpleasant atmosphere not conducive to care and healing. As part of holistic and ethical treatment of a patient, and support of family/caregivers, the home care nurse has a responsibility to try to ameliorate the abusive situation.

Four Categories of Abusive Behavior

1. Physical abuse—any forceful physical behavior that inflicts pain or injury; may be life-threatening. The atmosphere of intimidation defines the behavior as abusive, not the degree of injury.
2. Sexual abuse—any nonconsensual sexual behavior or act, not simply forced sexual contact. In its many forms, sexual abuse demeans, humiliates, and shames.
3. Emotional abuse—involves hurt, anger, fear, and degradation. Emotional abusers bolster their self-esteem by creating relationships in which they are "one up." Emotionally abusive behavior creates a person with diminished self-worth and sense of powerlessness to escape further abuse. Often emotional abuse is perceived as more devastating than physical abuse.
4. Spiritual abuse—results when one is physically, sexually, or emotionally abused. The abuser becomes a "higher power" through hate or worship, or the person who is abused blames a "higher power" for the abuser's behavior, thereby losing a sense of the sacred. When another withholds decision-making power, enforces social isolation or confinement, deceives or corrupts, or exploits a person's money, property, or other resources, a person is spiritually abused.

Although most abuse is perpetrated by men against women and by family/caregivers against patients, there are cases of women abusing men and patients abusing their families/caregivers. Each state has laws regarding the reporting of abuse against older, dependent, and disabled adults mandating that the provider report the abuse.

PROBLEM IDENTIFICATION

Characteristics and Observable Behaviors

Physical Abuse

- Threatening or using a weapon, throwing an object at another, or use of implements (such as, belts, hairbrushes, irons, etc) on another
- Slapping, shaking, pushing, shoving, hitting, tripping, choking or strangling, banging, cutting, beating, punching, or burning another
- Biting, kicking, pinching, scratching, twisting, wrenching, or pulling of hair or other body part of another
- Holding someone down, tying, or otherwise physically or chemically restraining one from moving or leaving, including tickling against one's will
- Refusing to get medical attention for one who is sick, injured, or pregnant
- Forcing one to consume an excessive amount of food or fluid or denying one adequate food or liquid
- Forcing one to take medicine that is not prescribed or to take medication that is not on schedule or in amounts that are contrary to medical directions or health maintenance
- Denying and interfering with the meeting of one's basic needs, such as eating or sleeping
- Harming or threatening to harm someone or something important to another (such as, another family member, pet, or cherished possession)
- Watching physical abuse done to another person

Sexual Abuse

- Making demeaning remarks about a person's body or body parts
- Minimizing a person's feelings about sex
- Berating a person about his or her sexual history, including blaming the person for having experienced sexual abuse as a child or being raped
- Jealousy or anger associated with the assumption that one would be or has been sexual with any available person, or harassing one about imagined affairs
- Sexual name calling or being told sexually demeaning remarks or jokes against one's wishes
- Withholding sexual affection or forcing one to beg for sexual affection
- Forcing a person to have sex when he or she is sick or when it is dangerous to the person's health
- Having sex with someone when that person is asleep or otherwise of diminished capacity to consent to such activity
- Openly showing sexual interest in another in the home or in public
- Flaunting an affair after agreeing to be in a monogamous relationship
- Making demeaning remarks about a person's dress or insisting that one dress in a more sexual way than may be comfortable, or otherwise treating a person as a sex object

- Insisting on sexually touching a person when the individual does not want to be sexually touched
- Forcing someone to take off clothes either alone or in the presence of others, or forcing one to pose for sexual photographs or pornography
- Inappropriately exposing the self to another either alone or with others
- Forcing a person to engage in sex (rape) or particular unwanted sexual behaviors, including forcing one to watch or have sex with others, with objects or weapons, to engage in other sadistic acts, or to have sexual contact with animals
- Coercing a person to have sex after an abusive incident

Emotional Abuse

- Verbally by another through screaming, name calling, speaking sarcastically, excessive teasing or being made fun of, ridiculed, scorned, or harped at
- Demanding that one be perfect or being overcontrolling to another
- Being intolerant or ignoring another's feelings
- Ridiculing or insulting one as a member of a group or by calling the person crazy, sick, sinful, disgusting, stupid, etc
- Insulting someone's friends or family
- Humiliating or shaming someone in private or public
- Abusing one's pets or punishing and depriving family members when one is angry at another
- Blaming one for actual or perceived problems with other family members and threatening to hurt friends or family
- Regularly threatening to leave or being told to leave a relationship and threatening harassment or violence (self-abuse, suicide, or homicide) if one tries to leave a relationship
- Listening to it happen to another

Spiritual Abuse

- Being or having been physically, sexually, and emotionally abused
- Being neglected and exploited
- Rejecting, abandoning, or deserting one
- Leaving one unattended in a hostile environment
- Threatening to disclose information about someone that the person wishes to be kept confidential
- Telling one that it was his or her fault that physical, sexual, and spiritual abuse, or neglect and exploitation occurred
- Distorting, denying, or minimizing that behavior to one is abusive, neglectful, or exploitative
- Continually criticizing and conveying the message that no matter what, one is not good enough
- Controlling or limiting use of the telephone and seeing friends or family members
- Refusing to work or be responsible for monetary affairs or making decisions and acting in ways that are detrimental to one's economic and social well-being
- Intellectually, by telling one that he or she is stupid, ignorant, dumb, etc
- Locking one in the house or forcibly confining the person in a room, closet, or other area
- Locking one out of the house or in a shed, garage, or other area

- Enforcing a lack of or disregarding rules and one's own philosophy of life
- Enforcing inhuman rules or a skewed philosophy of living
- Demanding that one seek permission to do or have something
- Threatening one with abuse, neglect, exploitation, punishment, death, torture, or abandonment

Objective and Subjective Behaviors

Consider abuse when p/f/c presents with the following problems: depression, suicidal or homicidal behavior, self-mutilation, hostility, aggressive behavior, drug toxicity, withdrawn behavior, eating disorders, substance abuse behaviors, and personality disorder problems, which may be evidenced by:

- "Learned helplessness" with denial of abuse, passivity, depressive behaviors, fear, ambivalence, unrealistic expectations, low self-esteem, fatigue and apathy, poor grooming, inappropriate body weight, inappropriate clothing, and feeling totally out of control
- Flashbacks, dreams or nightmares, intrusive thoughts, and other reexperiencing of the abusive behavior
- Feelings of helplessness, hopelessness, powerlessness, and anxiety
- Sleep disturbances, headaches, gastrointestinal disturbance or ulcers, and other physiologic problems that are exacerbated by stress
- Feelings of shame and humiliation or feelings of guilt, despair, remorse, and an inability to experience pleasure
- Hostility, rage, anger, poor impulse control, a history of assaultive behavior, suicidal ideas, or a history of suicide attempts and gestures
- Sexual problems, lack of trust, inappropriate dependency needs, economic or physical dependence, manipulative behavior, social isolation, and other difficulties in interpersonal relationships, including complaints of family conflict and substance abuse
- History of frequent urinary tract infections, congestive heart failure, and fatigue and weakness
- Presence of fractures, contractures, sleep or speech disorders, poor hygiene, patches of missing hair, eye injury, septal deviation, missing teeth, inappropriate clothing, lack of necessary assistive devices, burns, bruises or hematomas, skin rash or urine burn, difficulty walking or sitting, decreased sphincter tone or stool impaction, and habitual (eg, sucking, biting, etc) or antisocial or destructive behaviors and problems
- History or presence of vaginal discharge or bleeding, torn, stained or bloody underwear, itching or pain in the genital area, and discharge, bruises, lesions, or discharge of the perineal or rectal area
- History or presence of, with no other etiology or diagnosis, confusion, change in mental status, depression, fear and anxiety (especially in the f/c's presence), and obsessions, compulsions, and phobias

Factors Related to the Problem

- Pts over the age of 75 and female with only one, exclusive caregiver
- Low income, underemployment, or unemployment

- High level of family conflict, a strong power differential, and lack of trust between or among family members
- Role reversal with a family member, feeling forced to care for the patient, family/caregiver financially dependent on the patient, or patient dependent on the family/caregiver
- Partnership strain from keeping an ill, dependent, impaired, or disabled person at home
- Excessive concern or underconcern among family members regarding each other
- Excessive number of stressors, including the stress of caregiving, marital conflict, economic stress, multiple responsibilities, recent life crisis or transition, and substance abuse
- Presence of verbal aggression, hostility, or indifference
- History of being abused or witnessing abuse in family of origin
- Chronic illness, developmental delay, complex disabilities, dependence, or disability, including impaired impulse control, a personality disorder, or other psychiatric problems
- Low self-esteem and inappropriate dependency needs
- Patient history of repeated visits to health care providers for various injuries; going from health care provider to health care provider, being accompanied by someone other than the family/caregiver, not refilling medication prescriptions, or inappropriate medication use or polypharmacy
- Patient history of recent abuse or injury, especially with inconsistent observation of and explanation for injuries or statements that the pt is accident prone
- Family/caregiver uncooperativeness, uninvolvement in community activities, lack of religious affiliation or spiritual connection, social isolation, with an inability to accept help appropriately
- Cultural values, myths, sex-role stereotyping, and negative attitudes regarding older adults and women, which support the perpetration and acceptance of abusive behaviors

Assessment Tool and Instrument (see Appendix I)

1. TRIADS Assessment Tool

PROBLEM LIST

- Apathy
- Body Image Disturbance
- Family/Caregiver Role Stress
- Grieving
- Hopelessness
- Nutrition, Less than Body Requirements
- Pain, Acute or Chronic
- Personal Identity Disturbance
- Post-Trauma Response
- Powerlessness
- Rape-Trauma Syndrome
- Sexuality, Altered Patterns
- Sexual Dysfunction
- Sleep Pattern Disturbance
- Social Interaction, Impaired
- Social Isolation
- Spiritual Distress
- Violence, Risk for, Directed at Self, Other(s), or Property

A

PROBLEM MANAGEMENT

Prevention, Maintenance, and Restorative Interventions

- In a nonjudgmental manner and in private, listen to the pt first and then listen to the f/c after regarding potential abusive behaviors.
- Provide information about the costs and potential risk of caring for a frail, dependent adult if the potential caregiver is also older, chronically ill, or has limited emotional and financial resources.
- Assess the p/f/c and home environment for the risk and signs of abusive behaviors.
- Educate yourself, peers, public, and the p/f/c about establishing methods of self-protection, alleviating abusive behavior-promoting social conditions, and ways to reduce opportunities for abuse.
- Support the development and maintenance of services and legal and legislative efforts to eliminate or prevent abusive behavior.
- Intervene when mistreatment occurs; if necessary, arrange for separation of the parties and for the parties to connect with their families of origin.
- Identify and develop a plan to deal with the identifiable, associated risk factors for abuse.
- Make plans in advance for providing care (abuse prevention planning) well in advance of a f/c becoming overwhelmed, fatigued, ill, or emotionally and financially strained.
- Develop plans, which include cultivation of personal resources; early recognition of abuse; referrals for counseling, personal assistance, respite care for the f/c, emergency shelters, hospitals, and foster homes, other community services, mental health programs, or crisis intervention; and for minimizing stressors and preventing further mistreatment, if abuse has occurred.
- Assist the pt to anticipate difficult circumstances and make preparations, such as writing a will and preparing powers of attorney.
- Assist the f/c to identify sources of support and how to ask for understanding and emotional support before caregiving responsibilities become a strain or stress.
- Teach that abusive behaviors are a spiritual problem and create spiritual pain.

DO teach the p/f/c to:

- Remain sociable
- Develop a mutual "buddy system" with someone outside of the home with a plan for regular contact
- Keep medical, dental, and other personal appointments
- Ask friends and family to visit
- Provide the pt with own telephone, if possible
- Provide the pt the opportunity to open and post own mail
- Keep belongings, records, accounts, and property neat and in a customary place
- Have the pt keep control over assets until pt determines that he or she cannot manage the assets any longer
- Keep cash, jewelry, or cherished belongings locked in a secure place

- Discuss in advance wishes regarding health care, terminal measures, and the disposition of assets
- Engage a lawyer or other trusted advocate before making arrangements to accept personal care in exchange for a transfer or assignment of property or assets
- Remain in contact with old friends and neighbors, even if living arrangements change
- Ask for help when it is needed
- Refuse to live with a person who abuses substances or has a history of abusive behavior and violence
- Develop ways to assist f/c through using emergency response systems, public awareness, respite services, Neighborhood Watch programs, etc (adapted from Douglas, 1987)

Medication Management

No specific medications are indicated for this behavior, although medications might be appropriate for problems associated with the behavior.

NURSING MANAGEMENT

Nursing Interventions and Rationales

⭐ **Behavioral**

- Monitor for factors that are associated with abusive behavior to provide baseline data for early recognition and intervention. *This promotes the integrity of the p/f/c relationships.*
- Document suspected abuse accurately and objectively. *Comprehensive documentation is necessary for diagnosis and possible legal or social intervention.*
- Provide or refer to individual, couple, group, or family therapy. *This action supports changes in f/c roles and behaviors and decreases isolation.*
- Provide or refer to appropriate support groups for information, effective use of existing resources, and long-term support. *Support groups may decrease patient isolation and provide information on skills used to prevent or change abusive behavior.*
- Teach, role play, or rehearse with the p/f/c "time outs." *This gives p/f/c a plan to prevent a tense situation from escalating to an abusive one.*

🖐 **Emotional**

- Use a nonjudgmental approach to talk about feelings with the pt and then f/c. *They may not have had a chance to talk about the situation previously and may welcome the opportunity to receive help instead of blame.*
- Teach how abuse differs from anger. *The distinction helps the p/f/c determine what is and what is not abusive behavior.*
- Encourage the pt, if willing, to talk about the abusive experiences. *Recalling experiences is part of the grieving process that needs to be expressed, and counters the misperception that one deserved the abuse or that abuse in a relationship does not negate caring and love.*

A

△ Cognitive

- Provide or refer for cognitive (eg, rational emotive therapy, self-talk, thought switching, etc) and other types of individual, couple, group, or family therapy. *This assists the p/f/c to prevent or admit and change their part in the abusive behavior, pattern, or cycle.*
- Obtain an understanding of the pt's perception of the threat of abuse. *This facilitates the development of interventions that directly address the pt's concerns.*
- Teach the p/f/c about abusive behavior to create a framework. *Such information helps the p/f/c to identify and express feelings and face the reality of the situation.*

⊓ Physical

- Observe the skin for bruises, hematomas, chafing, excoriation, fractures, burns, malnutrition, and dehydration and document and treat injuries. *Careful observation helps to minimize or prevent complications from physical abuse.*
- If indicated, obtain x-rays, serum electrolyte levels, serum drug levels, and other diagnostic studies to identify fractures, evidence of physical harm and sexually transmitted diseases, malnutrition, dehydration, etc. *Study results provide documentation for patient's health records and for authorities.*
- Determine risk for physical harm and report to the appropriate authorities if the risk is probable. *P/f/c safety is paramount.*

◯ Social

- Educate the p/f/c about appropriate legal services. *This helps to uphold the pt's rights and obtain orders of protection or custody or eviction of a person who is abusive.*
- Contact previous health care providers, health care settings, and f/c outside of the home (with the requisite permission). *Such action helps the nurse to determine if the information presented is congruent and complete.*
- Institute measures to include the pt in social or business activities. *This action helps to prevent potential abuse.*
- Intervene when criminal damage to a person or property is involved, when there is the potential for serious injury or death, and when there is a likelihood of damage to public health and safety. *These actions can preserve life and are caring, accountable, and lawful.*
- Provide the p/f/c with information regarding legal considerations and options. *The patient may obtain legal protection, prosecution, or have information for future use.*
- Provide or arrange for assistance for the p/f/c. *These arrangements help p/f/c to cope with the legal ramifications of abusive behavior.*
- Assist the pt to explore having neighbors call the police when they hear or see anything that may indicate abusive behavior is pending or is in progress. *This action provides the pt with additional defense against abuse.*

✦ Spiritual

- Teach the p/f/c about the connection between abusive behaviors and spiritual pain. *This information helps the p/f/c to understand depression stemming from abuse or abusing.*

- Discuss with the p/f/c beliefs and values about life related to abuse. *Such discussion provides the p/f/c hope-giving experiences.*
- Ensure that the patient has access to a telephone, personal items, belongings, etc. *These items increase the ability to take and maintain control over one's own life and aspects of care.*
- Institute measures to include the pt in spiritual or religious activities. *This enhances spiritual well-being and prevents mistreatment.*

Nursing Goals

- To promote the prevention, recognition of, and intervention in abusive behaviors
- To accurately assess the potential for abuse to the pt and others, institute measures to prevent it, and connect the parties with their families of origin
- To assist the p/f/c to identify choices and make future plans to develop alternative ways of dealing with unhealthy interaction patterns
- To teach about the connection between abusive behaviors and spiritual pain

Patient Goals

- The pt will state that the precipitating factors for abusive behavior have been reduced or eliminated.
- The pt will state that he or she feels safe in own home.
- The pt will state that incidents of abuse have not occurred or have stopped.
- The pt will state that he or she understands the connection between abusive behaviors and spiritual pain.

Patient and Family/Caregiver Outcomes

The patient will:

- Identify abusive behavior within _____ (specify)
- State that incidents of abuse have not occurred within _____ weeks
- Demonstrate decreased behavioral, emotional, cognitive, physical, social, and spiritual effects of abusive behavior by _____ (date) within _____ weeks
- Express an understanding of the right to be free from any form of abuse by _____ (date)
- Maintain control over (specify) the telephone, mail, personal belongings, and resources by _____ (date)
- Report _____ contact(s) from outside of the immediate home environment within _____ weeks
- Verbalize identification and acceptance of losses and changes associated with the abusive relationship(s) by _____ (date)
- Make future plans based on an awareness of abusive relationship patterns and recovery process as demonstrated by _____ by _____ (date)
- Make alternative plans for the future in the event that the caregiving situation changes by discharge
- Express an understanding of the right to remain free of and protected from all forms of abuse within _____ weeks

- Report satisfaction with the ability to maintain or increase social contacts outside of the home within _____ weeks
- Have a written plan for preventing or managing abuse by discharge
- Understand the relationship between abusive behaviors and spirituality as demonstrated by _____ within _____ (specify)
- If necessary, separate from the abuser immediately and connect with a member(s) of the pt's family of origin immediately

The family/caregiver will:

- Contact and attend a respite service, support group, social service, or self-help group (specify) by _____ (date)
- Report an increased ability to cope with the responsibilities of caring for an ill, dependent, disabled, or older adult as demonstrated by _____ within _____ (specify)
- Identify the provider as a person to contact when problems arise by verbalizing _____ within _____ (specify)
- Understand the relationship between abusive behaviors and spirituality as demonstrated by _____ within _____ (specify)
- If necessary, separate from the pt immediately and connect with a member(s) of the f/c's family of origin immediately

RESOURCES AND INFORMATION

1. National Coalition Against Domestic Violence
   1401 Virginia Avenue, NW
   Suite 306
   Washington, DC 20037
   202-293-8860
2. Local crisis intervention hotlines listed in telephone directory under "Crisis, Domestic Violence, Rape Crisis, Women's Shelter, or Women's Protective Services"
3. American Association of Retired Persons
   601 E. Street, N.W.
   Washington, DC 20049
   800-424-3410
4. National Domestic Violence Hotline (for shelter and information): 1-800-333-SAFE (7233)
5. Family Violence Prevention Fund (statistics and information): http://www.fvpf.org/fund/
6. Professional organization's position statements on violence against women and others
7. USENET:
   a. alt.abuse.recovery (recovery from all types of abuse)
   b. alt.sexual.abuse.recovery (recovery from sexual abuse)
   c. alt.support.abuse-partners (for partners of childhood sexual abuse)

REFERENCES

Douglas, R. L. (1987). *Domestic mistreatment of the elderly—Towards prevention* (PF3904 [487]D12810). Washington, DC: American Association of Retired Persons.

Mederios, M. E., & Prochaska, J. O. (1988). Coping strategies that psychotherapists use in working with stressful clients. *Professional Psychology Research and Practice, 1,* 112–114.

Zemsky, B., & Gilbert, L. (1988). *Family and children's service.* Minneapolis: Family Violence Network.

Activities of Daily Living (ADLs) Problems

PROBLEM DESCRIPTION

The activities of daily living (ADLs) are a set of self-care activities that include bathing and hygiene, dressing, feeding, grooming, elimination, and toileting. Assisting the pt in ADLs allows the pt to foster self-care, mental and physical well-being, and maintain functional independence.

Personal care often presents major problems for persons with mental illness, and their inability to function often reinforces their feelings of low self-esteem. Often pts are unable to follow task instructions, which complicates care. Some pts are resistant to self-care issues and are noncompliant with directions or tasks (see Apathy). At times, ADLs can become control issues or they can be affected by impaired thinking. Designing a structured program and organization provides a secure and consistent situation that strengthens coping skills and reinforces reality. Planning and scheduling activities keeps tasks manageable. Encouraging participation in self-care empowers the patient to be responsible. Creativity, ingenuity, and enlisting f/c support can assist the pt in maintaining and improving independent functioning.

PROBLEM IDENTIFICATION

Characteristics and Observable Behaviors

- Inability to dress, feed, or bathe self
- Inability to perform personal hygiene
- Urinary or fecal incontinence
- Foul body odor
- Poor hygiene
- Unkempt appearance
- Lack of appetite
- Lack of interest in eating
- Refusal to eat
- Difficulty eating
- Malnutrition
- Inadequate hydration
- Electrolyte imbalance
- Starvation
- Disturbance in elimination
- Difficulty swallowing

Factors Related to the Problem

- Clinical evidence of perceptual or cognitive impairment
- Depression
- Schizophrenia
- Fatigue
- Impaired memory
- Inability to regulate water temperature or flow
- Medical limitations
- Muscular weakness
- Physical limitation
- Inability to ingest food
- Lack of awareness of need for food and fluids
- Delusions and other psychotic symptoms
- Anorexia nervosa
- Alzheimer's disease and other cognitive disorders

Assessment Tools and Instruments (see Appendix I)

Consider administering:

1. Barthel Index
2. Instrumental Activities of Daily Living

PROBLEM LIST

- Activity Intolerance
- Family/Caregiver Role Strain
- Functional Incontinence
- Incontinence, (Specify: Bowel, Stress, Total, Urinary)
- Mobility, Impaired Physical
- Noncompliance with Self-Care
- Nutrition, Altered
- Self-Care Deficit, (Specify: Feeding, Bathing/Hygiene, Dressing/Grooming, Toileting)
- Skin Integrity, Impaired
- Swallowing, Impaired
- Thought Processes, Altered
- Tissue Integrity, Impaired
- Urinary Elimination, Altered
- Urinary Retention

NURSING MANAGEMENT

Nursing Interventions and Rationales

Behavioral

- Consistently apply _____ therapy to aid the pt's independence. *Reinforcement and rewards may encourage the pt to perform self-care.*

- Give written instructions on bathing and hygiene techniques to f/c. *This helps to ensure correct and therapeutic technique.*
- Supervise return demonstration of hygenic techniques. *A return demonstration identifies problem areas and increases f/c self-confidence.*

Emotional

- Allow the pt to express frustration, anger, or feelings of inadequacy. *These expressions help the pt cope with the emotional consequences of functional deficits.*
- Provide privacy to enhance the pt's compliance. *The pt may not be comfortable being observed.*
- When the pt is bathing, reassure the pt with statements about the temperature, depth, and tasks to be performed. *This guards against panic or anxiety and establishes trust.*

Cognitive

- Promote pt participation in decision making about when ADLs will be accomplished. *Patient participation promotes compliance.*

Physical

- Plan treatment at the pt's convenience whenever possible. *This accommodates treatment to the pt's schedule and provides a sense of control.*

Social

- Ask for and be sensitive to pt preferences. *Such actions promote recognition and respect.*
- Eliminate secondary gains pt receives from not taking care of own ADLs (such as, negative attention or codependence). *This stops the benefits and satisfactions the pt receives from not providing self-care.*
- Provide family therapy for f/c discord regarding pt's illness. *Therapy helps reduce conflicts that may contribute to noncompliance.*
- Avoid a maternalistic or paternalistic relationship with the pt. *This action prevents relating to the pt as a child who needs mothering or fathering.*

Spiritual

- Promote a sense of value to life despite illness and self-care deficits. *This helps the pt value life rather than give up.*

Nursing Goals

- To assist the p/f/c maintain and improve the pt's ability to perform ADLs

Patient Goals

- The pt will maintain adequate routines for physiologic well-being.
- The pt will demonstrate independence in self-care activities.

A

Patient and Family/Caregiver Outcomes

The patient will:

- Develop a positive or therapeutic relationship with provider as demonstrated by _____ by _____ (specify)
- Describe _____ consequences of noncompliance with prescribed treatment regimen as shown by _____ within _____ (specify)
- Communicates _____ (specify) feelings related to _____ (specify) self-care deficits within _____ weeks

The family/caregiver will:

- Assist with the pt's ADLs (specify) as demonstrated by _____ within _____ (specify)

RESOURCES AND INFORMATION

1. Help for Incontinent People, Inc. (HIP)
   PO Box 544
   Union, SC 29379
   803-579-7900 (1-800-BLADDER)
2. National Institute on Aging (NIA)
   Public Inquiries re: Incontinence
   Federal Building, Room 6C12
   Bethesda, MD 20892
   301-496-1752
3. Simon Foundation (for . . .)
   PO Box 835
   Wilmette, IL 60091
   847-864-3913
   1-800-23SIMON (Incontinence)
4. International Hearing Society
   20361 Middlebelt Road
   Livonia, MI 48152
   810-478-2610
   Hearing Aid Helpline: 1-800-521-5247

Adverse Reactions

PROBLEM DESCRIPTION

All medications and treatments have the ability to produce results other than those desired. Side effects and adverse reactions are the result of medication or treatment interactions with other medications and physical, metabolic, or clinical variables. They may be harmless, bothersome, dangerous, or life-threatening. Side effects may pass with time and are tolerable. Adverse reactions are usually unexpected occurrences that require discontinuation of medication or treatment and often require other treatment interventions. Adverse reactions are reportable incidents to the prescriber and agency.

PROBLEM IDENTIFICATION

Characteristics and Observable Behaviors

Side effects and adverse reactions interact with all body systems.

Cardiovascular (CV)
- Angina
- Arrhythmias
- Blood pressure changes
- Cardiac arrest
- Circulatory collapse
- Electrocardiograph (ECG) changes
- Hypertension, hypertensive crisis
- Hypotension, orthostatic
- Palpitations
- Tachycardia
- Thrombocytopenic purpura

Central Nervous System (CNS)
- Akathisia
- Blurred vision
- Clonic movements
- Confusion
- Convulsions
- Dizziness
- Drowsiness
- Dyskinesia
- Dystonia
- Extrapyramidal symptoms (EPS)
- Fatigue
- Headache
- Hyperactivity
- Insomnia/sleep disorders
- Memory loss
- Neuroleptic malignant syndrome
- Nightmares
- Numbness
- Paradoxical reactions in elders
- Paresthesia
- Pseudoparkinsonism
- Restlessness
- Seizures
- Slurred speech
- Stimulation
- Stupor
- Tardive dyskinesia
- Tremors
- Twitching
- Weakness

Eye, Ear, Nose, Throat (EENT)
- Blurred vision
- Dry eyes
- Glaucoma
- Laryngospasm
- Mydriasis
- Tinnitus

Endocrine (Endo)
- Growth retardation

A

Gastrointestinal (GI)

- Abdominal pain
- Anorexia
- Appetite, increased or decreased
- Constipation
- Cramps
- Diarrhea
- Dry mouth
- Epigastric distress
- Hepatitis
- Hepatotoxicity
- Incontinence
- Jaundice
- Metallic taste
- Nausea
- Paralytic ileus
- Stomatitis
- Weight loss
- Vomiting

Genitourinary (GU)

- Acute renal failure
- Albuminuria
- Amenorrhea
- Decreased libido
- Edema
- Enuresis
- Glycosuria
- Gynecomastia
- Impotence
- Nephrotoxicity
- Polydipsia
- Polyuria
- Proteinuria
- Uremia
- Urinary frequency

Hematologic (Hema)

- Agranulocytosis
- Anemia
- Blood dyscrasias
- Leukocytosis
- Leukopenia

Integumentary (Integ)

- Erythema multiforme
- Exfoliative dermatitis
- Hair loss
- Photosensitivity
- Pruritus
- Rash
- Sweating
- Urticaria

Miscellaneous (Misc)

- Arthralgia
- Fever

Factors Related to the Problem

Contraindications, precautions, interactions, and incompatibilities must be addressed.

Assessment Tools and Instruments (see Appendix I)
1. Medication Education Evaluation Form
2. History and Physical Examination Report

PROBLEM LIST

- Ineffective Management of Therapeutic Regimen
- Noncompliance with Medications
- Poisoning, Risk for
- Thought Process, Altered
- Violence, Risk for, Directed at Self

PROBLEM MANAGEMENT

Prevention, Maintenance, and Restorative Interventions

- Observe for signs and symptoms (s/s) of side effects or adverse reactions.
- Assess body systems each visit for potential adverse reactions.
- Assess laboratory reports for therapeutic medication levels.
- Draw laboratory specimens to analyze therapeutic medication levels.
- Teach medications, actions, side effects, adverse reactions, and compliance management.
- Teach recognition of s/s of toxicity with medications.
- Observe for EPS and administer medications as necessary.
- Observe changes in behaviors for medication compliance.

Symptom Management, Categories, and Techniques

- Akathisia: observe and instruct pt for s/s: continuous restlessness and fidgeting; instruct pt that symptoms may occur 50 to 60 days following initiation of therapy
- Akinesia: observe and instruct pt for s/s: muscular weakness; instruct pt that symptoms may appear one to five days following initiation of antipsychotic and other medications
- Blood dyscrasias: instruct p/f/c in s/s of hematologic reactions and when to call prescriber and agency; teach pt to observe for sore throat, fever, malaise, easy bruising, or unusual bleeding; monitor lab values
- Blurred vision: explain symptoms will likely subside after a few weeks; instruct f/c to assist with tasks requiring visual acuity; maintain safe environment to prevent accidents
- Constipation: teach pt to consume foods high in fiber; increase physical activity and fluid intake

- Delayed onset: observe and instruct p/f/c that medications often have a lag time between first dose and therapeutic level for effect
- Dry mouth: teach pt to use sugarless candy, ice, frequent sips of water; teach oral hygiene
- Dystonia: observe and instruct pt for s/s: involuntary muscular movements or spasms of the face, arms, legs and neck; instruct pt that symptoms occur most often in men and patients under 25 years of age
- Extrapyramidal symptoms (EPS): Observe for s/s and administer antiparkinsonism drugs as ordered; instruct pt in s/s and when to call prescriber and agency; educate pt on plan for as needed (prn) or prophylactic medication schedule
- Hand tremors: observe and instruct pt in s/s and to notify prescriber and agency; prescriber may decrease dose of medication
- Hormonal effects (decreased libido, retrograde ejaculation, gynecomastia, amenorrhea): instruct in s/s and causes of problems; provide reassurance of reversibility; discuss with pt and prescriber alteration in medication
- Hypertensive crisis: observe and instruct p/f/c about s/s: severe occipital headache, palpitations, nausea, vomiting, nuchal rigidity, fever, sweating, marked increase in blood pressure, chest pain, and coma; instruct pt to discontinue medication immediately; instruct pt to call prescriber and agency; instruct p/f/c that if pt is taking a monoamine oxidase inhibitor (MAOI) to avoid foods high in tyramine, such as aged cheese, overripe or fermented foods, broad beans, pickled herring, beef or chicken liver, sausage, beer, wine, yeast products, chocolate, caffeinated drinks, canned figs, sour cream, yogurt, soy sauce, and over-the-counter cold medications and diet pills
- Hypotension: observe and instruct p/f/c for s/s: pulse irregularities or arrhythmias; prescriber may decrease dose of medication
- Lithium toxicity: observe and instruct p/f/c in s/s: blurred vision, ataxia, tinnitis, persistent nausea and vomiting, severe diarrhea, excess output dilute urine, increasing tremors, muscular irritability, psychomotor retardation, mental confusion, giddiness, impaired consciousness, nystagmus, seizures, coma, oliguria/anuria, arrhythmias, myocardial infarction, cardiovascular collapse; instruct p/f/c importance of laboratory blood draws to monitor serum lithium levels; instruct p/f/c to notify prescriber and agency of any s/s, and to call 911 if instructed
- Nausea, GI upset: review with pt and prescriber the possibility for antiemetic or antacid; dilute medication with juice, other liquid or food if appropriate; plan medication schedule before, during, or after meals if possible
- Neuroleptic malignant syndrome (NMS): observe and instruct p/f/c for s/s: severe parkinsonism muscle rigidity, hyperpyrexia up to 107°F, tachycardia, tachypnea, fluctuation in blood pressure, diaphoresis, rapid deterioration of mental status to stupor or coma; instruct p/f/c to discontinue medications immediately and to call prescriber, agency and 911
- Oculogyric crisis: observe and instruct pt for s/s: uncontrolled rolling back of the eyes; instruct pt that s/s may look like seizure or dystonia; instruct p/f/c that this is a potential emergency and to call prescriber and agency immediately; instruct p/f/c to stay with pt and offer reassurance and support during this frightening time
- Orthostatic hypotension: instruct pt to rise slowly from lying or sitting position; monitor blood pressure (B/P) lying or sitting and standing; instruct pt in safety while dizzy or lightheaded

- Paradoxical excitement: observe and instruct p/f/c in s/s: agitation, excitation, or sleeplessness when medication is intended to calm pt; instruct p/f/c to withhold medication and contact prescriber and agency
- Paralytic ileus: observe and instruct pt to recognize s/s: abdominal distention, absent bowel sound, nausea, vomiting, epigastric pain; instruct p/f/c to report symptoms to prescriber and agency immediately, and call 911 if instructed
- Photosensitivity: instruct p/f/c to use sunscreen on exposed skin and use sunglasses; instruct p/f/c to report any burns
- Polyuria and dehydration: observe and instruct p/f/c of s/s: decreased thirst, decreased liquids, decreased/increased urine output, sudden weight loss/gain; instruct pt to notify prescriber and agency immediately if s/s occur
- Pseudoparkinsonism: observe and instruct pt for s/s: tremor, shuffling gait, drooling, rigidity, instruct pt that symptoms may appear one to five days following initiation of antipsychotic and other medications
- Sedation, drowsiness, dizziness: discuss possibility of medication administration at bedtime; assess and discuss possible decrease in dosage; instruct safety while sedated: not to use heavy or complicated machinery or participate in activities that require alertness
- Seizure: instruct p/f/c in seizure protocols and safety, instruct to call prescriber and agency
- Skin rash: instruct pt to report any rash
- Tachycardia, arrhythmias: observe and instruct p/f/c to report significant changes; monitor blood pressure and pulse rate/rhythm at each visit
- Tachycardia, decreased sweating, elevated temperature: observe and instruct pt to recognize s/s and to call prescriber and agency immediately; instruct p/f/c that this adverse reaction shows that the body is not able to cool itself
- Tardive dyskinesia: observe and instruct pt for s/s: bizarre facial and tongue movements, stiff neck and difficulty swallowing; instruct p/f/c that pts receiving long-term antipsychotic medication therapy are at risk; instruct p/f/c that drug should be discontinued until the prescriber and agency are notified; instruct p/f/c that prompt action may prevent irreversibility
- Tolerance: observe and instruct p/f/c about s/s: physical and psychological dependence; instruct pt not to quit taking drug abruptly
- Urinary retention: observe and instruct pt to report any difficulty urinating; instruct pt to note any color changes or smell of urine; instruct pt to note amount voided and liquids taken
- Weight gain: instruct pt to weigh per schedule; educate pt about diet, exercise, and sodium

NURSING MANAGEMENT

Nursing Interventions and Rationales

☆ Behavioral

- Set up a schedule for medications. *A schedule monitors compliance and maintains therapeutic medication levels.*

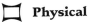 **Emotional**

- Provide supportive environment. *Patient needs to feel safe taking medications.*
- Instruct the f/c in the importance of providing positive reinforcement for the patient's positive actions. *Positive feedback enhances the success of further positive actions.*

Cognitive

- Instruct the p/f/c in s/s of adverse reactions and interventions for each medication. *Such instruction prevents untoward medication reactions.*
- Assess p/f/c knowledge of information presented. *This builds on p/f/c strengths and allows instruction in areas of knowledge deficit.*

Physical

- Administer and monitor laboratory draws for therapeutic medication levels. *This determines the best dose of medication for each particular pt and prevents or minimizes untoward medication effects.*
- Observe for s/s of side effects and adverse reactions. *Such observations help to prevent complications.*

Social

Instruct the p/f/c to:

- Keep a written record of all medications, including nonprescription and vitamins, herbs, etc
- Follow directions for taking medications
- Store medicine in original container
- Keep caps tightly closed
- Keep medicine out of the reach of children
- Recheck labels for instruction each time they take medicine
- Not take medicine left over from a previous illness
- Not share prescription medicines with friends or relatives
- Not stop taking medication just because they begin to feel better
- Not mix medicine in containers
- Not take medication beyond its expiration date
- Not store drugs in extreme heat, humidity or light
- Not refer to drugs as "candy" when talking with children
- Not take medicine at night without turning on a light
- Keep a chart of medications and when they are scheduled to be taken
- Understand that over-the-counter medications and other preparations can also cause side effects and adverse reactions
- Not be afraid or embarrassed to ask the prescriber any questions about medications
- Minimize or prevent adverse reactions

These instructions aid in correct self-administration of medications, ensure that medications are the correct ones to be taken, and ensure that medications are not abused or taken by other parties.

✦ Spiritual

Teach the p/f/c about the importance of taking medications, positive feedback, and realistic expectations. *These actions assist the patient.*

Nursing Goals

- To convey to the p/f/c an understanding of the pt's medication schedule, and possible side effects and adverse reactions
- To assist the p/f/c to comply with the medication schedule

Patient Goals

- The pt will verbalize an understanding of the medication schedule and possible side effects and adverse reactions.
- The pt will exhibit compliance with medication schedule.
- The pt will verbalize s/s of disease process, s/s of exacerbation, s/s of side effects, adverse reactions, and management techniques.
- The pt will notify the prescriber and agency of any s/s of side effects and adverse reactions.

Patient and Family/Caregiver Outcomes

The patient will:

- Verbalize understanding of medication schedule, side effects, adverse reactions, and rationale by _____ (date)
- Be compliant with _____ and understand medication complications (specify) by _____ (date)
- Verbalize signs and symptoms (s/s) of _____ disease process, s/s of exacerbation of _____, and management techniques (specify) by _____ (date)
- Exhibit ability to take medications on schedule with or without (specify) assistance within _____ (specify)
- Take medications without evidence of mistrust as demonstrated by _____ by _____ (date)

The family/caregiver will:

- Assist the pt with medication schedule and compliance by _____ by _____ (date)
- Set up medications as necessary within _____ (specify)
- Verbalize an understanding of side effects and adverse reactions to medications by _____ (date)

- Verbalize understanding of s/s disease process, s/s exacerbation, and management techniques by _____ (date)

RESOURCES AND INFORMATION

1. AHCA Publications (Module 9–Psychotropic Medication)
   PO Box 96906
   Washington, DC 20090-6906
   1-800-321-0343
2. American Association for Retired Persons (AARP)
   601 E. Street, N.W.
   Washington, DC 20049
   800-424-3410
3. Public Citizen Health Research Group (for the books, *Worst Pills/Best Pills* and *Over the Counter Pills That Do Not Work*)
   2000 P Street, NW
   Suite 300
   Washington, DC 20036
4. Council on Family Health (for *Medicines and You: A Guide for Older Americans*)
   225 Park Avenue South
   Suite 1700
   New York, NY 10003
   212-598-3617

Aggressive Behaviors

PROBLEM DESCRIPTION

Aggression is a forceful, generally inappropriate and nonadaptive verbal or physical action. Anger is a feeling of extreme displeasure, annoyance, indignation, exasperation, or hostility. The feeling of anger and aggression is both physical and emotional and may be directed toward self or others. When the attainment of a goal is frustrated and a person feels inadequate, anger surfaces.

Aggression is related to anger. Aggression manifests itself in destructive behaviors. Anger and aggression can be described on a continuum from mild to violent rage. Anger can be both positive and negative. Positive aspects are energizing, motivate change, and give a sense of control over the situation. Negative anger is often expressed in depression, physical illness, passive-aggressive behavior, or violence.

The continuum of aggression includes:

- Mild—actions conveying displeasure or tension (eg, sarcasm)
- Moderate—direct expression of anger or displeasure (eg, verbal abuse, threatening physical violence, harassment)

- Extreme—physical acting out of verbal threats, anger, or displeasure; destruction of property (physical force)

Anger is a normal human emotion that is crucial for individual growth and a factor present in all relationships. Anger is a normal response to something a person perceives as a frustration of desires or a threat to one's needs. It is a derivation of anxiety and includes feelings of powerlessness and helplessness that may be rational or irrational. Anger may be justified or unjustified, conscious or unconscious, intentional or unintentional. When handled appropriately and expressed assertively, it is a positive creative force leading to problem-solving and productive change.

When channeled inappropriately and expressed as verbal or physical aggression, it is a destructive and potentially life-threatening force. Physical aggression is also called assault, battery, or violence. Anger may also be expressed indirectly as passive aggression (sarcasm) or internalized, and it may lead to unpleasant emotional and physical problems.

In assessment it is necessary to determine the history of aggressive behaviors, intensity, targets, degree of inner control, and degree of unpredictability. Determine prior coping methods and meaning behind the aggressive behaviors.

PROBLEM IDENTIFICATION

Characteristics and Observable Behaviors

- Agitation
- Argumentative
- Assaultive
- Bragging about prior violence
- Crying
- Damage to property
- Demanding, arguing, belligerent
- Domination
- Feelings of failure, violation, alienation, demoralization, depression, powerlessness, frustration, exasperation
- Homicidal ideation
- Hostility
- Impatience
- Increased motor tension (eg, pacing, agitation)
- Inappropriate forceful verbal action, without consideration of others
- Inappropriate forceful physical action, directed to self or others, including assault/injury
- Inappropriate forceful physical action against property

- Intimidation
- Irritability, rage, fury
- Jealousy
- Negativism
- Overconfident, grandiose
- Overt defiance
- Passive aggressive behavior
- Physical threat
- Rage
- Resentment
- Sarcasm
- Scapegoating
- Screaming
- Self-mutilation
- Suicide
- Swearing
- Temper tantrums
- Threatening nonverbal body language (eg, glaring, angry facial expression, clenched fists, strained or raised voice)
- Violation of others' rights
- Withdrawn, self-isolative

A

Factors Related to the Problem

- Acceptance of aggressive behavior as a norm by members of subculture
- Auditory and visual hallucinations
- Brain tumors
- Confusion, delusions, disorientation
- Difficulty in learning from past mistakes
- Endocrine or metabolic disorders
- Environmental factors
- Fear, anxiety, hostility
- Frustration of needs or wants
- Grief (anger phase)
- Guilt
- Helplessness
- History of violence or abuse; family violence
- Inferiority and low self-esteem
- Interpersonal conflicts
- Invasion of personal space
- Lack of trust
- Loss of dignity, relationships, possessions, inhibitions
- Manic excitement
- Misinterpretation of environment/interpersonal stimuli
- Need to test reality
- Overwhelming stress
- Panic attack
- Paranoid ideation
- Perceived threat
- Perceptual or cognitive distortion
- Physical disorder/impairment (minimal brain dysfunction)
- Poor impulse control
- Powerlessness
- Prolonged insomnia
- Repressed resentment, hostility, or hate
- Social milieu rejection
- Suspiciousness
- Threats to self-esteem, health or safety, sense of control, sense of security, needs
- Threatened goal progression or achievement
- Threatened or poor self-concept
- Thwarting of goals, needs, power, control, authority, autonomy, attention
- Toxic reactions
- Use of disinhibitors
- Victimization

Assessment Tools and Instruments (see Appendix)

Administer the:

1. Modified Overt Aggression Scale

PROBLEM LIST

- Activity Intolerance, Risk for
- Communication, Impaired Nonverbal
- Communication, Impaired Verbal
- Grieving, Dysfunctional
- Hopelessness
- Mobility Impaired, Physical
- Noncompliance
- Parental Role Conflict
- Post-Trauma Response
- Powerlessness
- Rape-Trauma Syndrome
- Self-Esteem, Disturbance in
- Sensory/Perceptual Alteration
- Sexual Dysfunction
- Sleep Pattern Disturbance
- Social Interaction, Impaired
- Social Isolation
- Spiritual Distress
- Thought Processes, Altered
- Violence, Risk for, Directed at Self, Other(s), or Property

PROBLEM MANAGEMENT

Prevention, Maintenance, and Restorative Interventions

See common general interventions.

Medication Management

Medications and drugs associated with aggression:

- Alcohol
- Hypnotic and antianxiety agents
- Analgesics
- Steroids
- Antidepressants
- Amphetamines and cocaine
- Anticholinergic drugs including over-the-counter sedatives

Currently, no single medication is indicated specifically for the treatment of aggression. However, some medications decrease s/s of aggression as they relate to the underlying diagnosis (eg, agitated depression, psychosis, manic behaviors). Medications used in aggression management include antipsychotics, stimulants, anticonvulsants, lithium, and the serotonin-norepinephrine reuptake inhibitor antidepressants.

Antipsychotics are indicated when aggression is directly related to psychotic ideation or in acute management of violence or aggression using sedative side effects. The standard doses of antipsychotics are used to treat aggression. Oversedation and multiple side effects including risk of tardive dyskinesia should be considered in long-term treatment of chronic aggression.

Carbamazepine (Tegretol) is used for aggression as it relates to complex partial seizure disorder; 600 to 1200 mg/d in divided doses is recommended. Blood levels between 4 and 12 μg/mL are therapeutic. The pt must be monitored for evidence of bone marrow suppression or hematologic abnormalities.

Lithium is indicated when aggression and irritability are related to manic excitement or cyclic mood disorders; 300 mg three times a day and a serum level of 0.6 to 1.2 mEq/L are recommended. This regimen has been shown to be effective for aggression in prisoners and the mentally retarded.

Buspirone (BuSpar) is used for aggression associated with severe anxiety. The recommended dosage is 10 to 20 mg orally three times a day. It may take 4 to 6 weeks for onset of action.

Propranolol (Inderal) is used in chronic or recurrent aggression in pts with organic brain disease or injuries; 200 to 800 mg/d in divided doses is recommended. It may take 4 to 6 weeks for onset of action.

Paroxetine (Paxil), fluoxetine (Prozac), and sertraline (Zoloft) act on aggression by changing the levels of serotonin in the brain to provide a balance. Serotonin levels are low in persons with frontal injury who may be having difficulty expressing anger and aggression. These medications improve membrane integrity of the injured neurons and reduce the "kindling response" that expresses itself in anger and aggression.

Medications used for acute aggression include lorazepam, trazodone (Desyrel), and clonidine. Medications for acute and persistent management include antiseizure medications (eg, carbamazepine [Tegretol]), valproic acid, propranolol, serotonin agonists, and lithium carbonate.

NURSING MANAGEMENT

Nursing Interventions and Rationales

⭐ Behavioral

- Observe for indicators of agitation. *Such signs may indicate that anger is escalating.*
- Work with the pt on alternatives to aggression, such as stress reduction, physical exercise, expression of angry feelings. *These measures reduce the energy and feelings of power that accompany anger.*
- Work with p/f/c to decrease environmental stimuli when pt's behavior escalates. *This action decreases external threats or overstimulation.*
- Teach f/c to respond in a low, calm voice, to reorient the pt and to provide a safe environment. *Calmness decreases the threat of aggressive behavior.*
- Teach f/c to find alternative methods of dealing with stress of threatening behaviors. *Such methods provide p/f/c with productive alternatives to angry outbursts and aggressive behavior.*
- Teach p/f/c consistency in setting limits and interventions. *Consistency gives p/f/c a framework of what will happen in advance of stressful situations and promotes trust.*
- Do not rush the pt through activities or overly structure environment. *This decreases tension from feelings of being forced or pushed to act a certain way.*

♡ Emotional

- Communicate warmth, empathy, respect, and genuineness to encourage verbalization of angry feelings. *This brings feelings into awareness and prompts other coping skills.*
- Encourage the pt to choose socially acceptable methods of managing aggressive and angry feelings. *These methods reinforce positive behaviors.*
- Inform pts that they are responsible for controlling their own behavior, recognizing feelings, and choosing the appropriate method to deal with threats. *This information creates a sense of responsibility for their feelings and responses.*
- Help the pt identify consequences of anger. *This assists pt in developing an awareness of effects of anger on self and others.*
- Provide feedback on nonverbal behaviors. *This identifies anger and behavior when angry.*
- Instruct f/c to not convey fear when the pt is out of control, but to appear to be in control and set limits. *Such actions promote security.*

△ Cognitive

- Encourage positive self-statements. *This increases self-worth.*
- Help the pt identify alternative coping strategies for anger and tension. *New strategies increase coping skills.*
- Encourage the pt to verbalize angry feelings to f/c or supportive other when escalating. *Verbalization allows f/c to assist in coping skills and de-escalation of behaviors.*

- Assist the pt in identifying sources of anger or frustration. *Pt can learn to handle the situation causing anger, avoid it, or accept it.*
- Confront the pt about behaviors after a therapeutic relationship is established. *Such action helps to maintain a trusting relationship with pt.*
- Set limits on inappropriate angry behaviors. *Limits prevent injury to self, others, or property and clarify expectations.*
- Help the pt to discuss conflicts objectively. *Discussion lessens the intensity of the emotions.*
- Develop goals for appropriate expression of anger. *Goals increase self-concept and participation in decision-making.*
- Explore past experiences with anger and aggression and reward/secondary gains from behavior. *This determines how gains are perceived.*
- Take threats of physical aggression seriously. *This prevents injury to self, others, or property and lets the pt know the pt was heard.*
- Rehearse situations that may result in anger and what methods would be used to cope. *Such action builds confidence in methods of expressing anger.*

◯ Social

- Protect yourself; keep a safe approach distance. *This avoids injury and promotes your own safety.*
- Do not try to physically touch the pt; wait until the pt has calmed down, and then offer verbal reassurance. *Such action prevents or minimizes harm and damage due to pt misinterpretation of caregiver actions.*
- Determine if the pt is responding to hallucinations or delusions or if something is wrong or being misinterpreted. *This decreases or prevents aggressive behavior.*
- When the pt is aggressive, do not overreact or talk too much. *This minimizes aggressive behavior and prevents harm or injury to others or property.*
- Calmly talk about what happened and possible consequences. *Referring to patient's anger calmly avoids shaming the pt for behavior.*

✦ Spiritual

- Communicate acceptance of the pt through actions. *Acceptance gives recognition that the pt is a unique individual who has a problem with anger.*

Nursing Goals

- To prevent physical aggression or acting out that can cause danger to pt or others
- To provide a nonthreatening environment
- To deal safely and effectively with pt's aggression
- To deal safely with pt who has a weapon
- To provide an outlet for pt's feelings, physical tension, and agitation
- To decrease psychotic symptoms

Patient Goals

- The pt will demonstrate ability to exercise internal control over behavior.
- The pt will be free of psychotic behavior.
- The pt will seek help immediately when beginning to feel out of control.

- The pt will have fewer violent responses and decrease acting out behaviors.
- The pt will experience decreased restlessness, agitation, fear, anxiety, or hostility.
- The pt will identify and follow through with ways to deal with tension, aggressive feelings, fear, anxiety, hostility in a nondestructive manner.
- The pt will express anger in ways that are not injurious to self or others.
- The pt will develop the ability to deal with tension without becoming combative.
- The pt will identify ways to deal with tension and aggressive feelings in a nondestructive manner.
- The pt will be able to verbalize understanding of aggressive behavior, associated disorder(s) and medications, if any.

Patient and Family/Cargiver Outcomes

The patient will:

- Demonstrate congruency between the feeling of anger and behavior as shown by _____ within _____ (specify)
- Gain control over angry impulses through verbalizing _____ feelings by _____ (specify)
- Gain control by venting frustration through _____ feelings by _____ (specify)
- Gain control through _____ nondestructive channels by _____ (specify)
- Gain control through _____ taking time-outs by _____ (specify)
- Gain control by taking medications by _____ (date)
- Discuss source(s) of angry feelings and appropriate ways to handle frustration by _____ (specify)
- Exercise internal control over behavior as demonstrated by _____ by (date)

The family/caregiver will:

- Set realistic goals, such as learning stress-management strategies or _____ by _____ (date)
- Establish limits on the pt's behavior and uphold them within _____ (specify)

RESOURCES AND INFORMATION

1. Crisis Prevention Institute, Inc. (for training programs, videotapes, consultations regarding violence prevention)
   3315-K North 124th Street
   Brookfield, WI 53005
   1-800-558-8976
   Fax: 1-414-783-5906
   E-mail: cpi@execpc.com
   Resource Center: http://www.execpc.com/-cpi

REFERENCES

American Psychiatric Association. (1994). *Diagnostic and statistical manual of mental disorders* (4th ed.). Washington, DC: Author.

Esser, A. (1989). *Mental Illness: A homecare guide.* New York: Wiley.

Aging

PROBLEM DESCRIPTION

Aging is a multiple process of decline that can be separated into primary and secondary aging. Primary aging is intrinsic to the organism and is influenced by inherent or hereditary factors. Secondary aging refers to the appearance of defects and disabilities caused by hostile factors in the environment including trauma and acquired disease.

All living organisms age, but the rate of aging can vary among individuals and groups. Aging differences are, in part, genetically determined but are substantially influenced by nutrition, life-style, gender, and environment. Some changes occur gradually and are barely noticed; others may be sudden or marked by events that can change an individual's life. Aging can affect role function, relationships, responsibilities, skills and abilities, work, leisure, levels of social and economic status, self-image, independence, and dependence. Changes in physical, emotional, mental, and spiritual aspects of life also occur.

PROBLEM IDENTIFICATION
Characteristics and Observable Behaviors

- Difficulty with own ADLs
- Anger
- Anxiety
- Apathy
- Altered cognitive functioning
- Altered communication patterns
- Altered level of consciousness
- Decreased attention span
- Changes in appetite, energy level, motivation
- Change in ability to perform social, vocational, and family roles
- Change in mental or physical capacity that affects ability to perform usual roles
- Complaining
- Difficulty making decisions
- Disorientation
- Fear
- Frustration
- Grief
- Guilt, sorrow
- Helplessness
- Hopelessness
- Impaired reality
- Insomnia
- Loneliness
- Memory loss
- Impaired motor activity
- Negative view of self
- Overwhelmed caregiver
- Panic
- Physical deterioration
- Psychosis
- Sleep disturbances
- Somatizing
- Speech problems
- Substance use
- Visual, hearing problems
- Weight loss
- Withdrawn

A

Factors Related to the Problem

- Chronic medical illness
- Cancer
- Hearing and visual deficits
- Elimination and incontinence problems
- Dementias
- Sleep disturbances

- Medical illness and complications
- Fractures
- Sexual dysfunctions
- Somatization
- Schizophrenia
- Substance abuse

PROBLEM LIST

- Body Image Disturbance
- Caregiver Role Strain
- Communication, Impaired Verbal
- Decisional Conflict
- Grieving, Anticipatory
- Hopelessness

- Poisoning, Risk for
- Powerlessness
- Relocation Stress Syndrome
- Social Isolation
- Thought Process, Altered

PROBLEM MANAGEMENT

Prevention, Maintenance, and Restorative Interventions

- Assist the pt in dealing with aging issues
- Educate and discuss importance of the aging process
  1. Understand the facts: separate facts about aging into three categories—positive facts, negative facts, and uncertainties. Look at each fact and keep it in its proper perspective.
  2. Reject unnecessary limitations: carefully probe each uncertainty. Accept the negative facts (ie, arthritis) while rejecting the idea that it will limit activity.
  3. Create positive expectations: positive expectations allow mental and emotional growth and health.
  4. Develop an action plan: a good understanding of the situation and positive expectations for the future will enhance the quality of life. An action plan is needed to help make those expectations happen. Action plans place the pt in control.
- Educate pt about creating positive expectations. (Assist pt to decide what is important at this time, eg, exploring new interests, taking control of own life, making new friends, lending support to a cause or campaign, taking time to think about problems and possible solutions, creating a bright new vision of the road ahead, finding ways to reward self daily, making time for play, taking care of health, saying yes to life).
- Educate pt on visualization techniques. (Using the pt's imagination, consciously create a clear image of something pt wishes to make happen. Creative visualization helps replace negative imagery with positive mental pictures, which reduce stress effects.)

- Educate pt in creating positive self-talk affirmations. (Affirmations allow creation of positive thoughts and subconscious integration. Positive affirmations allow pt to raise expectations about life and change and improve the reality.)
- Assist pt to implement memory enhancements at home. (Teach that the first step toward improving memory is to learn to protect memory.)
- Six specific actions that can protect memory are:
  1. Eat well
  2. Exercise
  3. Minimize medications
  4. Limit intake of alcohol
  5. Laugh and smile
  6. Use memory or lose it
- Teach that memory training improves memory. Use improved attention techniques, relaxation techniques, visual imagery, name–face visualization, and grouping of like items to stimulate memory. Teach use of memory aids—calendars, daily reminders, notepads, chalkboards, alarm wrist watch, eyeglass keeper, special place for keys, cooking timer, bill collection box, medical insurance notebook, address book, and medication box.

Medication Management

Guidelines for use of medications with older adults:

- Start with a small dose and gradually increase until therapeutic effect or adverse side effects occur. This is usually one-third to one-half of the younger adult dose.
- Use the smallest does that will produce relief.
- Each pt needs individual attention to effects and reactions.
- Gradually taper medications; do not stop abruptly.
- Determine if the aging pt is able to manage without any medications.

Older adults demonstrate altered responses to drug therapy and increased adverse effects. The aging process produces numerous bodily changes that affect absorption, distribution, metabolism, and excretion of drugs:

- Increased gastric pH—decreases absorption
- Increased body fat—decreases fat-soluble drug concentration
- Decreased body water—increases water-soluble drug concentration
- Decreased serum albumin—increases unbound drug leading to increased drug activity
- Decreased cardiac output—decreases metabolism of drugs
- Decreased renal function—decreases metabolism of drugs
- Decreased liver mass, blood flow—decreases metabolism

Special considerations for medications and older adults:

- Antidepressants cause hypotension.
- Amitriptyline produces the most anticholinergic side effects.
- Desipramine, trazodone, and fluoxetine produce the fewest anticholinergic side effects.

- CNS symptoms of toxicity include disorientation, confusion, and memory loss.
- Give antidepressants cautiously to pts with history of CV disease.
- Haloperidol, fluphenazine, and thiothixene cause more EPS than most other antipsychotics.
- Older adults are more prone to EPS due to age-related CNS changes.
- Thioridazine and clozapine have a low incidence of EPS.
- These pts are particularly susceptible to tardive dyskinesia.
- Agranulocytosis is most common in women, especially with clozapine.
- Long-acting or depot antipsychotics are not usually prescribed because of their long half-life.
- Long half-life of benzodiazepines is lengthened by age-related changes that prolong sedation, cause poor coordination and disorientation, and may lead to misdiagnosis.
- Benzodiazepines not usually ordered include chlordiazepoxide (Librium), clorazepate (Tranxene), diazepam (Valium), and prazepam (Centrax).
- Benzodiazepines with shorter half-lives that are typically prescribed include lorazepam (Ativan), oxazepam (Serax), clonazepam (Klonopin), and alprazolam (Xanax).
- Lithium is excreted from the kidneys more slowly and increases the chances for prolonged side effects.
- Sodium depletion from diet or diuretics will increase serum lithium levels.
- A lower blood level of lithium may be appropriate.
- NMS may be potentiated with a combination of lithium and antipsychotics.
- Alcohol increases potential side effects when used with medications.
- Use of medications involves risks associated with polypharmacy, noncompliance, and altered pharmacokinetics.

NURSING MANAGEMENT

Nursing Interventions and Rationales

☆ Behavioral

- Give p/f/c information about developmental tasks of aging by accepting changes in mental and physical capacities, giving up past roles, creating new social relationships, substituting new activities and interests, and revising goals, values, and self-concept. *This information helps p/f/c understand that these tasks are a normal part of the aging process and enhances coping abilities.*

♡ Emotional

- Provide an open and accepting environment and encourage the p/f/c to express feelings about the illness. *This helps them work through emotions, such as anxiety, denial, fear, depression.*
- Encourage pt to help make health care decisions. *Such action promotes the pt's autonomy.*
- Encourage the pt to express feelings about physical changes associated with aging. *This conveys a caring and accepting attitude.*

- While conversing with the pt, focus on the pt's strengths; emphasize the positive aspects of aging. *Such focus increases self-esteem.*
- Assess the effects of the pt's disease on p/f/c functioning. *Assessment helps in planning interventions.*
- Maintain objectivity when dealing with family conflicts or becoming involved in dynamics of the dysfunctional family. *This assists the nurse in intervening effectively because dysfunctional family coping patterns evolve over many years and are unlikely to change just because the pt is older.*

△ Cognitive

- Encourage the pt to reminisce. *Reminiscing helps recall past challenges and successful coping strategies.*
- Provide the pt with information about the aging process, how to cope with stress, and techniques used by other older adults to meet the demands of daily living. *Such information enhances coping strategies.*
- Discuss with the pt the possibility of making life-style changes. *Adjustments can improve the pt's ability to cope.*

⊟ Physical

- Educate the p/f/c about age-related changes, such as atrophy, loss of protein, decreased liver and kidney functions, and change in body mass, that can influence how medications affect the body. *This increases their knowledge and prevents drug interactions or toxicity.*
- Monitor the pt's urine and serum drug levels as necessary. *Such observations monitor age-related changes and chance of toxicity or increased risk of drug interactions.*

◯ Social

- Encourage f/c to express their feelings about caring for the pt and reason for anger toward pt. *Such expression minimizes or prevents abuse, neglect, and exploitation.*

✴ Spiritual

- Identify factors that make the pt feel powerless. *This helps realign expectations.*
- Guide the pt through life review to reflect on past achievements. *This fosters a sense of satisfaction and promotes acceptance of current status.*
- Explore ways in which the pt can contribute to society (ie, volunteer work). *Such actions restore a sense of purpose.*
- Provide the pt with opportunities to express grief over unresolved conflicts with family members. This assists in identifying problems and planning interventions.

Nursing Goals

- To promote self-confidence and independence
- To facilitate development of social skills
- To help pt identify choices and make future plans

A

Patient Goals

- The pt will report increased success in meeting demands of daily living.
- The pt will report improved ability to cope with changes associated with aging or illness.
- The pt will maintain an environment that is enhanced to help cope with memory deficits.
- The pt will participate in activities that provide mental stimulation.
- The pt will be allowed to reminisce about the past as a means to stimulate communication.
- The pt will review and update advance directive annually.
- The pt will show decreased physical s/s of fear.
- The pt will report improved communication patterns.
- The pt will participate in decisions about own care and life-style.
- The pt will express increased acceptance of changes caused by chronic illness or aging and increased self-esteem.
- The pt will obtain information about volunteer activities or other opportunities for increased involvement in community.
- The pt will report improvement in social relationships.

Patient and Family/Caregiver Outcomes

The patient will:

- Modify life-style by _____ to minimize disability by _____ (date)
- Discuss physical changes caused by aging by _____ (specify)
- Identify at least one positive aspect of aging within _____ (specify)
- Describe how aging process can affect prescribed medication dosages within _____ (specify)
- Express grief related to unresolved conflicts with family members and others within _____ (specify)
- State plans to adjust to changes in health status by _____ (date)

The family/caregiver will:

- Listen to suggestions for dealing with unresolved issues from their past without expressing anger or denial within _____ (specify)
- Verbally express willingness to provide emotional support as the pt adjusts to altered role performance within _____ (specify)

RESOURCES AND INFORMATION

1. Aging Network Services
   4400 East West Highway
   Suite 907
   Bethesda, MD 20014
   301-986-1608

2. Children of Aging Parents (CAPS)
    Woodbourne Office Campus
    Suite 302-A
    1609 Woodbourne Road
    Levittown, PA 19057
    215-945-6900
3. Family Caregiver (for "The Family Caregiver," send a large self-addressed, stamped envelope)
    PO Box 16329
    Stamford, CT 06901
4. Lighthouse National Center for Vision and Aging
    800 Second Avenue
    New York, NY 10017
    212-808-0077
    1-800-334-5497
5. National Council on Aging (NCOA)
    409 Third Street, SW
    2nd floor
    Washington, DC 20024
    202-479-1200
    Fax: 202-479-0735

Agitation (See Aggressive Behaviors and Delirium)

Alcohol Abuse (See Substance Abuse Behaviors)

Anger (See Aggressive Behaviors)

Anxiety

PROBLEM DESCRIPTION

Anxiety is a subjective, emotional experience that is not linked to a specific object or source. It is not directly observable but is communicated through behaviors and physiologic symptoms. Fear is different from anxiety in that it is a response to identifiable, external threats. Anxiety is a response to perceived threats to self-concept, self-esteem, or identity. It is often associated with punishment, disapproval, withdrawal of love, disruption of a relationship, isolation, or loss of bodily functioning. Anxiety is an essential emotion of life and is part of our internal system that warns us when things are wrong. The symptoms of anxiety are an exaggeration of the normal bodily responses, have both mental and physical components, and can be adaptive or maladaptive. Everyday anxiety assists the person in developing a stronger sense of self and courage and provides an impetus for learning and change. Intervention becomes necessary when anxious behavior or anxiety becomes maladaptive.

Anxiety can be defined on a continuum of four levels—from mild to panic—as follows:

- Mild—normal anxiety that motivates individuals on a day-to-day basis. Stimuli are readily perceived and processed. The ability to learn and solve problems efficiently is enhanced.
- Moderate—perceptual field is narrowed; person hears, sees, and grasps less. Learning can occur with the direction of another. The individual may fail to attend to environmental stimuli but will notice things that are brought to his or her attention.
- Severe—individual focuses on small details or scattered details. The perceptual field is greatly reduced. The individual is unable to solve problems or use the learning process.
- Panic—most extreme form of anxiety. The individual is disorganized and may be dangerous to self. The person may be unable to act or speak or may be hyperactive and agitated.

Anxiety is the most widespread and frequently diagnosed of all psychological problems. It affects individuals of all ages; the amount of anxiety increases with age, and it is roughly the same for all socioeconomic groups. Recent studies have shown that 8% of adults living in U.S. cities have experienced one or more periods of severe anxiety in the past 6 months. Women are twice as likely to be severely anxious as are men. Recurring anxiety attacks may start at any age, but most frequently begin between the ages of 15 and 35, and may persist through old age. Some individuals suffer a higher than average level of anxiety all their lives, whereas others experience repeated, brief episodes of severe anxiety.

Categories of anxiety include:

1. Generalized anxiety disorders: a state of uneasiness of mind with a vague sense of undefined danger affecting both mental and physical factors. A combination of worrying thoughts and hyperventilation cause and maintain feelings of anxiety. Under stress, the body's fear reaction can become oversensitive and easily triggered. Older adults tend to deny or somaticize feelings either because of social desirability or projecting an image of self-reliance. It is difficult to distinguish the physiologic factors and assess whether they are related to depression or anxiety.
2. Obsessive-compulsive behaviors: reactions to recurring irrational ideas, thoughts, impulses, or images, it is the most common anxiety reaction in older adults. The compulsive behaviors seek to prevent, neutralize, or undo some dreaded event. Obsessive thoughts frequently lead to compulsive behaviors/repeated activities/rituals that are performed in a response to an obsessive thought; these behaviors may place restrictions or demands on others in the environment. Individuals experiencing obsessive thoughts recognize that they do not make sense but are unable to stop the ideas or images even if they cause discomfort or embarrassment. Individuals struggling for control are often likely to exhibit anxiety symptoms. Obsessions often involve dirt, contamination, disease, real or imagined trauma, or other

frightening or unpleasant themes. Two to 3% of adults experience marked OC behaviors that range from adaptive to maladaptive.

3. Phobic anxiety: a form of situational anxiety in which the primary method of coping is avoidance. This avoidance brings temporary relief, but increases the likelihood of further apprehension, negative thoughts, bodily symptoms, and the development of a phobic reaction. Agoraphobia is the phobia most often treated. Complex phobias develop as a response to feared objects that have a private, symbolic, or unconscious meaning. They are most likely to develop in the context of interpersonal conflict and involve coping mechanisms such as projection, displacement, and regression.

4. Traumatic anxiety: occurs in survivors of tragic, unanticipated experiences such as, but not limited to, war, rape, and physical-emotional-sexual abuse. It is associated with sleep disturbances, nightmares, restlessness, irritability, headache, overactive startle reflex, feelings of isolation, distrust, sense of inadequacy, social isolation, and restriction of activities.

5. Changes in brain function: increased nervousness and anxiety caused by changes in brain chemistry affect the individual's ability to understand the surroundings, placements of personal belongings, or what behaviors are expected. Individuals are fearful of "messing up" and doing something wrong. These people may not be able to tell you why they are upset. They are restless, often pacing or fidgeting. This is a difficult situation for the caregiver because the behaviors are annoying and can "get on your nerves."

6. Panic disorder: a diagnostic subtype, characterized by a spontaneous panic attack, lasting 5 to 30 minutes, of intense fear or discomfort that does not occur in association with a specific anxiety-provoking situation (see Panic).

Feelings of anxiety in themselves are not harmful and do not indicate anything seriously wrong. Interventions become necessary when the anxiety becomes disruptive or maladaptive. When the individual understands the anxiety and how to deal with it, then half the battle is won.

PROBLEM IDENTIFICATION

Characteristics and Observable Behaviors

- Agitation, pacing, hyperactivity, restless
- Easily startled
- Frightened
- Impending feeling of doom
- Giddy, jittery, jumpy, keyed up, shaky, wound up
- Increased muscle tension, stiff neck and back
- Preoccupied
- Scared for no reason
- Substance abuse
- Tense, terrified, worried
- Frequent complaints of GI, GU, CV, or respiratory distress
- Avoidance or escape patterns of behavior

- Attention span decreased and concentration difficulties; difficulty focusing on a single topic in conversation
- Chest pains or discomfort, choking or smothering fears and sensations, dyspnea, palpitations
- Altered cognitive function and altered mental status
- Decreased ability to communicate verbally and ineffective expression of feelings
- Compulsive, ritualistic behaviors, including self-mutilation or other physical problems related to ritualistic behaviors
- Fear of being left alone, dying, losing control
- Self-preoccupation, especially with physical status and fears of or rumination on disease or unspecified consequences
- Feelings of apprehension, guilt, inadequacy, or helplessness
- Feelings of weakness or failure and low self-esteem
- History of repeated visits to physicians or hospital admissions
- Sweating, hot and cold flashes, and paresthesia
- Inability to deal with or manage stress and poor impulse control
- Obsessive thoughts
- Panic attacks and phobia

Factors Related to the Problem

Anxiety can be secondary to medical conditions when the physical conditions produce all the symptoms associated with intense, prolonged anxiety. Medical conditions that may present with prominent anxiety symptoms include:

- CV/respiratory: angina, asthma, arrhythmias, COPD, CHF, hypertension, hyperventilation
- Endocrine: carcinoid, thyroidism, diabetes, menopause, premenstrual syndrome
- Neurologic: akathisia, arthritis, collagen vascular diseases, epilepsy, multiple sclerosis

Medications that produce anxiety:

- Antidepressants
- Blood pressure medications
- Caffeine-containing medications
- Cold medications
- Diet pills
- Sleeping pills
- Stimulants
- Thyroid supplements

Medications that when discontinued cause anxiety:

- Antianxiety medications
- Blood pressure medications
- Pain pills
- Sleeping pills

Miscellaneous causes of anxiety:

- Caffeine—high doses, more than 2 to 4 cups of strong coffee a day
- Alcohol

Differential Diagnosis

If s/s of anxiety are evident, it is necessary to rule out other causative factors before treating disorder.

If pt exhibits:

- Headache, facial flushing, pacing, hand wringing, check pulse and vital signs to rule out pre-existing physical problems
- Obsession with physical complaints, sleeplessness, and disturbing dreams, assess depression and mental status to rule out depression
- Verbal complaints of nervousness and muscle tension, assess stress and anxiety to rule out stress reactions
- Verbal complaints of dread or apprehension, assess pt awareness and identification of specific source of feelings to rule out fear as factor

Assessment Tools and Instruments (see Appendix)

Administer the:

1. Beck Depression Inventory
2. Geriatric Depression Scale
3. Modified Overt Aggression Scale
4. Sheehan Patient Rated Anxiety Scale
5. Spiritual Perspective Clinical Scale
6. Suicide Risk Assessment

PROBLEM LIST

- Grieving, Dysfunctional
- Powerlessness
- Social Isolation
- Thought Process, Altered
- Sleep Pattern Disturbance

PROBLEM MANAGEMENT

Prevention, Maintenance, and Restorative Interventions

- Try to understand the underlying anxiety to avoid threatening the person.
- Explore the causes for the anxious feelings and listen for the anxiety-causing event to plan interventions.

- A brief discussion of phobic thoughts and the accompanying feelings of fear help the person to put uncomfortable situations in perspective.
- Trying to get pt to explain what is troubling or arguing will only make the pt more upset.
- Nutritional measures relieve anxiety because much of anxiety is nutritionally caused (eg, by caffeine or alcohol); try using foods that contain the amino acid tryptophan to increase the brain serotonin levels; milk, cashew nuts, and turkey are good sources of tryptophan.
- Calm reassurances are good for adults with organic problems and changes in brain chemistry.
- Exercise and physical activity such as walking, jogging, and other large motor skilled activities can alleviate the anxiety and increase the ability to tolerate stress and discomfort.
- Allow the person to set the pace for activities to help avoid anxiety.
- Administer medications that may help alleviate the symptoms of anxiety by lessening the acquired avoidance response or diminish arousal and anticipatory responses to external or imagined danger or unpleasant situations.
- Teach stress reduction and relaxation techniques, which are often helpful in the mild and moderate stages of anxiety.
- Use simple objects, like worry beads, to shift focus away from the inner negative experience to turn it into a calming ritual.
- Allowing or encouraging avoidance and escape can be adaptive.
- Help the pt develop some perspective about the causes, manifestations, and consequences once the anxiety is manageable to put it into perspective and reduce the anxiety.
- Teach the anxious pt what secondary gains are produced from the anxiety to minimize the anxiety.
- Provide or arrange for cognitive and behavioral therapy to restore coping skills, increase self-confidence, decrease physical tension, decrease avoidance behaviors, and break through negative feedback.
- "The five Rs" are core concepts used in the reduction of anxiety or stress:
    1. Recognition of the causes and sources of the threat or distress; education and consciousness raising
    2. Relationships identified for support, help, reassurance
    3. Removal from/of the threat or stressor; managing the stimulus
    4. Relaxation through techniques such as meditation, massage, breathing exercises, or imagery
    5. Re-engagement through managed re-exposure and desensitization (Tupin, 1988)

Symptom Management, Categories, and Techniques

- Distraction—talking to friends, listening to music, prayer, dancing, watching television, working, writing, going to a nature setting, going for a ride
- Fighting back—positive self-talk, positive thinking, yelling at the voices, not paying attention to the thoughts in your head, avoiding situations that increase symptoms

- Help seeking—going to the hospital, going to the mental health clinic, talking with a health care professional, seeking the support of a family member
- Attempts to feel better—eating, using medications, taking a bath or shower, hugging a pillow or stuffed animal, using medication/relaxation
- Isolation—going to bed, staying home

Medication Management

Antianxiety medications are useful if:

- There is no reasonable cause for anxiety
- Anxiety symptoms are severe and interfere with daily functioning
- They keep pt from enjoying the ordinary pleasures of life
- Anxiety symptoms do not respond to other nondrug treatments

Caution should be used in medication treatment for anxiety. Antianxiety medications traditionally used are benzodiazepines: alprazolam (Xanax), diazepam (Valium), clorazepate (Tranxene), lorazepam (Ativan), oxazepam (Serax), prazepam (Centrax), chlordiazepoxide (Librium), and halazepam (Paxipam).

Buspirone (BuSpar), antihistamines, and β-blocking drugs are also frequently used. A second opinion may be warranted if the pt is prescribed antipsychotics or meprobamate.

Benzodiazepines can cause physical and psychological dependence within 2 to 4 weeks. Long-term use (more than 4 weeks) is not recommended. Use benzodiazepines with caution in older pts. If this medication is used to aid in sleep, the recommended dosage should be taken at bedtime. Adverse reactions to benzodiazepines include unusual feelings of intense anger, outbursts of unaccustomed rage, hostility or violence, intense feelings of depression, intense anxiety and irritability, and severe insomnia. A number of other drugs can interact with benzodiazepines, so carefully monitor for adverse reactions and side effects if combined with narcotics, barbiturates, other sedatives, other benzodiazepines, or antidepressants. Overdose on benzodiazepines is possible but often not fatal with the usual amounts ordered for a month. Caution must be taken to keep pt from hoarding, mixing other lethal medications, or taking alcohol with benzodiazepines; these combinations could cause death. Ativan (lorazepam) has less of an effect on the liver. Alprazolam (Xanax), lorazepam (Ativan), and oxazepam (Serax) are eliminated from the body more quickly, but are more likely to produce withdrawal symptoms when discontinued; they are also less likely to produce side effects of sedation, impairment of coordination, concentration, memory, and muscular weakness.

β-Adrenergic blockers have been used to relieve the physical symptoms of anxiety, such as increased heart rate, sweating, and nervous stomach. The side effects of β-adrenergic drugs are dizziness, low blood pressure, depression, respiratory distress, diabetes, slowed heart rate, and heart failure. These effects can be serious in the elderly. β-Adrenergic drugs are more effective in relieving anxiety symptoms in younger adults than in older adults.

Antihistamines have a mild effect on anxiety and work best on patients with COPD. The most often used are hydroxyzine or diphenhydramine.

Buspirone (BuSpar) is less sedating than the benzodiazepines. It does not impair coordination or cause memory loss and has little potential for addiction. BuSpar may be used for treatment periods longer than 4 weeks and has fewer complications or side effects for older adults. BuSpar is recommended to be taken two to three times a day, and it may take as long as 1 to 3 weeks to notice the desired response.

NURSING MANAGEMENT

Nursing Interventions and Rationales

Select and sequence interventions depending on whether an individual is experiencing a moderate, severe, or panic level of anxiety, and for what reason(s), to design appropriate interventions because intervening in one dimension will also affect other dimensions.

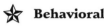 **Behavioral**

- Understand your own feelings toward the pt. *Self-understanding prevents prejudices from interfering with treatment.*
- Be aware that anxiety causes the pt's problem and accept pt's need to obsess or ritualize. *This minimizes the pt's guilt feelings.*
- Maintain a calm, nonthreatening manner while working with the pt. *Anxiety is "contagious" and may be transferred; pts develop feelings of safety and security in the presence of calm caregivers.*
- Avoid asking or forcing the pt to make choices. *Because the pt's ability to problem solve is impaired, the pt is not able to make sound decisions or often any decision at all.*
- Use short, simple, clear statements. *The ability to deal with abstractions or complexity is often impaired.*
- Assess the level of anxiety using the Sheehan Patient Rated Anxiety Scale (see Appendix). *This tool generates a baseline for reference in levels of anxiety and outcomes of interventions.*
- Assess and instruct the p/f/c to identify symptoms that are indicators of anxiety. *This minimizes or prevents harmful anxiety.*
- Instruct pt in practice breathing techniques by breathing through pursed lips and sitting over a table or chair during shortness of breath. *These techniques facilitate air passage and exchange and increase lung expansion.*
- Instruct in the importance of having and assist in the finding of a hobby. *Participation in such activities relieves anxious thoughts.*
- Instruct the pt to pair each anxiety-producing stimulus with a positive, calming quality such as muscle relaxation, deep breathing, imagery, or meditation. *This measure assists the pt in achieving physical and mental relaxation as the anxiety becomes less uncomfortable.*
- Instruct the p/f/c in problem-solving skills (define and allow appropriate time for ritualistic behavior; gradually decrease time for the behavior; explore more adaptive responses to stress). *This improves ability to perform skills more easily.*
- Instruct in the importance of undertaking new tasks. *This confronts the fear of failure and assists in improving self-esteem.*

- Instruct the f/c to offer recognition and positive reinforcement with successful endeavors. *Positive feedback decreases the chance of recurrence.*
- Instruct and assist the pt in developing one new task for the week. *This mechanism allows for change.*
- Instruct the p/f/c that positive feedback will be given for noncompulsive behavior and reinforcement for compulsive behavior will be avoided and ignored. *This approach will keep the pt from obtaining secondary gains from the ritualistic behavior.*
- Instruct the pt in a desensitization approach. *Gradual systemic exposure to the feared situation under controlled conditions allows the pt to begin overcoming the fear.*
- Instruct the pt to reduce excessive stimulation by providing a quiet environment, having selected and limited contact with others, and using no caffeine or other stimulants. *This assists in reducing anxiety by providing safety, security, and privacy.*
- Instruct the p/f/c to change the pt environment as little as possible. *This avoids increasing anxiety and causing a greater need for compulsive behaviors.*
- Provide simple structured tasks requiring concentration. *Simplicity helps the pt organize free time.*
- Instruct the pt on what needs to be done rather than asking the pt to make a decision during periods of increased anxiety. *This relieves the pt of decision-making anxieties and limits the time devoted to repetitive thinking.*
- Reduce anxiety promptly. *Chronic or intense anxiety tends to drive significant others away, at a time when they are needed most.*
- Assess the p/f/c's beliefs about and response to the pt's symptoms. *This assessment helps them modify their beliefs and behaviors and guides further interventions.*
- Instruct the f/c to discuss past experiences with crises and illnesses and invite comparisons with the current situation. *Comparisons heighten awareness, identify previous successful coping mechanisms, increase self-confidence, facilitate resolution of past events, and help in selecting which coping mechanisms to use this time.*
- Instruct the p/f/c to allow ample time to perform ritualistic activity, within reasonable limits. *This reduces anxiety.*
- Instruct the p/f/c to preempt behavior by helping the pt meet psychological needs that are motivating this behavior to reduce attention to or ignore the ritual but pay attention to the pt at other times. *Helps the pt realize that gains can be achieved without ritual behaviors, and if ignored, negative behavior is less likely to be repeated.*
- Instruct the p/f/c that stopping ritualistic behaviors, or forcing the pt to change behaviors, can lead to panic and possibly psychosis. *This avoids stress on pt.*
- Instruct the pt that if rituals interfere with nutrition, that a feeding schedule will be created to promote health and prevent indecisiveness about meals. *A schedule ensures proper nutrition.*
- Instruct the p/f/c that if rituals, such as washing hands, causes skin breakdown, that hand lotion, bandaging hands, or trimming nails may be necessary to prevent skin breakdown. *Such measures ensure pt's physical integrity.*
- Instruct the pt to not withdraw from situations, but instruct in small steps to overcome fear by interaction with a supportive other. *This avoids isolation.*
- Instruct the pt to channel ritualistic behaviors into constructive actions. *This will develop a sense of self-esteem.*

- Instruct the pt to evaluate the success of the chosen alternative and to continue to choose alternatives until one is successful. *This tells the pt that he or she can survive making a mistake and that making a mistake is part of the learning process.*
- Instruct the pt in recognizing areas of personal control, such as taking medications on time, following treatment regimens, controlling with self-care, choosing diets at mealtime, and choosing friends and providers. *These increase pt's autonomy.*
- Instruct the pt in identifying situations that precipitated onset of anxiety symptoms. *Creating awareness and recognition may be the first step in elimination of maladaptive responses.*
- Instruct the pt to recognize early signs of the anxious behavior. *The sooner the pt recognizes the onset of anxiety, the quicker the pt can alter the response.*

Emotional

- Instruct the pt to verbalize feelings of inadequacies, worthlessness, fear of rejection, and need for acceptance by others. *Verbalization allows pt to ventilate fears.*
- Assist the pt in understanding that negative feelings can create poor self-esteem, anger, hostility, aggression, anxiety, and depression. *The pt needs to understand the impact of negative feelings on his or her interactions.*
- Instruct the pt to express feelings more assertively. *Assertive expressions of feelings are self-enhancing and gives the pt power and control.*
- Instruct the pt to stop, wait, and not rush out of a feared situation as soon as it is experienced. *Pt needs to learn to tolerate uncomfortable feelings.*
- Instruct the pt that people with phobias fear "fear" itself, and the pt can wait out the beginnings of anxiety and decrease it with relaxation exercises. *Pt may be able to continue confronting fear.*
- Instruct the pt that negative evaluation by others may affect self-concept. *Hypersensitivity to others' comments must be recognized as negatively affecting the pt's health and self-esteem.*

Cognitive

- Instruct the pt in the definition and process of anxiety. *Continued confrontation of fears helps the pt gain control over thoughts.*
- Instruct the pt to observe anxious behaviors. *Observation helps the pt see the relationship between thinking and feeling and corresponding anxious behavioral response because the pt may be unaware of relationship between emotional issues and anxious behaviors.*
- Instruct the pt that anxiety and ineffective coping may occur. *This is a direct result of impaired thought processes and coping/adjustment skills resulting from the disease process.*
- Instruct the pt in maintaining a log (anxiety notebook) of events preceding, during, and after anxiety occurs. *A record helps the pt recognize themes in anxiety patterns and events that may have precipitated anxiety in the past.*
- Instruct the pt to write down coping strategies (and keep in possession on an index card). *Coping strategies will be available when needed for anticipated or potential future trouble areas.*

- Instruct the pt in problem-solving and coping strategies by identifying problems and treatment by: (1) identifying or recognizing the problem; (2) defining the problem; (3) exploring alternatives or formulating hypothesis or solution to the problem; (4) evaluating and then implementing hypothesis or solution to the problem; (5) formulating conclusions; and (6) making decisions. *Pt may be unaware of a logical process for examining and solving problems.*
- Instruct the pt that mild anxiety can be a positive catalyst for change and that the pt does not need to avoid anxiety. *Anxiety is and can be positive and useful for growth.*

☐ Physical

- Instruct the pt in physical symptoms of anxiety. *Symptoms are real although there may be no organic pathology.*
- Assess pt's level of oxygen and PO_2 saturation for adequate air exchange. *This decreases anxiety about breathing, or intervene, if necessary.*
- Assess and review results of pt's history, laboratory tests (especially: electrolytes, thyroid panel, glucose), physical examination, and observations of behavior. *These detect possible physiologic causes of anxious and phobic symptoms.*

◯ Social

- Instruct the pt regarding opportunities to interact with others. *This assists in maintaining reality orientation, decreases isolation, and lessens anxiety.*
- Instruct the pt in role play and rehearsals concerning behaviors, social contacts, and adapting new behaviors; give positive reinforcements and feedback to increase social skills and contact for the pt. *This relieves social isolation and lessens anxiety.*

✦ Spiritual

- Instruct the pt to set realistic goals to avoid setups for failure and to identify areas in life that are under pt's own control. *This promotes feelings of power and independence.*
- Instruct the pt regarding self-worth with positive affirmations. *This increases reinforcement to positively view self.*
- Instruct and assist the pt to recognize and accept areas in life situations that are not within pt's ability to control. *This aids in reality orientation toward feelings of powerlessness and fear of failure.*
- Instruct the pt that these skills will help to gain control over the ritualistic behaviors. *These skills allow the pt to control by understanding the meaning and purpose of them.*

Nursing Goals

- To help the pt overcome anxiety
- To assist the pt to recognize own limitations and capabilities
- To promote self-confidence
- To promote effective problem-solving techniques
- To facilitate verbal expression of feelings and identification of stress response

- To promote effective problem-solving
- To develop alternative ways of dealing with stress and anxiety
- To decrease the level of anxiety

Patient Goals

- The pt will verbalize understanding of the biologic and psychological components of phobic illness.
- The pt will set limits on phobic behavior, when ready.
- The pt will exhibit less guilt and anxiety related to phobias.
- The pt will maintain autonomy and independence without being handicapped by phobic behavior.
- The pt will demonstrate use of relaxation techniques to maintain anxiety at a manageable level.
- The pt will be able to recognize events that precipitate anxiety and intervene to prevent disabling behaviors.
- The pt will be able to maintain the anxiety level below the moderate stage, as evidenced by absence of disabling behaviors in response to stress.

Patient and Family Caregiver Outcomes

The patient will:

- Identify and demonstrate alternative ways to deal with stress, anxiety, or other (specify) feelings as demonstrated by _____ within _____ (specify)
- Respond to relaxation techniques with a decreased anxiety level as demonstrated by _____ by _____ (date)
- Objectively demonstrate decreased anxiety, fears, guilt, rumination, aggressive, or other (specify) behavior (see Assessment Tools section) by _____ (date)
- Describe successful use of direct communication to have needs met by _____ (date)
- Describe one difficult interpersonal situation that was solved by identifying the problem, choosing alternative ways to communicate and taking action by _____ (date)
- Describe at least two ineffective coping behaviors and appropriate alternative behaviors by _____ (date)
- Participate in _____ new activity(ies) without exhibiting extreme fear of failure as demonstrated by _____ within _____ (specify)
- Manifest no symptoms of depersonalization
- Interpret the environment realistically
- Reduce the amount of time spent each day on obsessive and ritualistic behaviors _____ by (specify) within _____ (specify)
- Make _____ fewer attempts to exert control over self and environment by _____ (date)
- Cope with stress without excessive obsessive-compulsive behaviors as demonstrated by _____ within _____ (specify)
- Identify _____ situation(s) that precipitate phobic reactions within _____ (specify)

- Connect life events to current problems with anxiety as demonstrated by _____ (specify)
- Discuss _____ feelings and _____ behaviors related to phobia and phobic triggers by _____ (within)

The family/caregiver will:

- Assist the pt to manage factors contributing to anxiety by _____ within _____ (specify)

RESOURCES AND INFORMATION

1. The Anxiety Disorder Association of America (ADAA) (advocacy and support for improved care, education, and research in the area of anxiety disorders)
   6000 Executive Boulevard
   Suite 513
   Rockville, MD 20852
   301-231-9350
   Fax: 301-231-7392

REFERENCES

Tupin, J. (1988). *Handbook of clinical psychopharmacology* (pp. 73–96). Northvale, NJ: Aronson.

Apathy

PROBLEM DESCRIPTION

Apathy is a behavior exhibited by lack of feeling or emotion or lack of interest or concern. It is often identified as spiritlessness, indifference, impulsiveness, or hopelessness.

Hopelessness is a subjective state in which the individual sees limited or no alternatives or personal choices available and is unable to mobilize energy on his or her own behalf.

Apathy and hopelessness work together to describe the pt who has given up on everything in life. The turning point for the pt experiencing these symptoms is to reach a level of willingness to act. Hope is an expectation of goal attainment and the probability of attaining it. When these pts finally see that a goal is attainable and they can achieve an end point, then hope comes into view.

The most common sources of hope are family, friends, and religious beliefs. Strategies to alleviate hopelessness and apathy include getting busy and doing something, praying or being involved in religious activity, thinking about other things, and talking to others. The pt willing to try and alleviate this problem will need to assume responsibility for taking action. The provider listens and is physically and emotionally available. Encouraging, setting attainable realistic goals, and monitoring progress assist the pt in taking action.

A pt experiencing apathy or hopeless is difficult to work with and does not communicate easily. Creativity, imagination, and patience are necessary to move this pt toward action.

PROBLEM IDENTIFICATION

Characteristics and Observable Behaviors

- Expression of hopelessness
- Lack of motivation
- Past suicidal history
- Poor compliance with medical regimen
- Presence of risk factors for hopelessness, including experience of multiple losses, isolation, physical deterioration, tenuous family connections
- Sleep disturbances
- Decreased affect and verbalization
- Decreased appetite
- Decreased initiative and involvement
- Increased sleep or sleep pattern disturbances
- Nonverbal cues, such as minimal eye contact, shrugging in response to questions
- Verbal cues, including frequent sighing and hopeless responses, such as "I can't," "What's the use?" or "There's no point"
- Anhedonia (no experience of pleasure)
- Suicidal ideas or feelings
- Depression
- Sorrow
- Despair
- Passivity
- Decreased communication
- Lack of initiative
- Anergy (lack of energy)
- Impaired social interaction
- Sleep disturbances
- Changes in eating habits
- Lack of feeling about anything
- Feelings of inadequacy and despair

Factors Related to the Problem

- Chronic or terminal illness
- Physical problems related to the illness
- Neurologic problems related to the illness
- Feelings of being overwhelmed, despair
- Chemical dependence

Assessment Tools and Instruments (see Appendix)
Administer the:

1. Beck Depression Scale
2. Geriatric Depression Scale
3. Brief Psychiatric Rating Scale
4. Spiritual Perspective Clinical Scale

PROBLEM LIST

*   Grieving, Dysfunctional
*   Noncompliance
*   Post-Trauma Response
*   Powerlessness
*   Sexual Dysfunction
*   Sleep Pattern Disturbance
*   Social Interaction, Impaired
*   Social Isolation
*   Spiritual Distress
*   Thought Process, Altered
*   Violence, Risk for, Directed at Self, Other(s), or Property

NURSING MANAGEMENT

Nursing Interventions and Rationales

☆ Behavioral

*   Assess pt for apathetic behaviors. *Assessment helps nurse and p/f/c design and intervene effectively.*

♡ Emotional

*   Encourage pt to express feelings verbally and nonverbally, in nondestructive ways. *This lessens feelings of despair.*

△ Cognitive

*   Teach pt steps for problem-solving process. *These steps may alleviate or eliminate apathetic behaviors.*

◯ Social

*   Provide pt with a therapeutic companion and a community network. *This provides a continuum of services.*

✦ **Spiritual**

- Refer pt to religious or other spiritual person to discuss hopelessness. *Such a referral provides an advisor who shares the pt's belief system.*

Nursing Goals

- To promote expression of feelings, especially anger, self-blame, anxiety, sadness, despair, spiritual distress, and alternative behaviors

Patient Goals

- The pt will manifest no symptoms of depersonalization.
- The pt will interpret the environment realistically.
- The pt will show reduced apathetic behaviors.
- The pt will demonstrate maximum level of decision-making in planning care.
- The pt will demonstrate the ability to identify choices or alternatives.
- The pt will have more energy.
- The pt will express both positive and negative feelings.
- The pt will express less negative thinking.
- The pt will make positive statements about self and others.
- The pt will express optimism about the future.
- The pt will exhibit a positive self-concept.

Patient and Family/Caregiver Outcomes

The patient will:

- Discuss feelings of hopelessness within _____ (weeks)
- Express improved feelings about self and begin to feel hopeful within _____ (specify)
- Show increased feelings of self-worth as demonstrated by _____ by _____ (date)
- Demonstrate decreased noncompliant behavior as demonstrated by _____ by _____ (date)

The family/caregiver will:

- Assist with reactivating the pt as demonstrated by _____ by _____ (date)
- Assist with remotivating the pt as demonstrated by _____ by _____ (date)

RESOURCES AND INFORMATION

1. See Social Withdrawal Resources and Information

Assaultive Behavior

PROBLEM DESCRIPTION

Assaultive behavior is the unlawful and intentional touching or injuring of another person, and includes spitting, biting, kicking, shoving, and hitting, as well as throwing objects and destroying property. The claim of assault or attack arises when one person assaults another person. Assaultive behavior, the pursuit of one's own interests by force, is violent acting out at the extreme end of the aggressive behaviors continuum. Assaultive behavior can develop slowly or occur suddenly, and it involves a significant degree of danger to f/c and providers (see Section 1). Assaultive behavior is difficult to predict.

PROBLEM IDENTIFICATION

Characteristics and Observable Behaviors

Profiles that lead to assaultive behavior:

- Excessive alcohol intake or substance abuse (especially PCP and amphetamines)
- Toxic reactions to medications and withdrawal syndromes (especially from sedative-hypnotics)
- History of previously assaultive or violent behavior with arrests and criminal activity
- History of childhood abuse
- Current or recently observed assaultive behavior or threats of assaultive or violent behavior
- Men of advanced age (over 85)
- Psychomotor agitation (eg, pacing, rocking, etc), aggressive, hostile, and restless behaviors
- Assaultive or violent fantasies, ideation, or feelings
- Confusion and impaired cognition and organic brain conditions
- Physical disorders, seizure disorders, and sensory loss and immobility
- Schizophrenia, bipolar disorder, borderline personality disorder with psychotic or disorganized thought process, intense paranoia, suspiciousness, delusions, or hallucinations, or fear, rage, panic state, or manic excitement
- Low self-esteem and loneliness
- Verbalized feelings of helplessness, hopelessness, and powerlessness
- Low frustration tolerance and poor impulse control
- Feelings of fear, guilt, anxiety, grief, rejection, tension, or irritability
- Taking medications that have been associated with violence (eg, fluoxetine)
- Inability to trust other people and need for control, autonomy, and personal identity

Conditions and situations that lead to assaultive behavior:

- Invasion of a pt's personal space
- Limiting a pt's behavior, especially with restraints

A

- Limited social support
- During the provision of personal care
- Sarcastic or defensive attitude of the provider toward the pt
- Dysfunctional subculture and family modeling of assaultive behavior

Assessment Tool and Instrument (see Appendix)

1. Administer the Modified Overt Aggression Scale (MAOS). When assessing the pt's mental status, the affect of a pt with assaultive behavior will be termed aggression, anger, rage, or hostility that is excessive; it may be unrelated to the pt's current situation.
2. Brief Psychiatric Rating Scale

PROBLEM LIST

- Anger
- Diversional Activity Deficit
- Powerlessness
- Self-Concept Disturbance
- Sleep Pattern Disturbance
- Social Interaction, Impaired
- Social Isolation
- Thought Process, Altered
- Violence, Directed at Self, Other(s), or Property

PROBLEM MANAGEMENT

Prevention, Maintenance, and Restorative Interventions

- Review agency or program policies and procedures regarding assault and battery.
- Avoid using or experiencing threatening body language, such as clenched fists, quick movements, hands on hips, or arms crossed.
- Avoid arguing or trying to reason with a pt who is exhibiting assaultive behavior.
- Ensure that the f/c do not use aggression or make threats when interacting with the pt.
- Institute close observation and preventive interventions (see Aggressive Behaviors).
- Do not be alone with an escalating pt, stay in control of yourself and the situation, remain calm, and obtain assistance as soon as possible.
- Deal safely with the pt who has a weapon, and if you are not properly skilled in this instance, do not attempt to intervene; rather avoid personal injury (leave and put something in between you and the weapon), summon help, leave the home, and protect f/c.
- Document observations and preventive measures in the pt's record, and inform other team members regarding the incidence of assaultive behavior.

- Identify, and if possible eliminate, factors in the home setting that may potentiate assaultive behavior.
- Assist the p/f/c in feeling safe in the home setting from factors that may potentiate assaultive behaviors.
- Be alert to increasing levels of anxiety and aggressive behaviors as precursors to assaultive behaviors and intervene early with a reduction of environmental stimuli (see Anxiety and Aggressive Behaviors).
- Eliminate any causes of discomfort or increased agitation, such as side effects or responses to medication.
- Assist the p/f/c to recognize and cope with assaultive behaviors.

Medication Management

The medications appropriate for aggressive behavior, the precursor to assaultive behavior, are indicated. Appropriate sedative or antipsychotic medications are most effective.

NURSING MANAGEMENT

Nursing Interventions and Rationales

☆ Behavioral

- Use the pt's preferred name, get eye contact, and give specific directions. *This gains the pt's attention.*
- Assess and record any assaultive behavior, as well as that which preceded the assaultive behavior. *Such assessment aids in developing a plan to minimize or prevent assaultive behavior in the future.*
- Present consequences of assaultive behavior to the pt in a matter-of-fact, nonblaming manner. *This preserves human dignity.*
- Assess effectiveness of medication order for aggressive behavior. *This determines the need for discontinuance, continuance, increase, or change in the medication(s).*
- Assist the pt to alter the behavior that led up to the assault. *This minimizes or prevents assaultive behavior in the future.*
- Refrain from using any type of restraints, which often lead to increased behavior difficulties and injury. *This minimizes or prevents assaultive behavior.*

♡ Emotional

- Accept verbal hostility without retaliation, sarcasm, or defensiveness. *This avoids escalating the situation.*
- Encourage ventilation of anger through verbalization of feelings. *Verbalization minimizes or prevents assaultive behavior.*
- Assist the pt to alter the feelings that contribute to assaultive behavior. *This minimizes or prevents assaultive behavior.*
- Assist the pt in role-playing management of anger in situations that precipitate assaultive behavior. *Such actions replace maladaptive responses with healthier, constructive responses.*

- Assess the match of the provider and pt, especially providers assisting with personal care and assistance with ADLs. *During personal care activities, assaultive behavior might be more likely to occur.*
- Support the p/f/c in adjustments that may be required, which are factors related to the assaultive behavior. *These adjustments may minimize or prevent assaultive behavior.*

Cognitive

- Assess the degree of assaultive behavior intent and intervene as indicated. *This minimizes or prevents harm, injury, or damage.*
- Assist the pt to alter the beliefs that contribute to assaultive behavior. *This minimizes or prevents assaultive behavior.*
- Discuss the assaultive behavior after the episode. *Discussion analyzes the factors that contributed to the episode and minimizes or prevents it from happening again.*
- Teach anger management skills with educational materials. *These materials assist the pt in developing alternative coping skills.*

☐ Physical

- Teach muscle relaxation and deep breathing. *These exercises may minimize or prevent assaultive behavior.*
- Structure the home milieu to reduce or eliminate the availability of potential weapons. *This minimizes or prevents assaultive behavior.*

◯ Social

- Identify environmental factors that may contribute to assaultive behavior and discuss and change these with the p/f/c. *Such changes may minimize or prevent assaultive behavior.*
- Set, and teach the f/c to set, firm nonthreatening yet enforceable limits stating what is and what is not acceptable behavior. *Limits provide an understanding of the boundaries of the therapeutic relationship.*
- Schedule enjoyable activities into the pt's day and evening. *This eliminates blocks of "empty time" that can contribute to the development of assaultive behavior.*
- Provide, and teach f/c to give, attention to the pt in response to positive, nonassaultive behaviors. *Such attention reinforces desired behaviors.*
- Refer to community resources and assist the f/c to participate in group, peer, or an assault "victim's" group. *These actions can provide support and efficient and effective use of existing resources.*
- Assist the p/f/c to determine when to involve law enforcement officials or providers. *This provides for early intervention and possibly prevention of assaultive behavior.*

✦ Spiritual

- Reassure the pt who is having threatening or frightening thoughts or perceptions that the pt will be kept as safe as possible. *Such assurances provide a sense of security.*

- Acknowledge the pt's distress and your intention to help. *This furthers a trusting relationship.*
- Strengthen the pt's sense of responsibility, security, and control by having the pt assist with scheduling, accepting responsibility for own actions without confronting or blaming, validating the pt's feelings, and providing positive feedback when behaviors change. *All these measures reduce the risk of assaultive behavior.*
- Ensure and maintain a familiar, predictable, and nonthreatening environment (including visitors). *This minimizes or prevents assaultive behavior.*
- Ensure that the p/f/c's feelings, dignity, and rights are considered. *The pt is a worthwhile person regardless of the assaultive behavior.*

Nursing Goals

- To remain safe, unharmed, and uninjured during an assaultive incident
- To evaluate and treat any personal harm or injury done during the assaultive episode
- To evaluate any property damage done during the assaultive episode
- To demonstrate relaxation and alternative aggression-release techniques
- To perform nonviolent conflict resolution skills
- To assist the p/f/c to prevent assaultive behavior
- To provide a nonthreatening, therapeutic home environment
- To deal safely and effectively with assaultive behavior

Patient Goals

- The pt will gain insight into sources of anger.
- The pt will cease from engaging in assaultive behavior.
- The pt will understand that choices for behavior are available.
- The pt will desire that incidents of assaultive behavior are reduced or eliminated.

Patient and Family/Caregiver Outcomes

The patient will:

- Cease from engaging in assaultive behavior by _____ (date)
- Verbally, and in written form, agree to a non-assaultive behavior contract as evidenced by _____ within _____ (specify)
- Demonstrate self-control and nonassaultive behavior by _____ within _____ (specify)
- Demonstrate increased control over angry impulses, fear, anxiety, and hostility by _____ within _____ (specify)
- Verbalize an understanding that the pt has choices for behavior by _____ (date)
- Demonstrate at least one alternate means of dealing with anger and frustration other than with assaultive behavior by _____ (date)

The family/caregiver will:

- Assist with gathering of assessment data related to episodes of assaultive behavior, especially if there is a pattern of assaultive behavior, by _____ (date)
- Identify serious risk factors for further assaultive behavior and implement assaultive behavior prevention strategies specific to the home setting by _____ (date)

RESOURCES AND INFORMATION

1. The National Victim Center for support groups: 1-800-394-2255
2. National Organization for Victim Assistance for a 24-hour crisis line: 202-232-6682

B

Bathing and Hygiene Problems (See Activities of Daily Living Problems)

Body Image Problems and Behaviors

PROBLEM DESCRIPTION

Body image is an individual's perception of physical self and functioning. Body image includes physical appearance, emotional reactions, and sensations. Feelings of self-esteem and self-worth can have positive or negative affects on body image.

Altered body image is a change in perception and attitude about the physical self. This often occurs during a growth period, maturation, stressful situations, or a major physical change and involves a loss with grieving.

Therapeutic interventions include dealing with grief and loss with resolution to adaptation to the change. Often a change in body image is more traumatic when the change is external, occurs suddenly, or is unforeseen, uncontrolled, or unwanted. Each person responds individually to life experiences. Before beginning any therapeutic intervention, it is important to assess the pt's self-concept, previous experiences, perceptions, and coping techniques.

PROBLEM IDENTIFICATION

Characteristics and Observable Behaviors

- Devaluation of self through criticism
- Fear or worries, especially of failure
- Feelings of disappointment and helplessness
- Feeling of fragility and inadequacy
- Minimization of own real strengths and abilities
- Sense of self-defeat
- Sensitive to negative information
- Denial of self-pleasure
- Hesitancy to offer own viewpoints
- Preoccupation with real or imagined past failures
- Ambivalence and procrastination
- Self-destructive behavior
- Failure to achieve goals and be successful
- Poor interpersonal relationships
- Inability to respect own opinion and opinions of others
- Difficulty in accepting positive reinforcement
- Seeking secondary gains from self-criticisms
- Lack of follow-through
- Failure to take responsibility for self-care
- Expecting the worst outcome for self
- Actual change in body structure or function
- Avoidance of eye contact and social interaction
- Denial of loss
- Inability to look at or touch the affected part
- Intentional or unintentional hiding of the affected body part
- Social isolation, withdrawal
- Denial of problem
- Not taking responsibility for self-care
- Feelings of hopelessness or worthlessness
- Self-deprecatory verbalization
- Lack of self-confidence
- Anxiety or fear
- Depression, despair
- Regression, dependency
- Fear of rejection
- Feelings of inferiority
- Fear of losing control
- Sense of self-diminution
- Inability to make decisions
- Impaired judgment
- Preoccupation with physical symptoms
- Sensitivity to criticism
- Lacking in assertiveness
- Negative statements about physical appearance

- Self-criticism, blaming others
- Denial of deformity, body change, and loss of function
- Grandiose thinking, boasting, and delusions
- Feelings of discomfort at social events
- Avoidance or responsibility for own behavior
- Chronic medical or mental health problems
- Hesitation to try anything new
- Need for excessive reassurance

Factors Related to the Problem

- Physical problems related to surgery, injury, illness
- Aging
- Weight loss or gain
- Physical change or illness
- Losses (body part, body function, health, role, or status)
- Separation or divorce
- Death of loved one
- Pregnancy
- Menopause
- Puberty
- Difficulty trusting
- Decreased self-esteem
- Guilt

- Problems with intimacy
- Gap between ideal and real self
- Conflicting cognitions and perceptions
- Perceptions of repeated negative experiences or traumatic events
- Perceived negative change in body structure or function
- Unrealistic demands on self or significant others
- Internalizing criticism of others
- Reliance on others for self-appraisal
- Abusive relationships
- Dysfunctional family relationships
- Conflicting cultural expectations

Assessment Tools and Instruments (see Appendix)

Administer the:

1. Beck Depression Scale
2. Geriatric Depression Scale
3. Mini-Mental Status Examination
4. Social Dysfunction Rating Scale
5. Spiritual Perspective Clinical Scale

PROBLEM LIST

- Body Image Disturbance
- Grieving, Dysfunctional
- Social Isolation

- Sexual Dysfunction
- Violence, Risk for, Directed at Self, Other(s), or Property

PROBLEM MANAGEMENT

Prevention, Maintenance, and Restoration Interventions

- Avoid minimizing the pt's change in body image.
- Acknowledge that the pt needs to feel normal.

- Acknowledge that the pt with body image problems often is embarrassed and feels social stigma.
- Assess and compare the pt's perception of self and ideal self.
- Assess the pt's goals and opportunities for and barriers to realistic accomplishment of changes regarding body image.

Medication Management

Medications will vary depending on the pt's concomitant condition(s).

NURSING MANAGEMENT

Nursing Interventions and Rationales

☆ Behavioral

- Reward those pt behaviors based on new insights. *Rewards increase desired behaviors likely to be repeated.*
- Focus on current behaviors and experiences. *This reduces self-criticism of blaming past events for present behavior.*
- Limit the pt's self-criticism. *This interrupts preoccupation with body image and self-blame.*
- Limit the pt's "worry time" to specific time each day. *Such a limit reduces preoccupation and teaches alternatives to worrying.*
- Teach the pt to give and receive compliments. *This increases self-confidence and social skills.*
- Reinforce positive body image self-statements. *Positivity reinforces behavior to be repeated.*

♡ Emotional

- Accept pt's perception of self. *Acceptance validates pt's feelings.*
- Encourage expression of grief about loss. *Grieving precedes acceptance of loss.*
- Encourage expression of feelings, including anger, resentment, guilt, self-blame, envy, fear of rejection, and inadequacy related to body image disturbance. *Such expression identifies feelings and works on grieving issues.*
- Encourage discussion of the pt's feelings regarding changes, perception, helplessness, and guilt. *Discussion assists pt to recognize that feelings are normal and part of the process for healing.*
- Teach the pt how to keep a journal. *A journal provides privacy and independence in identifying and expressing feelings and thoughts.*
- Discuss with pt specific feelings regarding self. *This helps pt to view self as a vital aspect of own personality.*
- Encourage pt to express emotions, fears, feelings of inferiority, sadness, and grief about body changes. *This expression provides catharsis.*
- Help the pt to accept body changes and losses in functioning and feel good about own body. *This improves the pt's body image.*

- Instruct pt to identify emotions and to explore physical manifestations of emotions. *This increases awareness of emotions and physiologic effects.*

△ Cognitive

- Encourage discussion on thoughts about changes, pt's perceptions, feelings of helplessness and guilt. *Discussion assists the pt to recognize that feelings are normal and part of the process for healing.*
- Explore pt's underlying negative assumptions about self. *Such exploration identifies causes of negative self-concept.*
- Provide anticipatory guidance. *This increases pt's ability and confidence in dealing with the self.*

☐ Physical

- Work with the pt toward acceptance of physical losses. *This shows connection between self-concept and body influence.*
- Explore ways the pt can maximize physical potential. *These show pt that a positive change in body image will have positive effects on self-concept.*
- Discuss with the pt that stress or anxiety can cause physiologic changes and lead to further feelings of negative self-image. *Discussion increases pt awareness of sources of negative self-image.*

◯ Social

- Use role playing and rehearsal. *These assist the pt to anticipate and prepare for the reactions of others.*
- Provide anticipatory guidance. *This increases the pt's ability and confidence in facing others.*
- Encourage the pt to identify and express feelings of isolation and fear of rejection and the reactions of others. *Helps significant others accept change and address their own feelings of fear, repulsion, and inadequacy.*
- Explore with the pt how negative self-concept affects relationships. *This establishes a cause and effect relationship.*

✦ Spiritual

- Educate the pt to learn to like body despite imperfection. *This helps pt to accept and value the self.*
- Discuss with the pt specific feelings regarding self. *Discussion helps patient to view self as a vital aspect of own personality.*
- Identify values and beliefs related to the pt's negative self-concept. *These help pt to determine rational and irrational aspects of beliefs.*
- Assist the pt to objectively review perceived past inadequacies. *This promotes reality testing.*

Nursing Goals

- To assist pt to acknowledge the loss of change of body
- To assist pt through grief process related to changes in body image and functioning

Patient Goals

- The pt will identify unrealistic personal expectations regarding body image.
- The pt will express positive feelings about body image.
- The pt will identify limitations and develop strategies to compensate for loss of body functions.
- The pt will discuss body image and change if confronted in a social setting.

Patient and Family/Caregiver Outcomes

The patient will:

- Verbalize feelings regarding the physical change, loss, or disability by _____ (date)
- Discuss altered body image within _____ (weeks)
- Acknowledge change in body image as demonstrated by _____ by _____ (date)

The family/caregiver will:

- Successfully provide needed emotional, physical, or social support (specify) regarding the pt's body image problems as demonstrated by _____ within _____ (weeks)

RESOURCES AND INFORMATION

1. National Association of Anorexia Nervosa and Associated Disorders (NANAD; for a partial listing of physical problems brought about by eating disorders, information on eating disorders, referrals, support groups, and crisis telephone counseling)
   Box 7
   Highland Park, IL 60035
   847-831-3438
2. Anorexia Nervosa and Associated Eating Disorders (ANERD; for publications regarding eating and exercise disorders, information support, and education)
   PO Box 5102
   Eugene, OR 97405
3. American Cancer Society (request publications related to body image problems)
   National Office
   1559 Clifton Road, NE
   Atlanta, GA 30329
   404-320-3333
4. National Cancer Institute (NCI) (request publications related to body image problems)
   Office of Cancer Communications
   Building 31, Room 10A24
   Bethesda, MD 20892
   1-800-4-CANCER

C

5. United Ostomy Association, Inc. (UOA) (call the 800 number for a list of publications)
   36 Executive Park
   Suite 120
   Irvine, CA 92714
   1-800-826-0826

6. Janelli, L. M. (1986). Body image in older adults: A review of the literature. *Rehabilitation Nursing, 11*(4), 6–8.

7. McBride, L. G. (1986). Teaching about body image: A technique for improving body satisfaction. *Journal of School Health, 56*(2), 76–77.

8. Food and Drug Administration (FDA; information on diet and nutrients)
   HFE-88
   5600 Fishers Lane
   Rockville, MD 20857
   301-827-4420

C

Caregiver Stress (See Family or Caregiver Stress)

Chemical Abuse Behaviors (See Substance Abuse Behaviors)

Codependent Behaviors

PROBLEM DESCRIPTION

Codependency is a condition of chronic dependency, a state that keeps an individual from self-fulfillment and personal freedom. "Codependency is a specific condition that is characterized by preoccupation and extreme dependence (emotionally, socially, and sometimes physically), on a person or object. Eventually, this dependence on another person becomes a pathological condition that affects the codependent in all other relationships" (Wegscheider-Cruse, 1985, p. 2).

Codependency is a life-style, a patterned way of relating to others, with low self-esteem at the core. Codependency often starts in childhood, being exposed to a family with substance abuse and other abusive behaviors. People with codependency usually maintain an intimate relationship with an addicted person, which intensifies with proximity and frequency of contact. Internal communications are dysfunctional and stunt or impede normal emotional and behavioral development. Anyone who lives in a family of denial, compulsive behavior, or emotional repression is vulnerable to codependency, even if no substance abuse is present. Family dynamics play a large role in grooming a person to become codependent (see Section 1).

Four characteristics set the stage for codependency:

1. Maintaining the family secret and "let's pretend."
2. Never openly discussing family traumas. Rather than face the pain the family members avoid and suppress it.
3. Rigid and dogmatic families that carry an overload of traditional dogma about the roles of family members breed people who may become codependent.
4. Families that use manipulation and control through intimidation, sarcasm, and finances to promote learned helplessness. The person learns to need or becomes dependent on the approval of others, to feel acceptable, resulting in reliance on others for external validation.

Denial or self-delusion involves a complex intermingling of love, fear, hate, and guilt. The person who is codependent then feels powerless to change his or her life and make important decisions. Stress, low self-worth, need for approval, and feelings of rejection and guilt lead to compulsive behaviors. People with codependency harbor deep emotional pain and guilt. No matter how hard they try to manipulate and seek approval, the approval never comes. They learn to keep their feelings inside and state that no one understands them, their loneliness, isolation, or fear. Anger erupts and the codependent person tries to regain control, but people are not controllable and this leaves them frustrated, irritable, and angry.

People with codependency play many roles to survive in this dysfunctional system. Depending on the time and situation they could be involved in collusion, using sickness as a tool for socially acceptable attention, procrastination, being late, being helpless, or being caught in the low self-worth cycle.

Cermak (1986 in Sullivan, 1995, p. 239) proposes the diagnostic criteria for codependency to include:

1. Continued investment of self-esteem in the ability to control both oneself and others despite serious, adverse consequences
2. Assumption of responsibility for meeting others' needs to the exclusion of one's own needs
3. Anxiety and boundary distortions concerning intimacy and separation
4. Enmeshment in relationships with personality disordered, chemically dependent, and impulse disordered individuals
5. At least three of the following: excessive reliance on denial; constriction of emotions; depression; hypervigilance; compulsions; anxiety; substance abuse; recurrent physical, sexual or emotional abuse; stress-related medical illness; or involvement in a primary relationship with an active alcoholic or other drug-addicted person for a least 2 years without seeking outside support.

PROBLEM IDENTIFICATION

Characteristics and Observable Behaviors

- Exaggerated sense of responsibility for the actions of other people
- Tendency to confuse love and pity, with the tendency to "love" people they can pity and rescue
- Tendency to do more than their share and become hurt when people do not recognize their efforts
- Unhealthy dependence on relationships, will do anything to hold on to relationship for fear of abandonment
- Extreme need for approval and recognition
- Sense of guilt when asserting self
- Lack of trust in self or others
- Fear of being abandoned or alone
- Rigidity and difficulty adjusting to change
- Problems with intimacy boundaries
- Chronic anger
- Poor communications
- Inability to have spontaneous fun
- Inability to let go of anything
- Inability to know what normal behavior is
- Confusion about making decisions
- Anxiety about making changes
- Black and white judgments
- Fear and denial of anger
- Lies and exaggeration, when it would be easier to tell the truth
- Tendency to look for people to take care of
- Needs to control self and others
- Easily angered and explosive
- Frequent feelings of disappointment in others with a feeling of being let down
- Avoiding relatives and friends
- Caretaker, people pleaser, workaholic, martyr, perfectionist

- Overcommitment
- Compelled to help others solve their problems
- Worthless when not productive
- Feels crazy and wonders what is normal
- Afraid of own anger
- Feels uncomfortable when a compliment is given
- Tries to control events and how other people should behave
- Finds it difficult to express emotions and make decisions
- Wish for more time for exercise, hobbies, and sports
- Anxiety, denial, compulsions, hypervigilance
- Evidence of physical, emotional, or sexual abuse
- Rigid or weak individual and family boundaries
- Depression or diminished self-esteem
- Enmeshment or isolation
- Substance abuse or abuse in home
- Limited insight
- Perceived responsibility for or need to control others
- Physical fights with partner
- Refusal of help from others
- Feels lethargic, depressed and becomes withdrawn and isolated
- Feels hopeless and begins to plan escape from a relationship they feel trapped in

Factors Related to the Problem

- Rapid weight gains, losses, fluctuations
- Chronic aches and pains—headaches, backaches, stomachaches, idiopathic/intractable pain
- Hypochondria
- Insomnia
- Hyperactivity
- Ulcers

Assessment Tools and Instruments (see Appendix)
Administer the:

1. Beck Depression Scale
2. Brief Psychiatric Rating Scale
3. Clinical Inventory-Withdrawal Assessment
4. Geriatric Depression Scale
5. Social Dysfunction Rating Scale
6. Suicide Risk Assessment Tool

PROBLEM LIST

- Caregiver Role Strain
- Communication, Impaired
- Fatigue

- Grieving, Dysfunctional
- Personal Identity Disturbance
- Post-Trauma Response
- Powerlessness
- Sensory/Perceptual Alterations
- Sexual Dysfunction
- Sleep Pattern Disturbance
- Social Interaction, Impaired
- Social Isolation
- Thought Processes, Altered
- Violence, Risk for, Directed at Self, Other(s), or Property

PROBLEM MANAGEMENT

Prevention, Maintenance, and Restorative Interventions

Twelve Steps for Codependents

1. Acknowledge and accept powerlessness in controlling the lives of others and that trying to control others makes life unmanageable.
2. Believe that a power greater than yourself can restore enough order and hope to create a growth framework.
3. Make a decision to turn your life over to this power to the best of your ability, and honestly accept that taking responsibility for self is the only way growth is possible.
4. Make an inventory of self, look for mental, emotional, spiritual, physical, volitional, and social assets and liabilities. Look at what you have, how you use it, and how you can acquire what you need.
5. Use the inventory as guide, and admit to self, to God, and to other caring persons, the exact nature that it is what is within that is causing pain.
6. Give to God as you know Him, all former pain, hurt and mistakes, resentments and bitterness, anger and guilt. Trust you can let go of the hurt caused and received.
7. Ask for help, support, and guidance and be willing to take responsibility for self and others.
8. Begin a program of living responsibly for self, for own feelings, mistakes, and successes. Become responsible for own part in relationship to others.
9. Make a list of persons to whom you want to make amends and commence doing so, except where doing so would cause further pain for others.
10. Continue to work program, each day checking out progress and asking for feedback from others in attempt to recover and grow. Do this through support groups.
11. See through own power and Higher Power, the awareness of inner self. Do this through reading, listening, meditation, sharing, and other ways of centering and getting in touch with inner self.
12. Having experienced the power of growing toward wholeness, find your body, mind, and spirit awakened to a new sense of physical and emotional relief that

leaves you open to a new awareness of spirituality. Seek to explore meaning in life by honest sharing with others; remember that becoming who you are is a lifetime task that must be done one day at a time (adapted from Wegscheider-Cruse, 1985).

Twelve Steps of Healing
1. Seek appropriate help.
2. Seek a wise therapist or sponsor
3. Dedicate yourself to the truth.
4. Become a choicemaker.
5. Accept responsibility for yourself.
6. Plan a self-care program
7. Love wisely.
8. Commit yourself.
9. Claim your personal power.
10. Assess your relationships.
11. Honor aloneness.
12. Open yourself to serendipity.

Remember: One choice at a time, one change at a time, and one day at a time (Wegscheider-Cruse, 1985, p. 162).

NURSING MANAGEMENT

Nursing Interventions and Rationales

✫ Behavioral

- Instruct the pt to look at problems in small steps. *Small increments help pt to avoid becoming overwhelmed.*
- Assist the pt to recognize lack of assertiveness. *This increases self-awareness and sense of responsibility for own behavior.*
- Support the pt's effort to change behavior. *Support provides encouragement and builds trust in the therapeutic relationship.*
- Instruct the pt that new behaviors can produce anxiety but will become comfortable with experience. *This helps sustain healthy behavior.*
- Instruct the pt in use of relaxation techniques, cognitive reframing, and thought stopping. *These increase control of own behavior.*
- Role play situations that encourage pt to use assertiveness skills. *Role playing increases proficiency in using skills.*

♡ Emotional

- Encourage each family member to express feelings and provide a safe environment in which they can do so. *When members feel safe, they are more likely to disclose true feelings, and this helps build self-esteem.*
- Introduce the f/c to the concept of codependency and the related feelings to explore ways in which they act as enablers; have them pay attention to their

own needs. *F/c may need assistance in becoming aware of their problems with codependency.*

- Discuss the quality of interpersonal relationships among the p/f/c. *Such discussion increases self-awareness and establishes goals for improved emotional relationships.*
- Discuss the fear of intimate relationships among the p/f/c. *This increases self-awareness and establishes goals for improved emotional relationships.*
- Instruct the pt to recognize guilt feelings for those responsibilities that cannot be met. *This allows the pt to understand that this is not an easy task, but it is healthy to allow others to meet some of one's own needs.*

Cognitive

- Complete a family genogram to identify family patterns of substance abuse, violence, victimization, and isolation. *A genogram helps p/f/c to accurately define the problem(s).*
- Instruct the p/f/c and other nuclear and extended family members about establishing rules for interactions, such as prohibiting violence, requiring treatment for substance abuse, and holding regular discussions. *Such action identifies specific learning goals for each member to improve interactions because by agreeing to basic rules, the members begin the therapeutic process of building a productive family unit.*
- Discuss history of codependent behavior. *History helps p/f/c understand how repeated codependent behavior patterns have affected life and allows them to design and evaluate interventions.*
- Instruct pt to make list of responsibilities pt has been meeting and compliment for being responsible. *This shows respect for productive, positive efforts.*
- Assist the pt to assume own responsibilities and not others. *This decreases anxiety and helps learn new ways of coping with stress.*
- Instruct the p/f/c about enabling behaviors and to use coping skills when anxiety becomes overwhelming. *This decreases anxiety and teaches new ways of coping with stress.*

Physical

- Assist the pt in determining respite care needs and taking care of self. *This decreases somatizations and related conditions.*

Social

- Instruct the pt to draw family floor plan of home and identify private spaces for each person. *A floor plan sets privacy boundaries.*
- When working with family members, do not allow one member to speak for the other. *This sets boundaries and decreases control.*
- Role play situations in which the pt is prone to exhibiting codependent behavior. *Role playing allows practicing alternative methods of responding to others.*

- Discuss the quality of interpersonal relationships among the p/f/c. *This increases self-awareness and establishes goals for improved social life.*
- Discuss the fear of intimate relationships among the p/f/c. *This increases self-awareness and establishes goals for improved social life.*
- Instruct the pt in identifying unproductive methods of social interactions. *This identifies areas of growth.*
- Help the pt differentiate between social and intimate relationships. *Such differentiation promotes healthy boundaries.*
- Discuss characteristics of healthy intimate relationship. *This helps form realistic expectations of self and others.*
- Support attempts to form intimate relationship. *Such support promotes personal growth.*

✦ Spiritual

- Instruct the pt to identify interests and strengths, identify what pt would like to do, and plan how to accomplish tasks. *This increases pt self-esteem by doing something enjoyable and following through with a wished for activity.*
- Instruct the pt to identify own priority needs. *Patients with codependent problems have difficulty identifying own need and will require assistance.*
- Instruct the pt to prioritize responsibilities and needs for self and others. *Prioritization allows pt to let go of responsibility over which pt has no control.*
- Reassure the pt that fears will be addressed gradually. *This lessens anxiety and maintains motivation.*
- Help the pt to identify personal strengths. *This increases hope of success.*

Nursing Goals

- To identify situations that may increase or decrease codependent behaviors
- To identify healthy social interactions and interpersonal relationships

Patient Goals

- The pt will begin to establish boundaries between self and family members.
- The pt will report reduced anxiety.
- The pt will agree to rules for safe, healthy interactions.
- The pt will gradually overcome the denial of family problems.
- The pt will express personal feelings without fear of reprisal.
- The pt will express satisfaction with the manner in which individual needs are addressed.
- The pt will exhibit improved self-esteem.
- The pt will report a reduction in level of depression and anxiety within the family.
- The pt will be able to recognize controlling behavior.
- The pt will be able to recognize lack of assertiveness.

Patient and Family/Caregiver Outcomes

The patient will:

- Acknowledge impairment in _____ social relationships as demonstrated by _____ by _____ (date)
- Discuss fears of changing codependent behavior by _____ (date)
- Discuss need to take greater interest in own life and activities by _____ (date)
- Discuss the relationship among level of self-esteem, emotional history, and current behavior by _____ (date)
- Act on information received about individual, group, and 12-step programs by _____ within _____ (weeks)
- Reduce codependent behavior as demonstrated by _____ by _____ (date)
- List own needs and family members' needs and identify those pt has power to meet by _____ (date)
- Identify and discuss irrational beliefs (specify) within _____ (weeks)
- Discuss the connection between social impairment and codependency by _____ (date)
- Demonstrate increased assertiveness as evidenced by _____ within _____ (weeks)
- Identify characteristics of positive intimate relationship through _____ by _____ (date)
- Attend _____ Al-Anon or ACOA meetings within _____ (weeks)

The family/caregiver will:

- Exhibit a reduction in abusive behaviors as demonstrated by _____ within _____ (weeks)
- Gradually overcome their denial of family problems by stating that _____ within _____ (weeks)
- Verbally express a commitment to maintaining a pattern of communication that encourages open expression of feelings by _____ (date)

RESOURCES AND INFORMATION

1. Adult Children of Alcoholics (ACOA) Interim
   World Service Organization
   2522 West Sepulveda Boulevard
   Suite 200
   PO Box 3216
   Torrance, CA 90515
   310-534-1815

2. Al-Anon Family Groups and Alateen Headquarters, Inc.
   PO Box 862
   Midtown Station
   New York, NY 10018-0862
   212-302-7240
   Fax: 212-869-3757
   1-800-356-9996 (24-hour, toll-free)

C

3. Alcohol, Drug Abuse and Mental Health Administration
    Parklawn Building
    5600 Fishers Lane
    Rockville, MD 20857
    301-443-4795
4. Alcohol Rehab for the Elderly
    PO Box 267
    Hopedale, IL 61747
    Hotline: 1-800-354-7089
5. Alcoholics Anonymous (AA)
    475 Riverside Drive
    11th Floor
    New York, NY 10115
    212-870-3400
    Fax: 212-870-3003
6. Families Anonymous (FA)
    PO Box 3475
    Culver City, CA 90231
    1-800-736-9805
7. National Clearinghouse for Alcohol and Drug Information (NCADI)
    PO Box 2345
    Rockville, MD 20852
    301-468-2600
8. National Council on Alcoholism and Drug Dependence (NCADD)
    Attn: Information Director
    12 West 21st Street
    New York, NY 10010
    212-206-6770
    Fax: 212-645-1690
    1-800-NCA-CALL

REFERENCES

Beattie, M. (1987). *Codependent no more.* Hazelden, MN: Hazelden Foundation.

Beattie, M. (1989). *Beyond codependency and getting better all the time.* San Francisco: Harper & Row.

Cermak, T. (1986). *Diagnosing and treating codependence.* Minneapolis: Johnson Institute.

Sullivan, E. (1995). *Nursing care of clients with substance abuse.* St. Louis: Mosby-Yearbook.

Wegscheider-Cruse, S. (1985). *Choicemaking.* Pompano Beach, FL: Health Communications.

Communication Problems

PROBLEM DESCRIPTION

Communication is the combination of speech (the mechanics of producing words) and language (the comprehension and expression of ideas). Communication problems are the lack of or decreased ability to send and receive verbal messages or use words correctly. Physical, psychological, social, and cultural conditions create or exacerbate communication problems.

PROBLEM IDENTIFICATION

Characteristics and Observable Behaviors

- Problems finding and naming words (anomia)
- Difficulty or inability communicating verbally (expressive aphasia)
- Difficulty or inability understanding verbal communication (receptive aphasia)
- Difficulty or inability communicating verbally and comprehending words (global aphasia)
- Difficulty and anxiety communicating in groups
- Problems with attention and concentration
- Repeatedly telling the same stories over and over
- Loss or impairment of writing ability (agraphia)
- Tendency to speak very little, use short phrases only, or give one word answers (poverty of speech)
- Rapid speech with little or no change in intonation between expressed ideas (pressured speech)
- Rapid switching from one expressed idea to another with little or no connection between them (flight of ideas)
- Sudden stopping in the middle of a sentence (thought blocking)
- Slow speech with little change in intonation between expressed ideas (halting speech)
- Little or no relation between the main point of the speech and the details presented (circumstantial speech)
- Disjointed or little or no connection between thoughts and ideas (loose associations)
- Repeating or echoing the words or phrases of another (echolalia)
- Stereotyped, meaningless repetition of the same words or phrase over and over (perseveration or verbigeration)
- Replacing facts with fantasy content or filling in forgotten information (confabulation)
- Putting words together that do not make sense or go together (word salad)
- Unintelligible, imprecise speech (dysarthria)
- Linking together sounds in a nonsensical manner or coining words that have meaning only to the speaker (neologism)

- Linking together two conflicting elements in the same communication (double bind)
- Lack of verbal speech (mutism)
- Repetition of words that have a similar sound (clang associations)
- Awkward, nonmelodic, and nonrhythmic speech (prosody)
- Others: stuttering; slurring words; garbled or incoherent speech; frequent gesturing; very low volume; very high volume; variations in voice quality; bizarre gesturing, facial expressions, and posturing; or unexplained incontinence

Factors Related to the Problem

Any number of physical, psychological, social, and cultural conditions can cause the pt to have verbal and nonverbal communication problems.

Physical Conditions Related to Communication Problems
- Decreased or interrupted blood circulation to the brain
- Brain tumor or brain injury (including normal pressure hydrocephalus)
- Intubation or tracheotomy
- Anatomic defects and neuromuscular changes
- Hearing impairment or visual impairment
- Medications, alcohol, and other noxious substances
- Fatigue
- Advanced pulmonary disease and dyspnea
- Over- or understimulating environment
- Cancer
- Decreased level of consciousness
- Age-related changes
- Infections
- Epilepsy
- Parkinson's disease
- Schizophrenia

Psychological Conditions Related to Communication Problems
- Severe anxiety or panic
- Psychosis
- Confusion, disorientation, and cognitive deficits
- Apathy
- Agitation
- Depression

Cultural or Social Conditions Related to Communication Problems
- Cultural differences
- Inability to read or write
- Educational level
- Inability to communicate in the dominant language
- Lack of or nonfunctioning appropriate assistive devices
- Social isolation
- Recent life changes

Assessment Tools and Instruments (see Appendix)

Administer the Mini-Mental Status Examination to detect the nature of the pt's verbal communication and anything remarkable about the pt's nonverbal communication.

Other Assessments

- Specialized hearing screening: spoken voice, Weber's test, Rinne's test, and an otoscopic examination
- Obtain other specialized testing and screening as indicated.

PROBLEM LIST

- Communication, Impaired Verbal
- Helplessness
- Hopelessness
- Powerlessness
- Self-Care Deficit (Specify)
- Sensory/Perceptual Alterations (Specify)
- Social Isolation

PROBLEM MANAGEMENT

Prevention, Maintenance, and Restorative Interventions

- Correct any defects or cause of communication problems (eg, fix eyeglasses or remove cerumen).
- Teach, attempt, and model trying to find the meaning behind the pt's behavior because usually the behavior is a response to the pt's environment and all behavior has meaning.
- Be aware of or learn about the pt's language patterns and cultural background.
- Educate the p/f/c regarding the nature of and ways to compensate for the pt's communication problem(s).
- Encourage the pt to speak slowly and at a volume of speech that is audible.
- Provide the pt with assistive devices and communication devices.
- Encourage the pt to use gestures, mime, pointing, devices, computers, etc.
- To avoid confusing the p/f/c, use the words I and you instead of we and us.
- Model and teach the f/c to frankly state when the pt's communication is not comprehensible rather than pretending to understand the pt.

Medication Management

No specific medications are indicated for this behavior, except for the medications necessary for the physical and psychological problems associated with this problem.

NURSING MANAGEMENT

Nursing Interventions and Rationales

☆ Behavioral

- Determine and devise alternative modes of communication (including drawing, singing, dancing, mime) for and with the p/f/c. *Alternative communication helps the pt in emotional expression and communicating basic needs and wants.*
- Use short sentences and observe the pt's behavior. *This determines level of comprehension and communication problems.*
- Repeat words as necessary, using the same words (not similar ones). *Repetition minimizes confusion and frustration.*

♡ Emotional

- Acknowledge and reinforce all attempts at communication. *This enhances self-esteem and future attempts at communication.*
- Ask how the pt is feeling and interact with the pt in a caring manner even though the pt may not currently be able to communicate with the provider. *This ensures the pt that communication channels remain open and the pt is not isolated.*

△ Cognitive

- Provide missing words, name objects, and post signs. *This assists with recollection or minimizes deficit.*
- Express one thought at a time with simple concrete words, and use names instead of pronouns. *These actions enhance comprehension.*
- Provide longer amounts of time for mental processing. *This decreases pt frustration.*
- Obtain input, if available, from specialists (eg, occupational therapists, psychologists, speech–language therapists) who are familiar with the pt, with the requisite authorizations. *Such input streamlines and efficiently provides for the pt's care.*
- Consider a referral or consultation to a specialist(s). *Referrals assist with functional adaptation and individualize the pt's care.*
- Provide or arrange for referral for psychotherapy for behavioral, coping, or social distress. *This referral will assist the pt to adjust to sensory/perceptual changes or other problems.*
- Teach the f/c regarding nonverbal communication techniques. *This reduces inappropriate behavior responses by the pt and decreases frustration.*

⬚ Physical

- Provide a consistent therapeutic environment (ie, free of noise and distractions, and safe, pleasant, clean, at the proper temperature, and with adequate lighting and ventilation). *This keeps the pt at ease and in the best environment to heal and recover.*
- Assess, monitor, and refer, if necessary, for specialized medical or dental evaluations regarding communication problems and consider a speech-language therapy, rehabilitation, audiology, or other consultation. *Such actions correct or decrease any problems.*

- Institute a planned walking program (suggest 30 minutes at least three times a week), which stimulates the motor cortex. *Walking improves communication and the quality of life of the pt* (Friedman & Tappen, 1991).

C 💬 Social

- Limit the number of people in the pt's immediate environment. *This lessens anxiety and facilitates communication.*
- Gain the pt's attention, use direct eye contact, and a calm reassuring voice tone. *This minimizes anxiety and frustration for the pt.*
- Identify underlying themes to repetitive stories. *The pt may be trying to convey a deeper meaning.*
- Request that the pt expand on part of the repetitive story or thank the pt for sharing and change the topic. *This lesses f/c stress.*
- Teach the f/c to maintain nonverbal emotional connection with the pt. *The pt still has needs and desires even though unable to verbally or directly express them.*

✦ Spiritual

- Respond to the pt's attempts at communication with actions and gestures. *This provides reassurance.*
- Include the pt in all conversations. *Such inclusion protects human dignity and provides a sense of belonging.*
- Express empathy for the pt's feelings regarding communication problems. *This provides a sense of human connection and understanding to the pt.*
- Provide reassurance, attention, and acceptance to the pt. *This conveys a sense of security.*
- Determine, if necessary, who can act as the pt's spokesperson (with the pt's permission). *A spokesperson may interpret the pt's communication in a more meaningful manner.*
- When appropriate, laugh with the p/f/c. *Laughter eases tension and provides a sense of shared humanity.*

Nursing Goals

- To assist the pt to improve communication
- To establish effective functional verbal and nonverbal communication with and for the pt
- To provide an environment that is understanding of and compensatory for the pt

Patient Goals

- The pt will have needs and wants met despite communication problems.
- The pt will develop alternative methods of communication.
- The pt will effectively communicate with others.
- The pt will communicate meaningfully with minimal frustration.
- The pt will be in a state of ease, comfort, and satisfaction.

Patient and Family/Caregiver Outcomes

The patient will:

- Respond to questions and make needs and wants known by _____ within _____ (specify)
- Improve the ability to communicate basic needs and wants as demonstrated by _____ within _____ weeks
- Establish an effective method of communicating with others through _____ within _____ weeks
- Verbalize satisfaction with _____ communication process by _____ (date)
- Communicate in a clear manner with _____ by _____ (date)
- Walk at least _____ minutes _____ times a week within _____ (weeks)
- Plan to contact a self-help, community, or support group within _____ weeks

The family/caregiver will:

- Assist with the identification of the pt's past and currently available communication skills and the pt's experience with and willingness to use the skills and devices by _____ (date)
- Write a list of the pt's interests, habits, and activities within _____ (weeks)
- Verbalize an understanding of the pt's behavior as a means of communication by _____ (date)
- Assist the pt to devise simple ways for the pt to communicate 24 hours a day as demonstrated by _____ within _____ (specify)
- Encourage and assist the pt to walk at least _____ minutes _____ times a week within _____ (weeks)
- Observe and document _____ gestures or _____ symbols that have communicative meaning for the pt within _____ (specify)
- Use appropriate methods and measures to communicate with the pt as demonstrated by _____ within _____ (specify)

RESOURCES AND INFORMATION

1. Lost Chord Club—see the white pages of the telephone book
2. New Voice Club—see the white pages of the telephone book
3. University centers with computer-aided communication departments
4. American Cleft Palate-Craniofacial Association
   1218 Grandview Avenue
   Pittsburgh, PA 15211
   412-481-1376
5. National Institutes of Health
   National Institute on Deafness and Other Communication Disorders
   9000 Rockville Pike
   Bethesda, MD 20892
   301-496-7243

6. United States Lighthouse for the Partially Sighted
   316½ East Mitchell Street
   Suite 4
   Petoskey, MI 49770
   616-347-1171

REFERENCES

Friedman, R., & Tappen, R. M. (1991). The effect of planned walking on communica-tion in Alzheimer's disease. *Journal of the American Geriatrics Society, 39,* 650–654.

Confusion (See Delirium, Dementias, and Depression and Depressive Behaviors)

D

Delirium

PROBLEM DESCRIPTION

Delirium, also known as acute or subacute confusional state, acute brain failure or syndrome, encephalopathy, toxic brain syndrome, or reversible dementia, is brief global cerebral nervous tissue or metabolism dysfunction. Primarily, the pt's ability to attend, receive, process, store, and retrieve information is impaired. Delirium always has a physical cause yet can mimic any and every conceivable psychiatric disorder. It has many potential causes and presents with many neuropsychiatric and motor abnormalities. Delirium usually develops within a matter of hours or days, but can be chronic and stable. The course of delirium rapidly fluctuates and the pt can have occasional lucid periods. Usually before the onset of delirium the pt has a prodromal stage with nonspecific symptoms of anxiety, nightmares, sleep and appetite disturbance, restlessness, and irritability. Pts with delirium are disoriented to time and place, but usually not to person; they have difficulty remembering recent events. A pt with delirium is easily distracted and usually the sleep–wake cycle is reversed, often worsening at night. A pt with delirium can be hyperactive, hypoactive, or both. Delirium often precedes the onset of medical complications and because delirium is *reversible*, the importance of early recognition and treatment cannot be overemphasized, since injury or death may result.

The neuropsychiatric symptoms of delirium are (Wise & Brandt, 1992, p. 294):

- Apraxia (loss of ability to carry out common purposeful movements, especially with objects)
- Delusions, illusions, and hallucinations
- Disorganized thinking and speech
- Dysgraphia (impaired ability to express self in writing)
- Dysnomia (incorrect naming)

The motor abnormalities associated with delirium are:

- Asterixis (motor disturbance with an assumed posture from muscle contractions, called "liver flap")
- Intention tremor
- Myoclonus (shocklike contractions of a muscle)
- Reflex and tone changes
- Intention tremor

PROBLEM IDENTIFICATION

Characteristics and Observable Behaviors

The following clinical features, which fluctuate, are prominent in delirium:

- Instability of arousal—decreased level of consciousness; "sundowning," "sunrising," and drowsiness; vigilance; clouded sensorium; stupor and coma when severe
- Abnormal beliefs—suspiciousness; paranoia; misperceptions; illusions; hallucinations (especially visual and tactile); does not recognize f/c and provider
- Psychomotor activity—incoherence; restlessness; agitation; posturing; reversal of sleep–wake cycle (sleeps during day and awake at night); calls out to f/c; climbs out of bed or remains in bed or huddled in a chair; pulls at tubes, etc; paces; gestures wildly; activities out of sequence
- Cognitive features—apathy; impaired cognition, especially attention; perplexed; disoriented; distracted; perseverates (says a word or a phrase over and over or repeats questions and answers); distracted by noise; responds to simple commands only; poor memory
- Mood and personality changes—labile; depressed; euphoric; apathetic; irritable; disinhibition; bizarre behaviors; appears frightened; wants to be with others; defensive
- Neurologic features—tremor; nystagmus; asterixis; myoclonus; hyperactive reflexes; bladder and bowel incontinence possible

Factors Related to the Problem

Consider the following pts at high risk for delirium (Wise & Brandt, 1992, p. 294):

- 60 years of age and older
- With pre-existing brain pathology
- With substance abuse and dependence

- Postcardiotomy
- With HIV-spectrum disorders

Other factors that contribute to the onset of delirium are chronic illnesses, multiple medications, excessive stress, exacerbation of underlying medical condition, psychiatric disturbance (usually depression with psychotic features, mania, and schizophrenia), rapid translocation from institution to home, postoperative sequelae (after cataract surgery, called "black patch delirium"), and seizure disorders.

Assessment Tools

A score of 20 or less on the Mini-Mental State Examination may indicate delirium. Pts with delirium usually are fearful and have general disorientation; perceptual, thought, and emotional disturbance; misnaming; and spatial displacement. They especially have difficulty with tasks requiring attention and concentration, such as counting backwards by sevens or recalling the three objects.

For additional assessments, consider administering the Suicide Risk Assessment Tool and screen for hearing and vision abilities.

PROBLEM LIST

- Aggression
- Bowel Incontinence
- Powerlessness
- Relocation Response
- Self-Care Deficit Related to Inability to Perform ADLs
- Sensory/Perceptual Alteration (Specify)

- Sleep Pattern Disturbance
- Social Isolation
- Suspiciousness
- Thought Process, Altered
- Urinary Incontinence
- Verbal Communication, Impaired
- Violence, Risk for, Directed at Self, Other(s), or Property

PROBLEM MANAGEMENT

Prevention, Maintenance, and Restorative Interventions

- Continually monitor the pt for subtle and overt changes in physical or mental status, appearance, and mood, and if detected, notify the physician.
- Correct any abnormality found during the mental status examination, physical examination, laboratory studies, etc.
- Provide adequate and appropriate pain relief measures.
- Call the pt by name and use simple words and short sentences to communicate.
- Place an easy-to-read clock, calendar, and other familiar objects in the pt's immediate surroundings.
- Provide a clearly indicated and lighted pathway to the bathroom.
- Provide adequate light, and close curtains or shades during the night to decrease the possibility of disturbing illusions.
- Close curtains or shades and turn on lights, plan a diversional activity, or schedule bedtime before the sun goes down, to minimize "sundowning."
- Obtain an order to discontinue all unnecessary medications.

- Review and correlate medication administration records with behavioral changes.
- Teach the f/c that the outcome is usually a full return to previous level of functioning, if intervention is done early.

Medication Management

No consensus exists regarding medication management for delirium. Haloperidol (Haldol) is usually the first drug of choice because it has almost no anticholinergic or hypotensive effects. However, because the high-potency neuroleptics are more likely to produce EPS, especially in older adults, it is important not to confuse EPS with worsening agitation and increase the medication, which often happens (see Adverse Reactions). It is important not to stop the medication immediately after the agitation or confusion has cleared. Rather it should be tapered off over a few days, with the largest (and sometimes only) dose of medication at bedtime, to normalize sleep patterns. (See Aggressive Behaviors; Psychosis; and Sleep Problems.) Pentobarbital is used if a pt is experiencing delirium due to withdrawal from some drugs.

Benzodiazepines are given as the drugs of choice for delirium tremens (see Anxiety and Substance Abuse Behaviors).

The following classes of drugs commonly cause delirium, even within normal adult or geriatric dosage ranges:

- Analgesics
- Antibiotics
- Anticholinergics
- Anticonvulsants
- Antihistamines
- Anti-inflammatory agents
- Antiparkinsonian agents
- Antitubercular agents
- Benzodiazepines
- Cardiac drugs
- Chemotherapeutic agents
- Sedative-hypnotics
- Sympathomimetics
- Tricyclic antidepressants
- Miscellaneous: amphetamines, baclofen, bromides, chlorpropamide, cimetidine, cocaine, disulfiram, ergotamines, insulin, lithium, metrizamide, metronidazole, podophyllin (by absorption), procarbazine, propylthiouracil, quinacrine, steroids, ranitidine, timolol ophthalmic

NURSING MANAGEMENT

Nursing Interventions and Rationales

☆ Behavioral

- Observe and assess for characteristic behavioral responses: confused behavior and agitation; inattention to self-care activities; apraxia; and exaggerated mannerisms. *Assessment helps the nurse to prevent or minimize the effects of delirium.*

- Approach the pt slowly and refrain from touching or restraining. *This minimizes the pt's irritability, agitation, and suspiciousness.*
- Refrain from making stressful demands and decisions of the p/f/c. *The course of delirium fluctuates rapidly.*
- Acknowledge the pt's statements by nodding your head when verbal communication is impaired. *Nonverbal communication lets the pt know you are listening.*

  ## ♡ Emotional

- Observe and assess for characteristic emotional responses: lability, inappropriate responses, irritability, defensiveness, and suspicion. *Observation helps the nurse to prevent or minimize the effects of delirium.*
- Institute and teach comfort measures, such as a back rub, soothing conversation, or soft music. *These help to decrease agitation and provide a safe, quiet environment.*

△ Cognitive

- Observe and assess for level of consciousness and characteristic cognitive responses: disorientation, memory and recall deficits, difficulty in reasoning ability and problem-solving, impaired judgment, decreased or short attention span, perceptual difficulties, perseveration, or fabrication. *This helps to prevent or minimize the effects of delirium.*
- Reorient the pt to date and the environment often. *During the course of delirium the pt's ability to be oriented to time and place rapidly fluctuates.*
- After the delirium has resolved, assist the p/f/c to understand the experience and put it into perspective. *After recovery some pts will remember part or all of the delirious experience, which can be bizarre, and often the p/f/c fear that the pt has dementia.*
- Provide verbal and printed descriptions of the phenomenon of delirium. *This helps to validate the p/f/c's experience and explain the pt's responses.*
- Educate the p/f/c regarding the predisposing factors and risks of delirium. *This helps to prevent or minimize the effects of delirium.*

☐ Physical

- Observe and assess for characteristic physiologic reasons that a pt may be delirious (eg, hypoxia, metabolic abnormalities, toxic states, infections, structural changes, vascular pathology, neurologic disease, self-care deficits, sleep patterns, sensory changes). *Monitoring vital signs can help the nurse prevent or minimize the effects of delirium.*

◯ Social

- Observe and assess for social manifestations of delirium: social withdrawal, diminished social skills, or interaction patterns and communication that might indicate the onset or presence of delirium. *This can help to prevent or minimize the effects of delirium.*
- If possible, arrange for a f/c to remain with the pt. *This provides pt with reassurance and monitoring.*
- Eliminate or decrease environmental stimuli. *This helps pt to focus attention.*

- Educate the f/c regarding the pt's inappropriate social interactions. *This provides reassurance and attends to the pt's self-esteem.*

✦ Spiritual

- Observe and assess for spiritual manifestations of delirium: loss of interest, detachment, or depression. *These observations can help to prevent or minimize the effects of delirium.*
- Provide brief continual reassurances, especially during lucid moments. *Reassurance helps to reduce anxiety and agitation.*
- Institute a consistent routine. *Consistency helps to support the pt's memory abilities and sense of safety and security.*

Nursing Goals

- To prevent the onset of delirium
- To identify the onset of delirium and intervene early to prevent or minimize complications

Patient Goals

- The pt will have a level of consciousness that is stable.
- The pt will exhibit an improved level of consciousness.
- The pt will exhibit an improved level of sensory function.
- The pt will demonstrate an improved communication ability.
- The pt will communicate thoughts and needs adequately.
- The pt will understand communication from others.

Patient and Family/Caregiver Outcomes

The patient will:

- Recover from a delirious episode within 1 week
- Establish a normalized sleep–wake cycle and experience a restful night within _____ weeks
- Have stable vital signs 2 weeks before discharge
- Demonstrate decreased levels of anxiety and agitation as demonstrated by _____ by _____ (date)
- Communicate thoughts and needs adequately
- Understand communication from others

The family/caregiver will:

- Assist with establishing a baseline for the pt's functioning and provide information about whether or not the pt has shown similar symptoms in the past within 1 week
- Identify possible causes of the pt's delirium within _____ (specify)
- Identify the pt's disorientation and provide reorientation within _____ (specify)

- Verbalize knowledge of levels of consciousness as demonstrated by _____ by _____ (date)
- Recognize the s/s of deterioration, possible causes, and appropriate actions to take as demonstrated by _____ by _____ (date)

RESOURCES AND INFORMATION

1. American Brain Tumor Association: 312-286-5571 or 1-800-886-2282
2. National Council of Patient Information and Education: 202-347-6711
3. National Library of Congress Referral Center: 202-287-5670

REFERENCE

Wise, M. G., & Brandt, G. (1992). Delirium. In R. E. Hales & S. C. Yudofsky (Eds.), *American Psychiatric Press textbook of neu-ropsychiatry* (2nd ed., p. 294). Washington, DC: American Psychiatric Press.

Delusions

PROBLEM DESCRIPTION

Delusional disorder, previously called paranoia, is an uncommon psychiatric condition characterized by delusions and relative absence of other psychopathology that differentiates it from other conditions. Delusions are false beliefs that have no true basis in reality. It is thought that the person with delusional disorder is meeting some need, such as self-esteem, security, reassurance, punishment, anxiety, fear, or guilt. The delusion is not easily corrected with reason or logic. The delusional thoughts are nonbizarre misinterpretations and distortions of reality that may be based on a portion of reality within the person's life.

According to the American Psychiatric Association (1994), to be considered as a clinical disorder, certain criteria must be met:

1. The delusions must be present for at least 1 month.
2. The delusions are not related to a schizophrenic condition.
3. Pt functioning is not markedly impaired and behavior is not obviously odd or bizarre.
4. If mood episodes occur concurrently, their total duration is brief relative to the duration of the delusional periods.
5. The disturbance is not due to direct physiologic effects of a substance or general medical condition.

Delusions may be a number of types:

1. Erotomanic: delusions that another person, usually of higher status, is in love with the individual

2. Grandiose: delusions of inflated worth, power, knowledge, identity, or special relationship to a deity or famous person
3. Jealous: delusions that the individual's sexual partner is unfaithful
4. Persecutory: delusions that the person (or someone to whom one is close) is being malevolently treated in some way
5. Somatic: delusions that the person has some physical defect or general medical condition
6. Mixed: delusions characteristic of more than one of the above types, but no one theme predominates
7. Unspecified

Delusions may be transient or fixed. Transient delusions develop with organic illness and disappear when the pathologic condition is eliminated. Fixed delusions persist over time. Three phases of delusional thinking have been identified:

1. The pt is totally involved in the delusion.
2. Reality testing and trust in others coexist with the delusions.
3. The pt no longer experiences the delusions or is not bothered by them.

Pts with delusional disorder tend not to see psychiatrists because they do not think they have a problem. They often approach police to report being followed or seek out their physician or other provider to treat an undiagnosed disorder. Commonly pts with a delusional disorder stay in the community, function, and often work and are thought of as peculiar or eccentric. They are oriented, their judgment is intact, and decision-making abilities are stable; they are able to make cognitive choices and the personality stays intact.

The onset of delusional disorder can occur at any age from adolescence onward, but is most often seen between ages 35 and 45. Both sexes are affected and the disorder is usually chronic and lifelong, but, the outlook for treatment is better than schizophrenia with one-third to one-half of delusional pts achieving remission. Etiology is unknown at this time. What is known is that a family history of psychiatric illness is common and organic factors may be relevant in inducing onset.

PROBLEM IDENTIFICATION

Characteristics and Observable Behaviors

- Angry, irritable, hostile
- Guarded, evasive, suspicious, secretive, mistrustful
- Hypersensitive
- Attention to small detail
- Litigious
- Self-righteous
- Sullen
- Malnourished
- Poor personal hygiene
- Affect flat, blunted, inappropriate
- Fears of being harmed, rejected, isolated, or mind control

- Guilty or embarrassed
- Distorted perception
- Impaired judgment and insight
- Inability to think abstractly
- Preoccupied with delusions
- Suicidal ideas, sexual preoccupation, or homicidal plans
- Use of defense mechanisms, especially denial, projection, and regression
- Fixed delusional system
- Lowered self-esteem, unrealistic perception of self
- Withdrawn and isolated
- Impaired capacity to perform social roles
- Excessive religiosity
- Lacks ability to enjoy pleasures in life, humorless
- Delusions of grandeur
- Nonreality-based thinking, disorientation
- Labile affect
- Short attention span, distractible
- Impaired judgment
- Feelings of persecution and victimization
- Erroneous somatic beliefs about alterations in body or bodily functions
- Resistive to treatment
- Preoccupation about belief(s)
- Impaired ability to evaluate own perceptions and thoughts
- Easily irritated when others do not believe delusions
- Impaired relationship with others
- Difficulties with work role

Factors Related to the Problem

- Sensory loss, deprivation, or overload
- Alcohol or drug withdrawal
- Renal or metabolic disorders
- Low neuroleptic levels
- Perceptual and cognitive impairment
- Organic illnesses caused by acute ineffective or metabolic disturbances
- Systemic illness
- Substance intoxication
- Severe psychosocial stressors
- Perception of personal inadequacy
- Anxiety
- Loneliness
- Aggressive feelings
- Major mental illness
- Schizophrenia
- Organic mental disorders
- Mood disorders

Differential Diagnosis

The diagnosis of delusional disorder is a process in which the patient is examined to determine if a delusion is present along with other paranoid features. It is necessary to rule out more common conditions such as a medical disorder (metabolic, endocrine, or infectious), substance abuse, or other psychiatric illnesses. Diagnosis is complicated in that the delusional disorder is often misdiagnosed as another disorder, particularly schizophrenia. Delusions are not related to any other disorder. Table II-1 differentiates delusional disorder from schizophrenia and depression.

Assessment Tools and Instruments (see Appendix I)

Administer the:

1. Beck Depression Inventory
2. Brief Psychiatric Rating Scale
3. Brief Psychiatric Schizophrenic Rating Scale
4. Geriatric Depression Scale
5. Global Assessment of Functioning
6. Mini-Mental State Examination
7. Short Portable Mental Status Questionnaire

PROBLEM LIST

- Loneliness, Risk for
- Personal Identity Disturbance
- Sensory/Perceptual Alterations
- Social Interaction, Impaired
- Social Isolation
- Thought Processes, Altered

Table II-1
Characteristics of Delusional Disorder Compared to Schizophrenia and Depression

Characteristic	Delusional Disorder	Schizophrenia	Depression
Delusions	Nonbizarre	Bizarre	N/A
Hallucinations	Olfactory	Auditory, visual	N/A
Functioning	Not impaired	Impaired	Impaired
Affect	Normal, usually	Flat and blunted	Variable
Depression	Mood changes with short occurrence schedule		Evident long term

PROBLEM MANAGEMENT

Prevention, Maintenance, and Restorative Interventions

Strategies for working with delusions (Harris, 1981; Stuart, 1995):

- Establish a trusting, interpersonal relationship: Do not argue or challenge delusion, ensure the pt that it is safe and no harm will come, use openness and honesty, encourage verbalization of fear and anxiety, center on pt as a person, remain calm, be consistent in all areas (ie, length of visit, limitations on behavior, and follow through).
- Identify the content or type of delusion: Assist pt in understanding purpose of delusion, clarify any confusion, and identify presence of central topic and feeling tone.
- Investigate meaning of delusion: Assess area of life pt is having trouble controlling, assess concrete ways delusion interferes with functioning, assess any action taken based on delusion, without agreeing, arguing, or questioning the logic or reasoning behind delusion.
- Assess the intensity, frequency, and duration of the delusion: Assess if delusions are fleeting or short, fixed, or long term; does pt start conversations with the delusion; are you able to redirect; if patient is intent on telling the delusion—just listen until there is no need to discuss it any longer.
- Identify what triggered the delusion.
- Place the delusion in a time frame: Identify all components of delusion by placing it in time and sequence.
- Identify current major stresses.
- Correlate the onset of delusion with the onset of stress: Help pt connect false beliefs to time of increased anxiety.
- If the pt asks directly if you believe the delusion, respect that this is the pt's experience: Present reality without listening or invalidating pt's perception.
- Identify emotional needs the delusions may be meeting: Respond to underlying feelings rather than the illogical nature of the delusion, use the process of conversation rather than content by reflecting feelings back to the pt.
- Meet the needs the delusion fulfills: Promote diversional activities to interrupt pathologic thinking, provide structured activities and time schedules.
- Once the delusion is understood, avoid and discourage repetitious talk of the delusion: Encourage responsibility for own behavior, give some measure of control regarding daily activities and decision-making, involve the f/c as possible.
- Clarify confusion surrounding the delusion.
- Be consistent in intervention.
- Avoid joking or teasing about delusion to prevent threatening pt.
- Do not be anxious or avoid the delusional person.
- Do not reinforce the delusion.
- Do not attempt to prove the person wrong.
- Do not set unrealistic goals.
- Do not become incorporated into the delusional system by being aware of verbal and nonverbal communication.
- Do not see the delusion first and the person second.

Medication Management

Until recently, pharmacologic therapy of delusional disorder had been unsatisfactory. Within the last 10 years there has been more success. Pimozide, a dopamine-blocking agent, has been used with some success in patients with somatic-type delusional disorder. Selective serotonin reuptake inhibitors have altered the course of delusional disorders, which raises the question of overlap with the pathophysiology of obsessive-compulsive disorders, mood disorders, and body dysmorphic disorder. Published reports indicate that risperidone and clozapine in low doses give beneficial responses (Manschreck, 1996).

NURSING MANAGEMENT

Nursing Interventions and Rationales

☆ Behavioral

- Refrain from discussing delusional material. *This avoids reinforcing delusional thinking.*
- Refocus conversation to another topic after listening to delusion. *Refocusing avoids reinforcement.*
- Enforce limit setting and elicit cooperation of others. *These measures promote continuity of care.*

🖤 Emotional

- Identify feelings, verbally and nonverbally, underlying delusions. *This helps pt understand fears and anxieties.*
- Facilitate pt expression of feelings. *This lets pt know that it is acceptable to feel and to express feelings.*
- Relieve anxiety by assisting p/f/c. *This creates a predictable environment to promote sameness and security and reduce anxiety.*

🔺 Cognitive

- Be sincere and honest when communicating and avoid vague or evasive remarks. *Pts with delusions are sensitive; they can recognize insincerity, plus evasive comments reinforce mistrust.*
- Interpret reality by stating facts clearly and concisely. *Facts prevents misinterpretation of reality.*
- Explore with the pt stimuli that cause stress. *This identifies anxiety and helps plan other approaches.*
- After a relationship has developed, gently question the pt's delusions. *This creates doubt about credibility of delusion.*
- Assist the pt in learning new ways to deal with stress without delusions. *Alternatives may improve coping skills.*
- Teach the pt ways to interrupt delusions by whistling, singing or other activity. *This prevents alienation from others.*

- Promote intellectual stimulation with items such as crossword puzzles or word games. *Such activities provide distraction.*

⊓ Physical

- Refrain from focusing on delusions of a somatic nature. *This avoids reinforcing delusions.*
- Monitor medication regimen. *Monitoring helps p/f/c to be certain that pt takes medication as prescribed.*
- Refrain from touching the pt. *This prevents misinterpretation of intent.*
- Instruct the pt to watch food and medication preparation if the pt thinks it is poisoned. *Such observation prevents suspiciousness and mistrust.*

◯ Social

- Provide a busy structured environment. *Activity reduces time for delusions and stimulates interest in real world.*
- Elicit support of f/c and others. *This provides a low demand, low stress level, consistent home environment.*

✦ Spiritual

- Avoid discussion of religion when delusions are religious in nature. *This prevents reinforcement or argument.*
- Instill confidence in pt's ability to control delusions with medications and supportive care. *Pt confidence increases pt's feelings of control over own life.*

Nursing Goals

- To promote reality orientation and contact
- To identify and relieve fears, anxiety and mistrust
- To promote completion of daily activities
- To facilitate compliance with medications

Patient Goals

- The pt will live with delusions.
- The pt will be free of delusions or demonstrate ability to function without responding to persistent delusional thoughts.

Patient and Family/Caregiver Outcomes

The patient will:

- Demonstrate decreased anxiety level, as evidenced by _____ by _____ (date)
- Interact with _____ on reality-based topics _____ (times) within _____ (specify)
- Identify events and situations in life that are threatening or stressful and cause anxiety by _____ (date)

- Verbalize what is real and what is fantasy by _____ (date)
- Focus on reality-centered discussion, as demonstrated by _____ within _____ (weeks)
- Validate thoughts with others _____ (times) within _____ (weeks)
- Participate in regularly scheduled activities to decrease time for delusional thinking at least _____ times within _____ (specify)
- Identify when thoughts become delusional by _____ and will _____ by _____ (date)
- Verbalize inability to cope with stressors by _____ (date)
- State relief measures for stressors are _____ by _____ (date)
- Relate ways, other than delusion, to cope with _____ by _____ (date)

The family/caregiver will:

- Identify s/s of delusion by _____ (date)
- Identify strategies for working with pt when delusional by _____ (date)
- Communicate and provide alternative coping skills and assistance when pt asks for help by _____ (date)
- Discuss delusions only in private with _____ or with an understanding person by _____ (date)
- Identify when thoughts become delusional within _____ (specify) and _____ within _____ (specify)
- Counteract delusional thinking by distractions or involvement with _____ activities or _____ (persons) by _____ (date)
- Use family or significant other for support and to reduce withdrawal and alienation within _____ (weeks)

RESOURCES AND INFORMATION

1. Psychiatric-Mental Health Nursing Psychopharmacology Project (PMH-13); List $25.95; State Nurses Association members $16.95
    American Nurses Publishing
    PO Box 2244
    Waldorf, MD 20604-2244
    1-800-637-0323
    Fax: 301-843-0159
2. Moller, M. D. (1989). *Understanding and communicating with a person who is hallucinating* [videotape]. Omaha, NE: NurSeminars, Inc. To order:
    12204 W. Sunridge Drive
    Nine Mile Falls, WA 99026
3. American Psychiatric Association (for publications, "Let's Talk About Mental Illness," "Let's Talk Facts About Mental Illness," and "Schizophrenia")
    Division of Public Affairs/Code P-H
    1400 K Street, NW
    Washington, DC 20005
    202-682-6220
4. National Institute of Mental Health (NIMH; for publications related to Alzheimer's disease, depression, and general mental health)

Information Resources and Inquiries Branch
Office of Scientific Information
5600 Fishers Lane, Room 7C02
Rockville, MD 20857
301-443-4513

REFERENCES

American Psychiatric Association. (1994). *Quick reference to the diagnostic criteria from DSM IV*. Washington, DC: Author.

Busse, E. (1989). *Geriatric psychiatry*. Washington, DC: American Psychiatric Press.

Harris, A.C. (1981). *Mental health for community nurses*. New York: Springer Publishing Co., Inc.

Manschreck, T. (1996, April). Delusional disorder. *Current Approaches to Psychoses, 5,* 7–9.

Stuart, G.W. & Sundeen, S.J. (1995). *Pocket guide to psychiatric nursing* (3rd ed.) St. Louis: Mosby Year-Book.

Dementias

PROBLEM DESCRIPTION

There are many different types and causes of dementia, which results from widespread cerebral dysfunction or damage. Dementia, also known as cognitive decline, degenerative dementia, or senile dementia, is a syndrome, an acquired, persistent condition, with great variation in clinical features. According to American Psychiatric Association (1994) criteria, there must be memory impairment, and at least aphasia (inability to communicate verbally or understand verbal communication), apraxia (inability, despite physical ability to, carry out purposeful motor functions), agnosia (loss of ability to recognize sensory impressions such as smell, taste, and familiar others and objects), or disturbance in mental function that is severe enough to noticeably interfere with social or work activities. If a pt has a diagnosis of dementia, it usually means that the pt has global deficits in intellectual function.

A dementia can occur secondary to medications, physical disorders, and psychiatric disorders (especially pseudodementia; see Depression and Depressive Behaviors). Generally, a dementia is characterized by a gradual onset with continuing, progressive decline. Like delirium, some types of dementia are potentially reversible, depending on the underlying cause and the effective application of treatment, if available.

Clinical Features of Dementia

- Cognitive changes: defects in orientation, intellectual function, reasoning, judgment and perception
- Emotional changes: lability of mood; catastrophic reaction (anxiety, restlessness, and irritability to rage from too much internal or external stimulation; agitation when the pt with dementia becomes aware of deficits under stressful circum-

stances; usually time limited); social withdrawal; dull or apathetic facial expression and manner; paranoia possible
- Behavioral changes: defects in impulse control; difficulty in performing everyday tasks; faulty orientation in space and time; vague, stereotyped, or imprecise verbal communication (may become mute); sudden outbursts of anger or sarcasm; verbal or physical attacks

More than half of all dementias are caused by dementia of the Alzheimer's type or DAT, about 13% arise from multiple cerebral infarctions ("multi-infarct dementia" or MID), and about 10% are associated with a psychiatric disorder. Some pts have both DAT and MID. An increasing number of cases of dementia are related to HIV.

Types of Dementia

Dementia of the Alzheimer's Type

With a thorough examination, DAT is now correctly diagnosed about 90% of the time. It is a leading cause of death in the United States. When no other cause can be found, and a pt has severe loss of intellectual function, a diagnosis of DAT is made. Although it can begin at any age, it is more common after age 65 and slightly more women than men are diagnosed with DAT.

Multi-Infarct Dementia

Compared to DAT, MID has a more abrupt onset with a stepwise but fluctuating (instead of a gradual) progression. More common in men than women, a history of strokes and more focal neurologic s/s (eg, weakness of an extremity) from vascular changes accompany MID. There are some changes in cognitive functioning, whereas others remain intact resulting in "patchy" cognitive deficits. The contributing risk factors to MID—hypertension, hyperlipidemia, heart disease, diabetes, cigarette smoking, and alcohol ingestion—must be identified and treated as early as possible to prevent further progression.

Other Major Types of Dementia

Alcohol Dementia. In the absence of any other cause, this type of dementia lasts at least 3 weeks after cessation of prolonged, consistent (not binge) alcohol intake of 10 years or more. It is more common in women than men. In addition to failing intellect, by definition, social and occupational functioning is impaired. This type of dementia can range from mild to severe.

HIV Dementia. Neuropsychiatric symptoms are common, but diverse and nonspecific, such as emotional liability, fear, rage, apathy, impulsiveness, hallucinations, and delusions. Impaired judgment and memory, aphasia, and overall cognitive defects, along with frustration and anxiety, even catastrophic reactions, are most common.

Potentially Reversible Causes of Dementia

About 10% to 15% of all dementias are reversible if treatment is initiated in a timely manner and before irreversible damage has occurred. Despite the variability of onset, course, and prognosis the importance of early recognition and treatment of potentially reversible dementias cannot be overemphasized because permanent injury or death may result.

The most common, treatable, and therefore reversible, causes of dementia are:

- Post-trauma
- Hypoxia
- Cardiac arrhythmias
- Infectious diseases and systemic illnesses
- Toxic materials and conditions
- Psychiatric disorders (especially pseudodementia; see Depression and Depressive Behaviors; see also: Anxiety; Manic Behaviors; Obsessive-Compulsive Problems; Paranoia; Personality Disorder Problems; Psychosis; and Somatization Problems)
- Alcohol and drug intoxications and interactions
- Metabolic and endocrine disturbances (eg, thyroid, parathyroid, and pituitary-adrenal)
- Normal pressure hydrocephalus (a triad of dementia, gait disturbance, and urinary incontinence)
- Cancers and tumors
- Parkinson's disease
- Sensory disturbances
- Vitamin and nutritional deficiency states

To quickly determine possible reversible or treatable causes of dementia, use this mnemonic:

- D = drug reactions, interactions, or overdose
- E = emotional disorders (eg, depression)
- M = metabolic and endocrine disorders
- E = eyes and ears, sensory loss of
- N = nutritional deficiency
- T = tumors and trauma
- I = infections
- A = arteriosclerotic conditions (eg, CHF)

Other Causes of Dementia

- Huntington's chorea
- Creutzfeldt-Jakob disease
- Kuru
- General paresis
- Multiple sclerosis
- Amyotrophic lateral sclerosis
- Systemic lupus erythematosus
- Transient global amnesia

PROBLEM IDENTIFICATION

Characteristics and Observable Behaviors

Generally, three stages of the dementias are recognized; they often overlap and vary.

Stage I—Mild or Early

This stage leads up to and includes the diagnosis, usually 2 to 4 years. The pt's symptoms and personality changes are subtle, often unnoticed, and usually attributed to stress, fatigue, or illness. When symptoms and changes are noticed they are first noted by the f/c, not the pt. Symptoms and personality changes of the stage I pt include:

- Easily tires, is forgetful, irritable, and anxious
- Poverty of ideas and speech
- Keeps to self and has a loss of initiative and spontaneity
- Intact capacity for independent living
- Personal hygiene and judgment relatively intact
- Increasing difficulty with complex familiar activities, such as playing card games
- Short-term memory loss, misplacing and losing objects, missing appointments, forgetting telephone messages, and getting lost on familiar outings
- Poor social manners and occasional bizarre behavior (eg, putting dishes in the clothes dryer)
- Disoriented to time and date and difficulty remembering thoughts, names, and words
- Retains control over coordination and motor skills, but may have slowed reaction time and driving an automobile may be questionable
- May be depressed
- Poorly tolerates alcohol and intake may precipitate disinhibited behavior

Stage II—Moderate or Middle

This is the longest stage and usually lasts 2 to 10 years after diagnosis. The pt's impairments are noticed by family, friends, employers, and others. The pt is likely to deny or be oblivious to the deficits but may make references about "losing my mind." Symptoms in this stage include:

- Personality traits exaggerated (eg, pt with a tendency toward paranoia becomes more paranoid) with frequent mood swings
- Restlessness and agitation; wandering and "sundowning" common
- Mistakes with money and financial and legal affairs
- Functions inefficiently at work, and with transportation and driving, cooking, housekeeping, and health and home maintenance
- Shorter attention span and becomes unaware of all recent events
- Gross difficulty with reading, writing, and numbers
- Sleeps often or may awake suddenly at night "to go to work"
- Perceptual-motor problems (eg, difficulty getting into a chair)
- Obsessive thoughts and compulsive rituals
- May exhibit agitation and psychotic behavior with delusions and hallucinations
- Gets completely lost in familiar surroundings and has difficulty functioning in new or strange environments
- Defects in judgment and difficulty grasping important concepts
- Needs some degree of supervision; independent living is hazardous and the pt needs instruction to perform tasks
- Often demonstrates inappropriate social behavior (eg, stealing or exposing self)
- Slowing and rigidity of movements with a slow shuffling gait and aimless behavior
- No new thoughts and more inflexible thinking
- Self-absorbed, insensitive to the needs of others, and displays little affection
- Uses broken speech to get needs met; perseverates; speaks slowly with many pauses; unable to complete sentences or continually revises speech
- Loss of impulse control
- Refuses or is afraid to bathe and has trouble dressing

- May be euphoric, silly, or teary at times
- May gain then lose weight; has big appetite for junk food or other people's food, then forgets last meal happened and loses interest in food
- Needs to pace and wander
- May have occasional muscle twitching or jerks

Stage III—Severe or Late

This is the terminal stage and usually lasts 1 to 3 years. The pt needs constant supervision and requires total care. Significant symptoms and personality changes of the stage III patient include:

- Indifference to food; may have difficulty swallowing or be unable to swallow
- Sleeps more
- Unaware of deficits and depression resolves; may still have lucid moments
- Cannot recognize self in mirror or f/c
- Does not recognize important people and is oblivious to others in the home
- Unable to maintain personal hygiene
- Uses few words, invents terms, cannot read, repeats words or phrases without understanding their meaning (echolalia), and loses all comprehension
- May be incoherent or mute; may return to primary language, which may still be distorted; may scream or yell spontaneously
- May be unable to smile
- May put anything in mouth or touch everything
- May experience grand mal seizures
- May be unable to walk or sit and have skin breakdown and be incontinent of urine and feces
- Stupor, then coma and death

Factors Related to the Problem

- Genetics may contribute to the development of both DAT and MID; hypertension is commonly associated with MID.
- Depression often precedes or accompanies the dementias and depression heightens the cognitive dysfunction of the dementias.
- Pts with parkinsonism often develop mild to moderate dementia.
- Pts with Down syndrome who live into their thirties usually develop DAT.
- About one-third of pts with DAT exhibit delusions.
- Anxiety in a pt with a dementia often results in increased physical complaints.

Differential Diagnosis

Normal memory changes that occur with aging do not interfere with the person's usual social and work life. With aging, there is some reduction in memory retrieval time and some difficulty in learning new material, which can be compensated for (Table II-2).

- A pt likely does not have dementia if there is a sudden onset in the absence of organic pathology, focal neurologic signs, and seizures or gait disturbances early in the course of the illness.

Table II-2
Differentiation Between Dementia of Alzheimer's Type
and "Normal" Forgetfulness

Problem	Pt with DAT	Pt with "Normal" Adult Forgetfulness
What is Forgotten	*The whole experience*	*Parts of an experience*
Delayed recall of missing items and names	Rarely	Often
Following directions	Gradually unable	Usually able
Ability to use reminders, cues, and notes	Gradually unable	Usually able

From Gwyther (1985)

- A trial with antidepressant medication is sometimes done to distinguish pseudodementia from dementia (see Depression and Depressive Behaviors). If the problem is indeed depression, the cognitive deficits usually resolve and mood improves.
- The apathy associated with subcortical dementias is often mistaken for a mood or a psychotic disorder.

Table II-3 differentiates dementia from delirium. It is imperative that a clear distinction be made among dementia, delirium, and depression.

Table II-4 differentiates DAT from MID. The Hachinski Ischemic Rating (Hachinski et al., 1975) is a useful tool for differentiating DAT from MID.

Assessment Tools and Instruments (see Appendix I)

The primary assessment tool is the:

- Mini-Mental State Examination (MMSE)

A score of 20 to 22 or less on the MMSE may indicate dementia. Pts with dementia usually do not have any psychiatric history and they attempt to hide their disabilities (eg, by making jokes or trying to change the subject). They will try hard to answer the questions and do the tasks tested by the MMSE, often with "near misses." The higher the pt's premorbid intelligence, the better able the pt will be to compensate for intellectual deficits. Usually pts with a dementia fail the cognitive tests, attention and concentration are impaired, and they especially have difficulty with recent memory testing (remote memory may remain intact) and copying the three-dimensional object. Usually memory for time and place is lost before that for the pt.

Additional assessment tools include:

1. Abnormal Involuntary Movements Scale
2. Beck Depression Inventory

Table II-3
Differentiation Between Dementia and Delirium

	Dementia	Delerium
Onset and course	Usually insidious (if sudden is after trauma, coma, or delirium); progressive deterioration	Acute, rapid, waxes and wanes abruptly
Duration	At least 1 month, usually longer	Usually <1 month
Orientation	In mild cases, may be correct; altered later in course	Faulty with tendency to mistake unfamiliar for familiar place and person
Thinking	Impoverished	Disorganized
Intellectual ability	Consistent loss and decline	Preserved during lucid intervals
Memory	Recent and remote impaired	Recent impaired
Speech	Usually slowed	Incoherent; severity of delirium determines degree of change
Attention	May be intact	Invariably disturbed, hard to direct or sustain
Awareness	Usually intact or decreased	Increased or reduced, fluctuates during day and worsens at night
Affect and mood	Flat or indifferent; depression	Fearful, perplexed, or bewildered, even at times panicky
Alertness	Normal or decreased	Increased or decreased
Paranoia	Less prominent	Prominent
Perception	Misperceptions often absent	Misperceptions often present
Sleep–wake cycle	Usually normal for age	Always disrupted
Appearance and behavior	Usually slowed responses	Possibly semicomatose; agitated
Prognosis	Usually irreversible	Usually reversible

Adapted from Bauer, Roberts, & Reisdorff (1991); Kaplan & Sadock (1994); Lipowski (1990); and Roth (1978).

3. Geriatric Depression Scale
4. Global Assessment of Functioning Scale
5. Modified Overt Aggression Scale
6. Obsessive-Compulsive Screening Checklist
7. Social Dysfunction Rating Scale
8. Suicide Risk Assessment Tool

Table II-4
Clinical Differentiation of Dementia of the Alzheimer's Type (DAT)
and Multi-Infarct Dementia (MID)

	DAT	MID
Course	Continuous, slow, gradual deterioration	Stepwise deterioration
Neurologic signs and symptoms	Usually absent or global	Focal signs and symptoms
Hypertension and cardiovascular disease	Not common	Common
Neuromuscular	Tremors, uncertain gait, muscular rigidity; incontinence	Paralyses; minor EPS
Gender	More women	More men
Age of onset	65 and older	45–65
Hereditary factors	Multiple factors likely	Some familial tendency
Orientation	Progressive disorientation	Episodes of acute confusion; lucid intervals
Patient awareness and depression	Less often	More often

Adapted from Gwyther (1985) and Lipowski (1990)

Screening for hearing, vision, and other physical abilities is appropriate. More sophisticated neuropsychological testing is helpful in the evaluation of the dementias (McKhann, et al., 1984).

PROBLEM LIST

- Abuse
- Activity Intolerance
- Role Strain
- Communication, Impaired Verbal
- Confusion, Acute or Chronic
- Diversional Activity Deficit
- Incontinence, Bowel
- Injury, Risk for
- Mobility, Impaired Physical
- Nutrition, Altered, Less than Body Requirements
- Powerlessness
- Relocation Stress Syndrome
- Self-Care Deficit Related to Inability to Perform ADLs (specify)

- Sensory/Perceptual Alterations (specify)
- Sleep Pattern Disturbance
- Social Interaction, Impaired
- Social Isolation
- Spiritual Distress
- Thought Processes, Altered
- Urinary Elimination, Altered
- Violence, Risk for, self-directed or directed at others

PROBLEM MANAGEMENT

Prevention, Maintenance, and Restorative Interventions

Generally, providers and the f/c must find what works with each particular pt at the time and share with each other what does and does not prove effective because although the cognitive decline of a person with dementia is progressive, the behavioral changes are not consistent.

- Ensure that diagnostic studies have been done to determine the cause(s) of cognitive decline.
- Call the pt by preferred name, gain eye contact, and use simple, specific words (and nouns, not pronouns), short sentences, and repeat communications frequently.
- Ask general questions, make general responses, and build on all attempts that the pt makes to communicate, whether based on current or past situations.
- Reinforce verbal communication with nonverbal communication.
- Assist the f/c to provide a consistent, safe, predictable environment (use calendars and a set place for important items) and to place familiar objects in the pt's immediate surroundings.
- Provide adequate light, close curtains or shades, turn on lights, plan a diversional activity, or schedule bedtime before the sun goes down to minimize "sundowning."
- Obtain an order to discontinue all unnecessary medications.
- Review and correlate medication administration records with behavioral changes.
- Teach the f/c that the outcome depends on the type of dementia as to whether or not it will be reversible.
- Teach the f/c that pts have "good" and "bad" days (eg, recall something at one time and be unable to do so at another time), instead of a single behavioral pattern.
- Teach the f/c that the use of gestures and exaggerated facial expression may enhance communication.
- Teach the f/c to repeat, as necessary, the same words (and not to use similar but different ones) to lessen confusion.
- Teach the f/c not to tire or push the pt; if the f/c is becoming frustrated or more than 5 minutes pass without success, leave the task and return to it later.

- Teach the p/f/c to focus on positive interactions rather than negative experiences and expectations.
- Teach the "ABC" approach by documenting the antecedents and behaviors before the problematic behavior, the actual problematic behavior, and the events occurring immediately after the inappropriate behavior to identify precipitant situations, target behaviors, and design interventions to modify behavior patterns (Alessi, 1991).
- Teach the f/c that they might unwittingly emotionally withdraw from the pt as a way to protect their own integrity.

Symptom Management, Categories, and Techniques

Target symptoms with specific interventions (Table II-5).

1. Appearance
   - Disheveled—see Self-Neglect
   - Inappropriate clothes—lay out two sets of clothing to allow for a choice; lay clothes out and hand each item of clothing to the pt in the order it is to be put on; use clothes without buttons and hooks; consider an OT consultation
   - Poor grooming—see Activities of Daily Living Problems
2. Behavior
   - Restlessness, agitation, impulsiveness—use distraction, change the topic, talk about former occupation, hobbies, interests; turn on (or off) the radio; hand the pt an object, etc
   - Wandering—see Wandering
   - Catastrophic reaction—prevention by noticing patterns and modifying environmental antecedents (the "ABC" approach); use distraction; remain calm; provide reassurance; do not argue; give directions one step at a time, and repeat word for word, if needed; assist with the next step of the task (if that is the precipitant); change the subject, or move the pt to a calmer environment; change or reduce expectations or activities to those that have success; limit the pt's decision-making; provide prompts; never restrain, instead move slowly and tell the pt what you are doing as you do it
   - Lack of cooperation—instead of arguing, tell the pt step by step what needs to be done; break down tasks into manageable, individual steps based on those that the pt can handle or initiate by self and assist with those that the pt needs help or prompting; establish a simple, regular, predictable routine (do the same thing at the same time every day); allow the pt to hoard safe objects
   - Impaired movement
     - Repetitive movement—use distraction; provide with a repetitive task to do (eg, folding napkins or screwing and unscrewing plastic pieces of pipe), or incorporate the repetitive movement into a satisfying activity; consider an OT consultation
     - Apraxia and loss of coordination—gradually remove unnecessary and confusing items from the environment, such as souvenirs and collections; consider a PT and an OT consultation
     - Rigidity, shuffling gait, stooped posture—assist with walking as needed; encourage walking if able; remove throw rugs and loose carpet; secure

Table II-5

General Principles for Managing Patients With Dementia

Principle	Interventions
Correct sensory impairment	Adequate vision and hearing examinations
	Correction of vision and hearing problems
	Speak and interact more closely
	Face pt when speaking to pt
	If acceptable, use frequent physical contact
Nonconfrontation	Note abilities and disabilities
	Matter of factly fill in or compensate for disabilities
	Answer questions briefly
	Remove potentially harmful or dangerous objects
Optimal autonomy	Determine pt's personal needs and coping ability
	Allow pt to do what pt wants to do as long as possible
	Provide supervision and suggestions, if accepted
Simplification	Find ways to reduce number and complexity of the demands in environment
	Introduce tasks as steps, one at a time
	Use convenience machines or services (eg, telephone answering devices or services)
	Use of one- or two-piece garments
Structuring	Determine the pt's need for and degree of structure
	Provide for predictability and constancy of daily activities
Multiple cueing	Use redundant cues (eg, say a word, make a gesture, draw a picture, make a sign, or demonstrate the same thing or activity)
Repetition	First engage pt's attention (eg, call the pt's name, or place a hand on the shoulder)
	Provide, repeating as necessary, step-by-step verbal and nonverbal cues of desired activity
Guiding and demonstration	Accompany requests and suggestions by pantomiming movements or with direct physical imitation or guidance
Positive reinforcement	Provide praise and recognition for desired behaviors
	Provide reminders or assistance to avoid undesired behaviors or incidents
Reducing choices	Give pt a choice of two alternatives and ask which one pt prefers

continued

Table II-5

General Principles for Managing Patients With Dementia Continued

Principle	Interventions
Optimal stimulation	Determine pt's need and preference for stimulation at various times of day, and schedule accordingly Provide or minimize amount of stimulation in environment, as indicated
Avoid new learning	Base new learning on already grasped principles or intact functions Respond to questions succinctly If new learning situation cannot be avoided, make it as familiar as possible
Determine and use overlearned skills	Based on pt's history, facilitate use of pt's skills and talents, with modifications as needed
Coupling learning with emotional arousal	Encourage or deter activity or behavior by saying and showing intent (eg, say "yes" and calmly clasp hands together while looking lovingly at the pt)
Minimizing anxiety	Keep environment simple; reduce choices; avoid new learning; keep focused on present day (avoid anticipation); keep surroundings familiar; use distraction
Distraction	Call attention to someone or something else
Adjust the environment	As the dementia progresses, make environment more predictable, less complicated and stimulating by removing unnecessary and decorative objects; create living space floors in one color without breaks in color; make appropriate barriers and cues; provide secured access to outside; strong or secured furniture; variety of sturdy chairs; thorough, continuous but varied lighting; remove mirrors, if indicated

Adapted from Chafetz (1991); Christner (1992); Jackson, Shroyer, & Pak (1994); Mace & Rabins (1991); and Weiner (1991)

cords; remove glass tables and other unsteady or delicate furniture; put bright reflector tape on steps; install gates on stairs with sturdy grab rails; install handrails; provide active and passive range-of-motion exercise; consider a PT consultation
- Difficulty writing—assess ability to write; consider an OT consultation
- Difficulty with or loss of ability to perform ADLs—see Activities of Daily Living Problems

- Speech Difficulties
  - Aphasia, slurred speech, few words, mutism—demonstrate effective communication techniques; say the word or name the feeling the pt may be trying to express and ask if the word or feeling is correct; guess at what the pt is trying to express; maintain a routine to lessen the need for communication; consider a speech-language therapy consultation
  - Repetitive questions, words, or phrases (perseveration or echolalia)—respond as if it is the first time you have done so and tell the pt that the pt will be cared for as the pt may be asking for reassurance; provide a simple, structured, nonthreatening environment and schedule; use distraction or redirection; ignore if possible; respond to the pt's feelings instead of the expressed verbal content; use an hourglass or timer when the pt loses the ability to perceive the passage of time
- Hypersexuality—try to determine the need or meaning of the behavior, and meet it if possible; protect from embarrassment; anticipate and prevent from self-embarrassment; remove or cover the pt as soon as possible; distract; consider use of neuroleptics or antipsychotic medication (see Sexual Problems)
- Difficulty sleeping—maintain activity level during the day; discourage, reduce, or eliminate naps during the day; see Sleep Problems
- Appetite changes—to best of pt's ability encourage balanced meals; finger foods if necessary; high-caloric diet, especially if pt is hyperactive; encourage fluids during the day; place a limited number of foods in front of the pt at a time at frequent intervals, including enhanced liquids; assist with eating, as needed; provide a quiet, nonstimulating meal time; determine causes if eating habits or appetite changes abruptly; observe for swallowing difficulties; teach aspiration precautions; consider general or parental feeding; consider a consultation from a registered dietitian or other provider as indicated

3. Emotions and mood
   - Instability, irritability, and lability—approach the pt slowly; use a low, calm voice; refrain from touching; do not confuse and frustrate the pt by providing explanations why something is to be done; allow ample time for a task to be done
   - Depression—see Depression and Depressive Behaviors
   - Suspicion, paranoia, and hostility—explore events that trigger the event; reflect back to the pt; learn the pt's hiding places; keep a reserve of items that pt commonly believes have been stolen; agree that the item is missing and help look for it; use distraction; help label the pt's feeling; repeat a brief explanation of everything that you do as you do it; label drawers; see Paranoia
   - Anxiety—see Anxiety

4. Cognitive processes (thoughts, beliefs, and perceptions)
   - Loss of recent memory—encourage discussion regarding the loss of memory; teach ways of coping with memory loss by using timers or beepers, lists, calendars, etc; put signs on items, doors, etc; use reflective tape to make arrows to indicate where the bathroom and other rooms are; write lists of daily activities and tasks for the pt; use old photos and music from the pt's past to prompt long-term memory; stimulate memory chains; summarize earlier events; repeat information often; focus on feelings underneath the behavior

and affirm with words and behavior; consider an OT and neuropsychological consultation

- Confusion and disorientation—do not attempt to reorient a pt who is continually disoriented; provide reassurance that the pt will be taken care of and kept safe; use validation therapy (Dietch, 1989; Feil, 1989); consider an OT and neuropsychological consultation
- Impaired judgment—assess for home safety (use the agency tool and see the Psychiatric Home Safety Tool in the Appendix) and assist the p/f/c to implement indicated changes; assist the p/f/c to evaluate the pt's ability to drive an automobile and perform other such activities; remove all dangerous items; reduce hot water temperature, cap electrical outlets, etc
- Impaired concentration—use short, simple sentences; ask only one question at a time; ask only questions that can be answered yes or no; try to elicit a response and praise attempts to respond; consider an OT consultation; see Depression and Depressive Behaviors
- Loss of abstract thinking and ability to calculate—provide slow and detailed information; make only one change a time; consider an OT consultation
- Inability to learn new things and information—do not introduce new topics, tasks, or decisions that the pt may not be able to process; eliminate all sources of distraction; use television quiz shows or radio talk shows to stimulate thought; do not substantially rearrange home and furniture
- Loss of ability to read words and know what they mean—assess ability to read and comprehend; put visual cues on items; try to understand the feeling tone of the communication; consider an OT consultation
- Confabulation (fabricating stories to conceal memory gaps)—accept the confabulation, but refrain from agreeing with ones that reflect memory impairment; acknowledge the plausible aspects of the story; if the pt cannot provide an answer give the answer and ask the pt to repeat it
- Loss of awareness of spatial relationships—concretely tell the pt where in space items, objects, etc, are, including the pt's body parts
- Illusions and misperceptions—assess the environment for any objects or situations that could be so construed and eliminate or change the situation; turn on lights before it gets dark outside and close curtains or shades
- Sensory problems
- Delusions and hallucinations—see Psychosis

5. Relationships and socialization
- Personality changes—personality traits will be accentuated (as the saying goes, "what was will be, only more so"); see Personality Disorder Problems
- Loss of social skills—observe and assess the pt's nonverbal behavior and look for cues in the pt's posture or facial expression to determine needs and wants; provide for social stimulation
- Social isolation—see Social Withdrawal
- Clinging, demanding behavior—reassure the pt that someone is near; reassure the pt that needs are and will be met; give the pt, if acceptable, a hug, pat, something to hold, or encourage the pt to move around; use humor; teach the f/c to use humor, to engage in self-care activities, and that the f/c is often viewed by the pt as the sense of security

- Loss of ability to sustain current relationships—encourage the pt to reminisce about past relationships and experiences with the aid of photos, music, etc
- Inability to recognize f/c, relatives, friends—give information to compensate for this inability (eg, "This is your daughter, Jane"); limit and schedule the number of people in the pt's immediate environment
- Hostility and combativeness—see Aggressive Behaviors; Assaultive Behaviors; Manic Behaviors
- F/c stress—see Family or Caregiver Stress

Medication Management

Medications for the dementias should be used only after behavioral, social, and the environmental therapies have been used, and then in conjunction with other therapies and modalities (Table II-6).

Tetrahydroaminoacridine (THA)

THA (Tacrine or Cognex) is the first FDA-approved medication (1993) for a pt with mild or early dementia. It prevents or slows the natural breakdown of the neurotransmitter acetylcholine, which is associated with memory, but does not alter the underlying dementia. In doses up to 160 mg/d, THA delays the progression of DAT, but only briefly. Its major side effect is liver toxicity; pts must be monitored for abnormal liver function through weekly determination of AST. Other side effects are nausea, vomiting, diarrhea, dyspepsia, anorexia, ataxia, and muscle aches. Pts should be monitored for abnormal liver function; elevated transaminase levels; induced bradycardia in pts with sick sinus syndrome; and occult or active GI bleeding.

Table II-6
Medication and Behavior Management in Dementia of Alzheimer's Type

Behaviors Usually Amenable to Drugs	Behaviors Usually Not Amenable to Drugs
Aggressive	Demanding
Agitated	Clinging
Anxious	Inappropriate actions
Deluded	Inappropriate verbalizing
Depressed	Inappropriate sexual activities
Hallucinating	Perseveration
Hyperactive	Social isolation
Impulsive	Inappropriate urination and defecation
Insomnia	Wandering
Restless	
Verbally hostile	

Drug interactions: increases the half-life and plasma concentration of theophylline; cimetidine (Tagamet) increases and prolongs blood levels of THA; synergistic effects with succinylcholine and cholinergic agents.

Antipsychotic or Neuroleptic Medications

These classes of medications can be effective in treating disordered behavior or thinking in pts with dementia, depending on the particular pt.

The high-potency antipsychotic medications such as haloperidol (Haldol), fluphenazine (Prolixin), and thiothixene (Navane) are usually chosen, especially for older adults, starting with a very low dose, because they have relatively less anticholinergic, sedative, orthostatic, and CV side effects. However, because the high-potency neuroleptics are more likely to produce EPS, especially in older adults, it is important not to confuse EPS with worsening agitation and increase the medication, which often happens (see Adverse Reactions).

Benzodiazepines and Buspirone

These drugs help with anxiety (see Anxiety). Buspirone (BuSpar), the anticonvulsant carbamazepine (Tegretol), and lithium carbonate (see Manic Behaviors) may help with agitation and aggressive behaviors, especially if neuroleptics have failed. The β-adrenergic blockers, like propranolol (Inderal) and pindolol (Visken), can also help with aggression in some pts (see Anxiety and Aggressive Behaviors).

Antidepressant medication is administered for concurrent depression (see Depression and Depressive Behavior).

Additional Medication Management

- For insomnia, short-acting benzodiazepines or a single, bedtime dose of a high-potency neuroleptic medication, are often used (see Sleep Problems).
- Ergoloid mesylate (Hydergine) and the psychostimulants methylphenidate (Ritalin) and dextroamphetamine (Dexedrine) can be used for apathy and withdrawal (see Apathy and Social Withdrawal), especially for the dementia associated with HIV, without the usual side effects of such drugs (Fernandez, Levy, & Galizzi, 1988).

CAUTION—NURSING ALERT—A patient with dementia is likely to develop delirium from any of the psychotropic or neuroleptic medications, so the provider must be alert for an exacerbation of symptoms. Often older adults can have idiosyncratic reactions (see Adverse Reactions) to medications.

Tissue plasminogen activator (Activase) helps prevent brain damage or death by dissolving blood clots that cause most strokes and is sometimes indicated for MID, as are anticlotting medications like warfarin (Coumadin), low-dose aspirin, and cholesterol-lowering drugs; proper precautions must be taken for these medications.

NURSING MANAGEMENT

Nursing Interventions and Rationales

★ Behavioral

- Observe and assess for uncharacteristic behavioral responses. *Assessment prevents or minimizes superimposed conditions on the dementia.*
- Approach the pt slowly and refrain from touching or restraining. *This minimizes the pt's irritability, agitation, and suspiciousness.*
- Use behavior prompts (eg, place a toothbrush in the pt's hand). *Prompts help the pt self-initiate behaviors, especially after the loss of verbal communication.*
- Use appropriate cues. *Cues enhance verbal communication (eg, "Do you want an apple" while showing the pt an apple).*
- Protect from injury during periods of agitation. *Catastrophic and other maladaptive responses usually involve sensory and perceptual disturbances that can threaten the pt's safety.*
- Ignore undesired behaviors that are safe. *All behavior has meaning and if no harm is being done it will be useful for the pt to engage in the behavior.*

♡ Emotional

- Observe and assess for uncharacteristic emotional responses. *This prevents or minimizes superimposed conditions on dementia.*
- Teach and practice calmness, gentleness, and patience. *One's emotional state is mirrored by pts with a dementia.*
- Institute and teach comfort measures, such as soothing conversation or soft music. *These measures decrease agitation and provide a safe, quiet environment.*
- Evaluate the emotional effects and changes (eg, emotional withdrawal of others, loss of loved ones, or reaction to the aging process) that can affect the progression of dementia and intervene as indicated. *Such evaluation lessens or prevents these factors from complicating the course of dementia.*
- Provide or arrange for supportive psychotherapy. *This focuses on changes in life-style and anxiety.*
- Assist the f/c to identify s/s (eg, wanting to leave a situation, purposeless movements, silence, fidgeting, etc) of increasing anxiety in the pt. *This prevents or minimizes anxiety, frustration, and catastrophic reactions.*

△ Cognitive

- Observe and assess for uncharacteristic cognitive responses. *This prevents or minimizes superimposed conditions on dementia.*
- Assess and identify skills and interests and provide a way to use them. *This will help the pt feel secure.*
- Provide information in a matter-of-fact manner with congruent nonverbal behavior. *Pts with a dementia are sensitive to the nonverbal behavior of others.*

- Provide verbal and printed information about dementia. *Such information validates the f/c's experience and explains the pt's behavioral responses and cognitive changes.*
- Evaluate the cognitive effects and changes (eg, perceptions of the aging process or overmedication) that can affect the progression of dementia and intervene as indicated. *Evaluation lessens or prevents these factors from complicating the course of dementia.*
- Patiently ask one question at a time (who, what, where, when, and why) and wait for each response. *Patience helps the pt assimilate information.*
- Assess if the pt is willing to discuss losses and changes and provide or arrange for cognitive psychotherapy to focus on anxiety, loss, changes in life, pending death, etc. *This reduces fear and anxiety.*
- Do not argue with a pt who has a dementia. *The pt's reasoning abilities are changed, which only results in frustration for the p/f/c and providers.*
- Cognitively challenge the pt with reversible dementia (eg, encourage the pt to correctly count change). *This stimulates attention, improves function, or helps pt learn to compensate for lost function.*

⊓ **Physical**

- Observe and assess for uncharacteristic medical and physiologic conditions. *Often infections and other medical problems go undetected in pts with dementia.*
- Evaluate the physical conditions and changes (eg, normal physical changes of aging or malnutrition) that can affect the progression of dementia and intervene as indicated. *This lessens or prevents these factors from complicating the course of dementia.*
- Reduce fatigue by scheduling 20- to 30-minute naps and alternate rest and activity. *Scheduling conserves the pt's energy for cognitive processes.*
- Instruct the p/f/c to restrict the pt's alcohol intake. *This minimizes or prevents confusion and disinhibition.*

◯ **Social**

- Observe and assess for uncharacteristic social interactions. *This prevents or minimizes superimposed conditions on dementia.*
- Evaluate the social conditions and changes (eg, loss of social contacts from death, relocation, and self-protection, or lack of money and transportation) that can affect the progression of dementia and intervene as indicated. *This lessens or prevents these factors from complicating the course of dementia.*
- If possible, arrange for a f/c or volunteer to be with the pt. *Companionship provides the pt reassurance and monitoring.*
- Teach the f/c that the pt leaving the home may precipitate anxiety or other behavioral problems if the setting is unfamiliar; eliminate or decrease environmental stimuli. *This prevents or minimizes anxiety.*
- Support the p/f/c in altered role performance. *This assists in the healthy adjustment of the f/c system.*

- Educate the f/c regarding the pt's inappropriate social interactions. *Such education provides reassurance and attends to the pt's self-esteem.*
- Teach the f/c to intervene as soon as possible if the pt engages in embarrassing behavior. *Intervention protects the pt's dignity and privacy.*
- Listen to the f/c and provide support regarding their frustrating experiences with the pt who is suspicious, has delusions, is forgetful, etc. *This minimizes or prevents the f/c displaying their frustration to the pt.*
- Provide the p/f/c with referrals to mental health professionals and other appropriate resources. *Referrals help reduce f/c stress (see Family or Caregiver Stress) and other effects of the pt's condition.*
- Assist the f/c to obtain identification for the pt (eg, an identification bracelet; name and address labels sewn in clothing). *These help identify the pt if the pt becomes lost.*
- Assist the f/c to schedule time away from the home. *The emotional strain and time placed on the f/c is considerable.*
- If indicated, refer to a partial hospitalization program. *Referral provides pt with socialization and group psychotherapy.*
- Encourage the f/c to evaluate long-term care facilities well before placement may become necessary; provide resources as indicated and consider a referral for medical social work consultation. *This provides f/c with advance warning and planning resources in case long-term care is needed.*

✴ Spiritual

- Observe and assess for uncharacteristic spiritual responses. *This reduces anxiety and agitation.*
- Evaluate the spiritual conditions and changes (eg, sense of own impending death) that can affect the progression of dementia and intervene as indicated. *This lessens or prevents these factors from complicating the course of dementia.*
- Respect the pt's right of wishing to die without agreeing with the wish. *Respect shares a sense of understanding.*
- Coordinate activities and visits in the home. *This promotes the pt's sense of self and feelings of belonging.*
- Communicate both verbally and nonverbally in such a way to convey positive regard for the pt. *Communication provides this human need.*
- Institute a simple, consistent, predictable routine. *A routine supports the pt's safety, security, and independence.*
- Teach and assist the p/f/c to make legal arrangements (eg, powers of attorney and living will) before the pt becomes incompetent. *This provides the most amount of control over the pt's affairs by the pt.*
- Suggest the condition (if irreversible) will worsen slowly and encourage continued reevaluation by the physician. *This offers hope.*
- Encourage continued reevaluation by the physician. *This validates the p/f/c's perception of the illness, the extent of the pt's disability, and provides f/c support.*
- Establish a trusting relationship and encourage independence. *This helps the p/f/c feel secure in the home setting and bolsters self-esteem.*
- Provide and model honest praise for accomplishments. *Recognizing accomplishments raises self-esteem.*

Nursing Goals

- To protect the human dignity of the pt
- To protect the identity, self-esteem, and respect of the pt
- To enhance the pt's sense of control, belonging, meaning and purpose, and intimacy and love
- To preserve the pt's spared functions and abilities
- To enhance the p/f/c's quality of life
- To assist the f/c manage the pt's cognitive and behavioral changes
- To provide for a consistent environment
- To support the p/f/c's safety and security

Patient Goals

- The pt will retain spared functions and function at an optimal level.
- The pt will respond appropriately without overreaction.
- The pt will have a decrease in episodes of decreased night wakening and an increase in hours of sleep at night.

Patient and Family/Caregiver Outcomes

The patient will:

- Interact with others in the home milieu as shown by _____ within _____ (specify)
- Identify and demonstrate _____ techniques for dealing with memory loss as demonstrated by _____ by _____ (date)
- Demonstrate less emotional agitation as displayed by _____ within _____ (specify)
- Display less behavioral agitation as demonstrated by _____ within _____ (specify)
- Identify _____ feelings regarding diminished capacity to perform usual roles as demonstrated by _____ within _____ (specify)

The family/caregiver will:

- Discuss _____ thoughts and _____ feelings regarding the pt's condition by _____ (specify)
- Assist with establishing a baseline for the pt's functioning and provide information about the pt's patterns of functioning by _____ (date)
- Use the "ABC" (antecedent, behavior, consequences; see Problem Management section) approach to understand and manage behavioral problems (specify) within _____ weeks
- Describe four health maintenance practices by _____ (date)
- Demonstrate healthy coping skills by _____ within _____ (specify)

- Recognize s/s of delirium, infection, and the like that can be superimposed on dementia, and take appropriate action as demonstrated by _____ within _____ weeks
- Identify and contact at least three sources of support by _____ (date)

RESOURCES AND INFORMATION

Aronson, M. K. (1988). *Understanding Alzheimer's disease.* New York: Scribners.

Christner, A. M. (Ed.). (1992). *Dementia and other mental impairment: Strategies for meeting the challenge.* Providence, RI: Manisses Communication Group.

Mace, N. L., & Rabins, P. V. (1991). *The 36-hour day: A family guide to caring for persons with Alzheimer's disease, related dementing illnesses, and memory loss in later life.* Baltimore: Johns Hopkins University Press.

For support groups, information on treatment, new research, and available facilities:

1. Alzheimer's Association
   919 N. Michigan Avenue
   Suite 1000
   Chicago, IL 60611-1676
   312-335-8700
2. "Alzheimer's Family Care" program of Parke-Davis, manufacturers of THA (Tacrine and Cognex): 1-800-600-1600
3. National Stroke Association
   96 Inverness Drive East
   Suite I
   Englewood, CO 80112-5112
   1-800-787-6537
   303-649-9299
4. American Heart Association: 1-800-242-8721
5. Stroke Connection: 1-800-553-6321
6. Agency for Health Care Policy and Research (AHCPR) for "What You Should Know About Stoke Prevention" fact sheet and the booklet "Recovering After a Stroke"
   AHCPR Publications Clearinghouse
   PO Box 8547
   Silver Spring, MD 20907
   1-800-358-9295
7. ComputerLink and other discussion groups on the Internet for caregivers of pts with DAT
8. United Parkinsons Foundation
   33 W. Washington Boulevard
   Chicago, IL 60607
   312-733-1893
9. National Parkinson Foundation
   1501 NW Ninth Avenue
   Miami, FL 33136
   1-800-327-4545

10. The Parkinson's Foundation
    UCI 366 Med-SurgII
    Irvine, CA 92697
    714-824-3870
11. Area Agency on Aging, Aging Information Office: in the white business pages of the telephone directory
12. American Health Assistance Foundation, Alzheimer's Family Relief Program
    15825 Shady Grove Road
    Suite 140
    Rockville, MD 20850
    301-948-3244
    1-800-437-2423
    Fax: 301-258-9454
13. National Institutes of Health/National Institute of Neurological Disorders and Stroke
    9000 Rockville Pike
    Bethesda, MD 20892
    301-496-5751

REFERENCES

Alessi, C. (1991). Managing the behavioral problems of dementia in the home. *Clinics in Geriatric Medicine, 7*(4), 787–801.

American Psychiatric Association. (1994). *Diagnostic and statistical manual of mental disorders* (4th ed.). Washington, DC: Author.

Bauer, J., Roberts, M. R., & Reisdorff, E. J. (1991). Evaluation of behavioral and cognitive changes: The Mental Status Examination. *Emergency Medicine Clinics of North America, 9*(1), 1–12.

Chafetz, P. K. (1991). Structuring environments for dementia patients. In M. F. Weiner (Ed.). *The dementias: Diagnosis and management* (pp. 249–261). Washington, DC: American Psychiatric Press.

Christner, A. M. (Ed.). (1992). *Dementia and other mental impairment: Strategies for meeting the challenge.* Providence, RI: Manisses Communication Group.

Dietch, J. T. (1989). Adverse effects of reality orientation. *Journal of the American Gerontological Society, 37,* 974–976.

Feil, N. (1989). *V/F validation the Feil Method how to help disoriented old-old.* Cleveland: Edward Feil Productions.

Fernandez, F., Levy, J. K., & Galizzi, H. (1988). Cognitive impairment of AIDS-related complex and its response to psychostimulants. *Psychosomatics, 28,* 38–46.

Gwyther, L. P. (1985). *Care of Alzheimer's patients: A manual for nursing home staff.* Chicago: American Health Care Association and Alzheimer's Disease and Related Disorders Association.

Hachinski, V. C., Iliff, L. D., Zilhka, E., et al. (1975). Cerebral blood flow in dementia. *Archives of Neurology, 32,* 632–637.

Jackson, K. M., Shroyer, J. L., & Pak, H. J. (1994). Adult day care environmental design strategies for persons with Alzheimer's disease. *Southwest Journal on Aging, 10*(1 & 2), 5—5-61.

Kaplan, H. I., & Sadock, B. J. (1994). *Synopsis of psychiatry: Behavioral sciences, clinical psychiatry* (7th ed.). Baltimore: Williams & Wilkins.

Lipowski, Z. (1990). *Delirium: Acute confusional states.* New York: Oxford University Press.

Mace, N. L., & Rabins, P. V. (1991). *The 36-hour day: A family guide to caring for persons with Alzheimer's disease, related dementing illnesses, and memory loss in later life.* Baltimore: Johns Hopkins University Press.

McKhann, G., Drachman, D., Folstein, M., et al. (1984). Clinical diagnosis of Alzheimer's disease: Report of the NINCD-SADRDA Work Group under the auspices of Department of Health and Human Services Task Force on Alzheimer's Disease. *Neurology, 34,* 939–944.

Roth, M. (1978). Diagnosis of senile and related forms of dementia. In R. Katzman, R. D. Terry, & K. L. Bick (Eds.). *Alzheimer's disease: Senile dementia and related disorders* (Vol. 7, pp. 71–85). New York: Raven Press.

Weiner, M. F. (Ed.). (1991). *The Dementias: Diagnosis and management.* Washington, DC: American Psychiatric Press.

D

Depression and Depressive Behaviors

PROBLEM DESCRIPTION

Depression is a normal human emotion that can become an illness with specific symptoms that affect the mind, body, and spirit. Depression involves disturbances in behavioral, emotional, cognitive, physical, social, and spiritual functioning and is the result of an interaction of several factors. Depression is one of the most common illnesses. Statistics show the enormous magnitude that depression plays in everyday life.

Facts About Depression

- Depression affects about 6% of all adults in the United States, more than 9 million people in any given 6-month period.
- At least one in five Americans will experience a major depressive episode during their lifetime.
- Women are twice as likely to develop depression as men.
- Between 80% and 90% of persons with depression can be successfully treated.
- An estimated 15% of those persons with depression commit suicide.
- Depression is considered to be the underlying cause in half of all suicides.
- Pts with major depression report substantially poorer relationships and less satisfying social interactions.
- Depression is highly prevalent in the primary care setting, affecting anywhere from 6% to 25% of pts, depending on the diagnostic criteria used.
- First degree relatives of an individual with a history of mood disorders (such as depression, dysthymia, or bipolar disorder) have an increased risk of developing a mood disorder.
- Major depression can begin at any age, but usually starts in the mid-twenties and thirties.
- Postpartum depression is prevalent in 10% to 15% of women within the first 3 to 6 months after childbirth.
- The presence of another medical condition increases the probability that a depressive syndrome may be present.

- Clinically significant depressive symptoms are found in 12% to 35% of pts with a nonpsychiatric general medical condition.
- The lifetime probability of at least one episode of major depression for any U.S. citizen is 6%.
- Between 50% and 85% of patients treated for one episode of major depression will have at least one subsequent episode in their lifetime.
- A medical outcomes study, involving more than 11,000 pts in three cities, found that depression impairs physical and social functioning more severely than hypertension, diabetes, angina, arthritis, GI disorders, or respiratory problems among the chronic diseases compared with depression (Wells, Stewart, & Hays, 1989).
- Heart disease is the only other condition that can cause as much impairment as depression.
- Older adults have the highest suicide rates of any group of Americans; it is 50% higher.
- Depression in the elderly can vary from 10% to 65% due to misdiagnosis with other illnesses (Carson & Arnold, 1996; Guze & Robins, 1970; Katon, Berg, & Robbins, 1986; NIMH/NIH, 1985, Reiger, Boyd & Burke, et al, 1988).

Depression is a mood or affective disorder with 11 major diagnostic categories (American Psychiatric Association, 1994).

Severity of Depression

Of the many ways to describe depression, one is by severity.

- Mild depression: brief, temporary sadness that is a normal reaction to stress, tension, frustration and disappointment. It does not seriously interfere with functioning or daily activities. Treatment may be emotional support and an opportunity to talk, or a change of situation. However, even mild depression needs to be closely observed because it can deepen or persist.
- Moderate depression: more intense and lasts longer. It is usually caused by a loss or an upsetting event. For moderately depressed persons, daily activities become harder but they still meet daily responsibilities. In addition to emotional support, professional support is necessary at this point.
- Severe depression: shows marked behavior changes and loss of interest. Often a chemical imbalance is involved. Ability to function is impaired and the person is unable to cope. Emotional support and professional treatment are necessary.

Individuals become depressed for different reasons. Different schools of thought attribute depression to many different factors; there has yet to be one cause defined or proven by research. Factors that influence depression are:

- Heredity
- Biochemical changes
- Psychodynamic issues
- Drugs
- Illness(es)

- Personality
- Sensory change and loss
- Stress
- Seasons

The good news about depression is that it is treatable. Over 80% of depressed people can be treated effectively and their symptoms are alleviated within weeks. A combination of emotional support, medications, and therapeutic interventions can work alone or in combination for treatment. Individuals with symptoms of depression consume higher levels of health care resources as well as suffer higher rates of unemployment and disability than do those who are not depressed. The NIMH (1985) has estimated that in the United States the cost of depression to society is over $27 billion each year, two-thirds of which is attributed to days lost from work. The tragedy is that when depression is ignored, undiagnosed, or untreated then persons with depression and society suffer the debilitating effects.

PROBLEM IDENTIFICATION

Characteristics and Observable Behaviors

- Recurrent thoughts of suicide or death
- Suicide attempts or talking about suicide
- Slowed mental processes, forgetfulness, and problem with memory and concentration
- Indecisive and unable to make decisions or take action
- Disordered thoughts, disorientation
- Denial
- Low self-esteem
- Complaining
- Paranoia and suspiciousness
- Anhedonia (decreased pleasure or enjoyment)
- Withdrawn and isolative behaviors
- Increased irritability, argumentativeness, or hostility
- Generalized restlessness, agitation, pacing, and hand wringing
- Anger or hostility
- Crying for no apparent reason
- Physical signs: aches and pains, change in appetite, change in sleep patterns, fatigue, lack of energy
- Pervasive sadness, anxiety, or "empty" mood
- Ruminations of inadequacy
- Delusions, hallucinations, or other psychotic symptoms
- Sexual dysfunction: diminished interest in sexual activity and inability to experience sexual pleasure
- Fear of intense feelings
- Apathy and indifference to others
- Feelings of hopelessness and pessimism
- Feelings of worthlessness, self-reproach, inadequacy, and helplessness
- Inappropriate or excessive guilt
- Neglect of personal appearance, hygiene, home, and responsibilities

- Difficulty performing daily tasks and doing ordinary tasks overwhelming
- Increased use of alcohol, drugs, or other substances

Factors Related to the Problem

Medical Conditions That Mimic or Cause Depression

- Hypoxia and COPD
- CV disease such as cardiomyopathy, CHF, or MI
- Neoplasms, especially of the pancreas, brain, and lung
- Endocrine disorders such as Addison's disease, diabetes, Cushing's syndrome, thyroidism, or PMS
- Infections such as Epstein-Barr virus, encephalitis, hepatitis, HIV, mononucleosis, pneumonia, post-influenza, and chronic fatigue syndrome
- Electrolyte imbalances
- Uremia
- Vitamin deficiencies
- Immune and collagen-vascular disorders such as multiple sclerosis, systemic lupus erythematosus, and rheumatoid arthritis
- Other CNS pathology such as Parkinson's disease, Huntington's disease, stroke, and subdural hematoma
- Alcoholism
- Anemia
- Hypertension
- Hemodialysis
- Postpartum affective disorder (onset within 4 weeks postpartum)

Drugs Associated With Depression

- Antihypertensives, especially methyldopa (Aldomet), reserpine (Serpasil), propranolol (Inderal), clonidine (Catapres), and hydralazine (Apresoline)
- Steroids, especially corticosteroids (cortisone, prednisone), anabolic steroids, progesterone (Femotrol), and estrogen (Premarin)
- Alcohol
- Amphetamines and related substances
- Cocaine, hallucinogens, inhalants, opioids, and PCP
- Sedatives, hypnotics, and anxiolytics such as benzodiazepines: alprazolam (Xanax); barbiturates: diazepam (Valium); chloral hydrate (Noctec); and ethanol
- Analgesics and NSAIDs such as indomethacin (Indocin)
- Anticholinergics
- Anticonvulsants
- Antiparkinson medications such as levodopa (L-dopa) and amantadine (Symmetrel)
- Antiulcer medications
- CV agents such as digoxin (Lanoxin) and procainamide (Procan SR)
- Oral contraceptives
- Psychotropic medications
- Muscle relaxants

- Stimulants and appetite suppressants such as amphetamines, or fenfluramine (Pondimin)
- Antimicrobials such as sulfonamides: sulfamethizole (Sulfasol), cycloserine (Seromycin), and gram-negative agents
- Heavy metals and toxins

Differential Diagnosis

It is sometimes difficult in the home care situation to distinguish whether someone is depressed or is grieving. Many of the same symptoms appear. Table II-7 shows how depression differs from grief.

Table II-8 shows a differential diagnosis, based on mental status examination findings, among delirium, dementia, mania, schizophrenia, and the depressive disorders.

Assessment Tools and Instruments (see Appendix I)
Consider administering the:

1. Beck Depression Inventory
2. Brief Psychiatric Rating Scale
3. Geriatric Depression Scale
4. Global Assessment of Functioning Scale
5. Mini-Mental State Examination
6. Modified Overt Aggression Scale
7. Social Dysfunction Rating Scale
8. Spiritual Perspective Clinical Scale
9. Suicide Risk Assessment Tool
10. TRIADS

PROBLEM LIST

- Activity Intolerance
- Bowel Incontinence
- Breathing Pattern, Ineffective
- Communication, Impaired Verbal
- Diversional Activity Deficit
- Fluid Volume Deficit
- Grieving, Anticipatory or Dysfunctional
- Growth and Development, Altered
- Hopelessness
- Incontinence, Functional
- Incontinence, Total
- Mobility, Impaired Physical
- Noncompliance (specify)
- Nutrition, Altered
- Pain (specify)
- Parenting, Altered
- Sensory/Perceptual Alterations (specify)
- Post-Trauma Response
- Powerlessness

Text continues on p. 173.

Table II-7

Differences Between Depression and Grief

Trait	Depression	Grief
Trigger	Specific trigger to depressive episode not necessary	Grief likely to occur as result of loss or mutliple losses
Active or passive	Depressed persons are passive and tend to remain "stuck" in sadness	Grief is active and person feels emotional pain and emptiness related to loss
Emotions	Generalized feeling of helplessness, hopelessness, pessimism, and emptiness	Grieving persons feel emotional pain and emptiness related to a specific loss; experience a range of emotions that are generally intense
Activities	Lack interest in previously enjoyed activities	Grieving persons can be persuaded to participate in activities, especially as they begin to heal
Self-esteem	Low self-esteem, low self-confidence; the person with depression feels like a failure, unattractive, and unloved	Self-esteem usually remains intact; person with grief does not feel like a failure, unless it relates directly to the loss
Ability to laugh	Person with depression is likely to be unresponsive, humorless incapable of being happy, or even temporarily cheered up and likely to resist help and support	Grieving persons will sometimes be able to laugh and enjoy humor and they are more likely to accept support
Description of feelings	Person with depression has difficulty identifying or describing their feelings, they may feel suicidal	Grieving people cry for an identifiable loss, and crying provides relief, not likely to be suicidal
Feeling of failure	People with depression may dwell on past failures and perceived shortcomings	Any self-blame and guilt the person with grief feels relates directly to loss, and are episodic and resolve as they progress toward healing
Grief to depression		Grief can turn into serious depression, especially when grief process is blocked or mourning over loss is increasingly turned inward. When they become "stuck" in the sadness or unable to function, is when further intervention will be needed

From: Harris (1981)

D

Table II-8
Differentiation of Mental Status Examination Findings

	Delirium	Dementia	Manic Episodes	Schizophrenic Disorders	Depressive Disorders
Appearance and Behavior					
	Fluctuating impairment of consciousness, restlessness	May show deterioration of personal habits but state of consciousness not clouded	Hyperactive, elated, assertive, boisterous, with rapid emphatic speech, may become suddenly angry or argumentative	Variable	Dejected, slowed, slumped, troubled
Mood					
	Anxiety, fear, lability	Irritability, lability	Elation, sometimes anger and irritability	Blandness, impoverishment of inappropriateness of affect	Depression, hopelessness
Thought Processes					
Coherence and relevance	May be confused, incoherent	May become confused	Rapid association of ideas that may seem illogical	Often incoherent, disorganized	Coherent

Thought content	May have delusions	May have delusions and confusion	May have delusions and feelings of persecution	May have feelings of unreality, depersonalization, persecution, influence and reference; delusions that are bizarre and symbolic	May have delusions often involving guilt, self-deprecation, somatic complaints
Perceptions	May have illusions, hallucinations	May misperceive environmental stimuli	May have illusions, rarely hallucinations	May have hallucinations and illusions, often bizarre and symbolic	May have auditory hallucinations
Cognitive Functions					
Orientation	May be disoriented	May be disoriented	Well oriented	Usually, but not always well oriented	May have illusions, rarely hallucinations
Attention and concentration	Poor	Poor	Distractible	Distractible	May be poor
Recent memory	Poor	Poor	May seem impaired	Usually well preserved but may be difficult to test because of inattentiveness and indifference	May seem impaired

continued

D

Table II-8
Differentiation of Mental Status Examination Findings Continued

	Delirium	Dementia	Manic Episodes	Schizophrenic Disorders	Depressive Disorders
Remote memory	May become poor	May become poor	May seem impaired	Usually well preserved but may be difficult to test because of inattentiveness and indifference	May seem impaired
Information	May misperceive information	Difficulty processing information	May misperceive information	May misperceive information	May be slow processing information
Vocabulary	Preserved until late	Preserved until late	Speech may be pressured	May make up own words	May be slow or slurred
Abstract reasoning	Concrete	Concrete	Abstract or concrete	Concrete, may be bizarre	Abstract or concrete
Perception	May be poor	May be poor	May be poor	May be poor	May be poor

From Stuart & Sundeen (1995)

- Rape-Trauma Syndrome
- Self-Care Deficit (specify)
- Self-Concept, Disturbance in
- Sexual Dysfunction
- Sexuality Patterns, Altered
- Sleep Pattern Disturbance
- Social Interaction, Impaired
- Social Isolation
- Spiritual Distress
- Swallowing, Impaired
- Thought Process, Altered
- Urinary Elimination, Altered
- Violence, Risk for, self-directed or directed at others

PROBLEM MANAGEMENT

Prevention, Maintenance, and Restorative Interventions

- Reflect and confirm if what the pt shares is correct to initiate conversations about reality and design possible action plans.
- Do not rush the pt for answers or ask difficult questions if the pt is having trouble coordinating thoughts or verbalizing in the beginning of treatment.
- Pace the therapeutic conversation based on verbal and nonverbal cues.
- Look beyond the loss to the meaning the pt attaches to the issues to see what other information the pt is trying to convey.
- Do not try to talk the pt out of the feelings but reflect and confirm if what you heard is correct.
- Use information confirmed in conversations to discuss reality and possible action plans.
- Educate the p/f/c that it is difficult to be around a depressive person who is sad, negative, and complaining.
- Educate the p/f/c to set up visits, telephone calls, and special focused time for the pt to increase or maintain social contacts.
- Work with the p/f/c to establish a structure and physical activities to engage the pt in large and small motor skills.
- Assist the pt in contributing ideas for events previously enjoyed and willing to try again.
- Reinforce strengths and plan activities that will be successful.
- Encourage the pt to exercise as much control and decision-making as they are able to handle.
- Do not push or intrude more than necessary.
- Respect the pt's autonomy.
- Be aware that holidays, birthdays, anniversaries, deaths, and other significant days can be triggers for a reaction of increased feelings of sadness, aloneness, vulnerability, anger, abandonment, and thoughts of suicide.

- Have pt identify anniversary days early in treatment, so that planning can be done ahead of date and the "what ifs" can be rehearsed so that the pt has alternative coping skills planned.

Medication Management

Depression is often treated with medications that include tricyclic antidepressants, SSRIs, lithium, and MAOIs. Most medications require a period of time to reach a therapeutic level. The time and level depends on various factors such as age, physical or medical problems, or other psychiatric issues. The pt might relate positive signs of medication effectiveness early in treatment. It is necessary to have the pt understand medication treatment, effectiveness, and interactions to report possible s/s of adverse reactions.

NURSING MANAGEMENT

Nursing Interventions and Rationale

☆ Behavioral

- If the pt expresses negativism during the conversation, assist the pt to use a specified time to continue discussing the negative feelings. *This allows the pt control in the situation.*
- If the pt expresses negativism during the conversation, after the time limit is set, restructure the conversation to another topic. *This teaches the pt how to use a diversion during negative thought patterns.*
- Observe closely for changes in depression baseline especially when beginning a new medication; after any sudden dramatic behavioral change; during interrelational conflicts; during periods of increasing obligations; when pt seems to be getting better. *Pt's reaction to changes are unpredictable.*

♡ Emotional

- Educate the pt to begin doing things to feel better, rather than waiting to feel better. *This initiates and motivates the pt to attempt further activities.*
- Give honest praise for accomplishments. *Praise increases self-esteem.*
- Encourage the pt to assume responsibility for own feelings by reinforcing positive behaviors. *Accepting responsibility prevents pt's dependence on others and pt gains a sense of control.*

△ Cognitive

- Educate the pt about the problem-solving process to explore possible options; examine consequences of each alternative; select and implement alternatives and evaluate results. *This teaches the pt systematic method of solving problems.*
- Assist the pt to identify illogical conclusions and painful feelings. *This promotes realistic thinking.*

- Instruct the pt to set aside a specific and limited time to worry. *A specific time prevents prolonged brooding and allows time for self-evaluation.*
- Teach the pt to set aside reflective time to address worries and concerns and to develop a realistic action plan to deal with the issues. *This assists the pt in seeing connection between problems and positive actions.*
- Encourage the pt to verbalize self-destructive thoughts. *This assesses risk for suicide.*

◻ Physical

- Take sitting/standing, lying/standing, or lying/sitting/standing blood pressures every visit. *Pt should be assessed for orthostatic hypotension.*

◯ Social

- Discuss with the pt the consequences of various behaviors exhibited in relationships and their effect on others. *Such discussion helps pt recognize the effects of behaviors and learn more effective ways to relate.*

✳ Spiritual

- Assist the pt in focusing on the present and not the past. *This allows pt to work on the current problem and immediate solutions.*
- Assist the pt to understand that past cannot be changed, but the pt can change the attitudes toward the past. *This helps pt to change negative thought patterns.*
- Teach the pt to replace self-criticism and negative thoughts with self-affirmations. *Self-affirmation helps pt to learn to be kind and gentle with self.*
- Assist the pt in clarifying values regarding the quality and meaning of life. *This allows pt to determine feelings and beliefs.*
- Encourage the pt to feel pleasure by enlisting the support of f/c. *Support of f/c assists pt in creating opportunities to enrich the quality of life.*

Nursing Goals

- To decrease disorientation, rumination, negative self-concepts, and withdrawn behavior
- To alleviate feelings of depression
- To facilitate realistic self-evaluation
- To assist the pt to cope with losses and work through the grieving process

Patient Goals

- The pt will make plans for the future consistent with personal strengths and reflect a will to live.
- The pt will be free of psychotic symptoms.
- The pt will demonstrate functional level of psychomotor activity.
- The pt will demonstrate an increased ability to cope with anxiety, stress, or frustration.
- The pt will verbalize and demonstrate acceptance of loss or change.

- The pt will assume responsibility for dealing with feelings and finding others with whom to talk.
- The pt will reestablish or maintain relationships.

Patient and Family/Caregiver Outcomes

The patient will:

- Participate in _____ (specify) activities by _____ (date)
- Demonstrate increased spiritual well-being as demonstrated by _____ within _____ (date)
- Discuss situations, events, or changes that seem to be associated with the depression as demonstrated by _____ within _____ (date)
- Acknowledge unrealistic or negative expectations of _____ (specify) and reflects positive expectations as demonstrated by _____ within _____ (date)
- Acknowledge own responsibility for getting needs met and practices assuming control of own behavior as demonstrated by _____ within _____ (date)
- Identify and verbalize irrational thoughts associated with self-criticism as demonstrated by _____ within _____ (date)
- Acknowledge personal strengths, assets and accomplishments, makes affirming self- statements as demonstrated by _____ within _____ (date)
- Accept compliments from others as demonstrated by _____ within _____ (date)
- Make statements that reflect self-confidence and optimism as demonstrated by _____ within _____ (weeks)
- Identify, verbalize, and recognize response of manipulative behaviors and impact on others as demonstrated by _____ within _____ (days)

The family/caregiver will:

- Verbalize an increased understanding of depression as demonstrated by _____ and the _____ (list) symptoms of depression within _____ (weeks)
- Verbalize the recognition that the family is not responsible for the cause or the healing of the depression as demonstrated by _____ within (weeks)
- Verbalize increased understanding of the treatment issues in depression as demonstrated by _____ within _____ (weeks)

RESOURCES AND INFORMATION

1. National Institute of Mental Health (NIMH)
    Information Resources and Inquiries Branch
    Office of Scientific Information, Room 15C
    5600 Fishers Lane
    Room 7-C02
    Rockville, MD 20857
    301-443-4513

2. National Institutes of Health (NIH)
    Office of Clinical Center Communications
    Building 10, Room 1C255
    Bethesda, MD 20892
    301-496-2563
3. American Psychiatric Association (APA)
    Division of Public Affairs, Code P-H
    1400 K Street, NW
    Washington, DC 20005
    202-682-6220
4. American Psychological Association (APA)
    750 First Street, NE
    Washington, DC 20002
    202-336-5500
    1-800-296-0272
5. National Mental Health Association (NMHA)
    1021 Prince Street
    Alexandria, VA 22314-2971
    703-684-7722
    1-800-969-NMHA
    Fax: 703-684-5968
6. Seventh-Day Adventist Community Health Services
    PO Box 5029
    Manhasset, NY 11040
    516-627-2210

REFERENCES

American Psychiatric Association. (1994). *Quick reference to the diagnostic criteria from DSM-IV*. Washington, DC: Author.

Carson, V. B., & Arnold, E. N. (1996). *Mental health nursing: The nurse-patient journey*. Philadelphia: Saunders.

Guze, S. B., & Robins, E. (1970). Suicide and primary affective disorders. *British Journal of Psychiatry, 117*, 437–438.

Harris, A. C. (1981). *Mental health practice for community nurses*. New York: Springer.

Katon, W., Berg, A. O., Robins, A. J., et al. (1986). Depression-medical utilization and somatization. *Western Journal of Medicine, 144*, 564–568.

National Institute of Mental Health/National Institutes of Health. (1985). Consensus Development Conference Statement. Mood disorders: Pharmacologic prevention of recurrences. *American Journal of Psychiatry, 142*, 469–476.

Stuart, G. W., & Sundeen, S. J. (1995). *Pocket guide to psychiatric nursing* (3rd ed.). St. Louis: Mosby-Yearbook.

U.S. Department of Health and Human Services, Public Health Service, Agency for Health Care Policy and Research. (1993). Depression in primary care: Detection, diagnosis, and treatment. *Journal of Psychosocial Nursing, 31*(6), 19–28.

Wells, K. B., Stewart, A., Burke, J. D., et al. (1988). One-month prevalence of mental disorders in the United States. *Archives of General Psychiatry, 45*, 977–986.

Detoxification (See Substance Abuse Behaviors)

Dressing Problems (See Activities of Daily Living Problems)

F

E

Eating Problems (See Activities of Daily Living Problems)

Elimination Problems (See Activities of Daily Living Problems)

Exploitation (See Neglect and Exploitation)

F

Family or Caregiver Stress

PROBLEM DESCRIPTION

In home health care, the pcg is usually a woman, but all family members are affected when a pt requires care. Furnishing an unpaid service to society, the pcg or f/c is responsible for providing the pt with emotional support, physical assistance, help with self-care, transportation, monitoring or administration of medications, identification and management of symptoms, and crisis prevention and intervention. When the pcg or f/c experiences difficulty or discomfort providing these needs or caring for a pt, for whatever reason, family or caregiver stress occurs; when the pcg/c or p/f/c relationship feels or becomes overwhelming, coping may have decreased or stressors may have increased. Each person in the pt's immediate and remote environment will have a unique response to the pt's condition and illness, which will affect the responses of all those in the pt's family system (see Section 1). A pt's illness disrupts the f/c's life and the f/c's attitudes and reactions toward the pt's condition affect the family dynamics.

The greatest needs of those who are responsible for a pt are psychological, emotional, tangible support and advice regarding pt care issues, social interaction, and information (about symptoms, medication, and treatment side effects, community resources, and what to expect) (Hileman, Lackey, & Hassanein, 1992; Jed, 1989). Family or caregiver stress is more apt to occur with a pcg or a f/c who is the same age at the pt, caring for a pt with a terminal, enduring, or progressive mental illness, for extended periods of time, with inadequate social support. If the pcg is a spouse, they are at heightened risk for overall decline in health, as well as physical and psychological disorders, and relationship and occupational difficulties.

PROBLEM IDENTIFICATION
Characteristics and Observable Behaviors

- Negative other and self-appraisals
- Abusive behaviors and evidence of injury
- Anxiety
- Depressive behaviors (especially inability to enjoy life and fatigue)
- Denial of personal needs and wants
- Report of lack of resources (time, energy, support, strength, etc) to provide caregiving
- Disruption of pcg and p/f/c life and routines
- Change in roles and responsibilities with a frequent need to change focus from, for example, home to work
- Lack of knowledge needed to provide pt care
- Lack of needed skills to provide pt care
- Excessive or overinvolvement of the pcg or f/c with the pt, with complaints about dependency
- Expressions of intermittent anger, hostility, irritation, resentment, pain, frustration, sadness, regret, or apathy
- Expressions of ambivalence (guilt and concern) toward the pt
- Expressions of hopelessness, helplessness, powerlessness, uselessness, entrapment, loss of control, pressure, unmet needs, and loss of freedom
- Current family and marital problems
- Inadequate problem-solving and judgment

- Lack of or poor communication among family members
- Multiple hospitalizations or calling of emergency services for the pt
- Psychosomatic and stress-related illnesses
- Unexpected, sudden illness
- Social and emotional isolation and withdrawal
- Alcohol or other substance misuse and abuse
- Rigid approach or reluctance to cooperate and participate with other f/c and providers

Factors Related to the Problem

Four main factors influence a pcg's or f/c's decision to provide care at home for a pt:

1. Mutuality (ability to find meaning and gratification in the relationship with the pt)
2. Management ability (to provide care and use resources)
3. Morale
4. Tension between unmet needs and perceived importance of the unmet needs (Hirschfield, 1983)

Patient/Family/Caregiver Conditions That Can Positively or Negatively Affect Family or Caregiver Stress
Physical
- Recreational and other opportunities for exercise
- Mobility and use of assistive devices, equipment, or aids
- Eating, appetite, sleeping, rest, and activity levels
- Complexity, severity, and prognosis of medical and mental illness(es)
- Medication regimen
- Alcohol or other substance misuse or abuse
- Gender, general health status, and functional ability (ie, strength, range of motion, and coordination)
- Stage of growth and development
- Modes of communication

Psychological
- Readiness to learn
- Willingness to use assistive devices, equipment, and aids
- Nature of the relationships
- Changes in motivation
- Memory capacity, intellectual level, and occupational history
- Self-esteem, trust, body and self-image, and control issues
- Presence of a medical or psychiatric disorder
- Psychological perception of the illness(es)
- Decision-making ability, problem-solving ability, and judgment
- Styles of communication
- Previous experiences and receptivity to counseling and caregiving
- The use of protective, defensive, and coping mechanisms (see Section 1)

Emotional
- Availability of confidants and friends
- Emotional resources, ability, and energy to care for self
- Emotional intelligence
- Mood changes
- Ability to deal with loss and change
- Ability to minimize or avoid guilt feelings
- Approaches to communication
- Capacity to create and maintain intimate, close relationships
- Perception of support from health care providers, others, and the community

Social

F

- Area of residence (ie, urban, suburban, or rural) and living arrangements
- Availability and accessibility of community support services, including volunteers, transportation, and respite services
- Economic status and financial arrangements
- Capacity to create and maintain relationships with family members and with those outside the home
- Role functioning and role conflict, including work attendance
- Any life changes, such as divorce, bankruptcy, job loss, etc
- The cultural or social perception of the pt's illness and health
- Degree of continued participation in diversionary or recreational activities and hobbies
- The presence and availability of a support network in and outside of the home

Spiritual
- Comfort with aging and mortality issues
- Participation in religious and spiritual activities
- Beliefs, rituals, and customs regarding aging, illness and health, and suffering and death
- Sense of self-esteem, self-worth, and adequacy
- Sense of control, dignity, pride, and autonomy
- Psychic ability and energy to care for pt and self

Assessment Tools and Instruments (see Appendix I)
Consider administering the:

1. Mini-Mental Status Examination
2. Social Dysfunction Rating Scale

Other assessment tools to consider include the:

1. Burden Interview (Zarit, Reever, & Bach-Peterson, 1980) to determine the pcg's current level of stress and to determine the effectiveness of interventions
2. Family APGAR (Smilkenstein, 1978)

3. Instrumental Activities of Daily Living (Lawton & Brody, 1969)
4. Multidimensional Functional Assessment Questionnaire (Lawton, 1971)
5. Caregiver Strain Questionnaire (Robinson, 1983)
6. Constructing a family ecomap or genogram (Wright & Leahey, 1984)

PROBLEM LIST

- Caregiver Role Strain
- Diversional Activity Deficit
- Grieving, Anticipatory or Dysfunctional
- Helplessness
- Hopelessness
- Injury, Risk for
- Pain (specify)
- Powerlessness
- Self Care Deficit (specify)
- Sleep Pattern Disturbance
- Social Isolation
- Violence, Risk for: self-directed or directed at others

PROBLEM MANAGEMENT

Prevention, Maintenance, and Restorative Interventions

- Involve all individuals who will be providing care to the pt in teaching sessions regarding the pt's disease and illness, management strategies, support groups, environmental modification, and monitoring.
- Interview the pt, pcg, and f/c alone to obtain a history of the home care situation.
- Discuss role, household rules, and routine changes to improve communication and cooperation among all people on the health care team.
- Encourage the pcg and f/c to make as few changes to the home and routine as possible.
- Assist the pcg and f/c to eliminate any unnecessary roles, rules, or routines.
- Correct or minimize any defects or causes of family or caregiver stress in the home environment.
- Teach the pcg about various body, emotional, cognitive, and spiritual therapies and refer as indicated.
- Communicate knowledge of the difficulty of the primary caregiving role to the pcg; caregiving to the f/c; and the receiving of caregiving role to the pt.
- Coordinate the provision of home care services and the visits of providers.
- Monitor the pcg and f/c for s/s of ineffective coping and for family or caregiver stress.

- Teach the pcg and f/c to identify those tasks the pt can and cannot do.
- Provide information about respite care, information and referral, long-term care planning, counseling and support groups, and state and federal aid.

Medication Management

No specific medications are indicated for this behavior, except for the medications indicated for the physical and psychological problems associated with this problem.

NURSING MANAGEMENT

Nursing Interventions and Rationales
☆ Behavioral

- Assist and encourage the pcg and f/c to maintain established roles, household rules, and routines. *Established roles, rules, and routines reduce family or caregiver stress and provide a sense of predictability.*
- Actively listen to the pcg describe the home care situation to provide support and elicit a history of the p/pcg and p/f/c relationship from the pcg's perspective; f/c describe the home care situation to provide support and elicit a history of the p/f/c and pcg's relationship from the f/c's perspective; and pt describe the home care situation. *Gathering information provides support and elicits a history of the p/pcg and p/f/c relationship from the pt's perspective.*

🝢 Emotional

- Provide an opportunity for the pcg and f/c to discuss their feelings regarding their needs. *This accurately determines the nature of the pcg's and f/c's emotional needs.*
- Assist the pcg and f/c to share their personal feelings about their own and the pt's needs. *These feelings determine their reactions to caring for the pt and the role reversal.*
- Arrange and facilitate a family conference to discuss rule change, role change, role reversal, etc. *Such discussions encourage sharing of feelings, open communication, and problem-solving.*
- Assess the pcg's and f/c's degree of comfort caring for the pt and provide here-and-now information. *Assessment precludes the pcg and f/c from gauging the current situation on a long history of emotional involvement.*
- Arrange, encourage, or reward the pt for speaking about concerns to _____ (specify) regarding their illness. *This allows pt to receive support from a more emotionally detached source.*
- Assess the pt's level of dependence on the pcg and f/c. *This determines the appropriate interventions and emotional support needed for the p/f/c and pcg.*
- Assess the pcg's and f/c's degree of emotional involvement with the pt and if it is adversely affecting the pt's care refer the f/c or pcg to a support group for people with codependency issues. *Such referral provides continuing support and education for the f/c and pcg (see codependency).*

△ Cognitive

- Teach and counsel the pcg and f/c about the effects of family or caregiver stress and effective coping strategies, especially positive thinking. *This provides information and prevents or minimizes health and coping problems* (Borden & Berlin, 1990).
- Assist the pcg and f/c to identify obligations that must be fulfilled from those that are limited or controllable. *This evaluates the pcg's and f/c's perceptions of the situation and identifies areas where professional and community referrals are indicated.*
- Obtain input, if available, from specialists (eg, an occupational therapist, psychologist, or speech–language therapist) who are familiar with the pt, with the requisite authorizations. *Input provides a basis to determine ways to lessen objective and subjective pcg and f/c stress.*
- Provide or arrange for case or care management and referral for psychotherapy for behavioral, coping, or social distress. *This assists the p/f/c to gain insight, define problems, and determine solutions regarding family or caregiver stress and the problems related to it.*

◻ Physical

- Consider a referral or consultation to a specialist(s). *Specialists can assist with functional adaptation, provide individualization of the pt's care, and support the pt's independence.*
- Assess the pcg's and f/c's personal health status and health care needs. *Assessment prevents or minimizes pcg and family or caregiver stress.*
- Encourage the pcg and f/c to engage in physical activities and exercise. *Physical activity enhances coping and decreases family or caregiver stress.*
- Teach the pcg about procedures, treatments, using appliances, etc. *This allows nurse to determine the physical ability and therapeutic competence of the pcg.*
- Teach the f/c about procedures, treatments, using appliances, etc. *This allows p/f/c to determine physical ability, therapeutic competence, and provide a backup for the pcg.*

◯ Social

- Assist the pcg and f/c to develop a plan to manage visitors in the home. *Planning lessens the pcg's, f/c's, and pt's fatigue, overstimulation, and possible confusion.*
- Role play and rehearse with the pcg and f/c to prepare them to interact with visitors and others regarding the pt's condition and caregiving situation. *Such actions lessens pcg's and f/c's feelings of embarrassment and prevents and minimizes social isolation.*
- Spend some nondirect care time with the pt, pcg, and f/c. *This encourages socialization and interaction.*
- Assess the pt's level of dependence on the pcg and f/c. *Assessment determines appropriate community resource referrals for caregiver support, education, and respite.*
- Provide information about community resources, respite services, financial assistance, mental health specialists, transportation, volunteers, and support group

meetings for caregivers. *Information enhances the pcg's and f/c's support and social networks.*

✦ Spiritual

- Develop a strategy for managing caregiving problems in advance. *This stabilizes the environment and gives a sense of control to all in the home care milieu.*
- Assess the pcg's and f/c's personal health status and health care needs. *Assessment focuses on the pcg's and f/c's well-being.*
- Teach the pcg and f/c to allow others to support the pt. *Support of others provides for emergencies.*
- Teach the c/f/c and pcg self-nurturing techniques. *This establishes self-worth and enhances self-esteem.*
- Express empathy for the pcg's and p/f/c's feelings regarding the stress of caregiving. *This increases feelings of control and offers hope.*
- Facilitate discussion of the pcg's and f/c's past caregiving experience(s). *Such discussion increases self-confidence and competency.*
- Assist the p/f/c and pcg to set individual goals and limits. *Goals and limits increase their individual and collective sense of control and hope.*
- Assist the pcg and p/f/c to determine which obligations are mandatory and which ones are optional. *Such determination enhances the p/f/c's sense of control and finds areas for formal and informal relief.*
- Encourage the pcg and f/c to discuss their beliefs about dependency, caregiving, and role reversal. *This preserves the pt's dignity.*
- Assist the pcg and p/f/c to determine ways to contribute to society. *This restores a sense of purpose.*
- Assist the pcg and p/f/c to determine ways to continue social and other activities. *Socialization maintains a sense of purpose and connection with self, others, and nature.*

Nursing Goals

- Teach the pcg and f/c cognitive, affective, and motor skills needed to care for the pt
- Provide necessary and supplemental information regarding caregiving and support groups to the pcg and p/f/c
- Accurately assess the actual and potential for family or caregiver stress in the home care situation

Patient Goals

- The pt will share household tasks and social responsibilities to the best of his or her ability.
- The pt will describe ways to maintain a sense of purpose in life in light of being cared for.
- The pt will make and adjust to changes in roles, household rules, and routines related to the illness.
- The pt will have needs and wants met despite pcg and family or caregiver stress.

- The pt will develop a realistic view of the home care situation and the pcg's and f/c's obligations.

Patient and Family/Caregiver Outcomes

The patient will:

- Verbalize how the _____ illness has changed previously established roles by _____ (date)
- Positively respond to the interventions of the pcg, f/c, and provider(s) as demonstrated by _____ within _____ (weeks)
- Speak about caregiving concerns with _____, who is someone outside of the home environment, by _____ (date)

The family/caregiver will:

- Participate in the care of the pt by _____ (date) as demonstrated by _____
- Review the plan of care for the pt at least _____ (specify), or when a major change occurs in the family
- Provide emotional support to the pt as demonstrated by _____ within _____ (specify)
- State _____ (specify number) of current obligations that must be fulfilled by _____ (date)
- Verbalize how the pt's _____ illness has changed previously established roles, household functions, rules, and routines by _____ (date)
- Verbalize how the pt's _____ illness has affected the goals, aspirations, and social interactions of the pcg and f/c within _____ (specify)
- Demonstrate the _____ (specify) skills needed to care for the pt
- Verbalize knowledge of the pt's multidisciplinary treatment plan, illness, and medications by _____ (date) as demonstrated by active participation or _____ during weekly treatment planning meetings
- Appropriately assess and intervene with the pt who is not effectively responding to caregiving as demonstrated by _____ within _____ (date)
- Maintain _____ (specify number of) relationships outside the home as shown by _____ within _____ (specify)
- Verbalize emotional response(s), including uncertainty about the future, about caring for the pt within _____ (weeks)
- State that there is less role stress or strain by _____ (date)
- Efficiently manage time by _____ (specify) within _____ (specify)
- Verbalize a need for _____ assistance and obtain it by _____ (date)
- Develop a plan to decrease family or caregiver stress by _____ (date)

RESOURCES AND INFORMATION

1. Local senior centers and government aging offices
2. State government aging offices

3. Children of Aging Parents (CAPS; for referrals, workshops, publications, and support)
   Woodbourne Office Campus
   Suite 302-A
   1609 Woodbourne Road
   Levittown, PA 19057
   215-945-6900

4. National Council on the Aging (NCOA; for advice and publications)
   409 3rd Street, S.W.
   Suite 200
   Washington, DC 20024
   202-479-1200

5. Family Caregiver Program—"Best Wishes Edith and Henry" (1984)
   Oregon State University Cooperative Extension Service
   Vicki L. Schmall
   Extension Home Economics
   161 Milam Hall
   Oregon State University
   Corvalis, OR 97331
   541-737-2711

6. Family Caregiver Program—"Hand in Hand" (1984) and "A Path for Caregivers" (D12957)
   American Association of Retired Persons
   AARP Program Department
   601 E. Street NW
   Washington, DC 20049
   202-434-2277

7. Description of a 6-week course with references: Ruppert, R. A. (1996). Caring for the lay caregiver. *American Journal of Nursing, 96*(3), 40–45.

8. Well Spouse Foundation—peer support, newsletter, support groups
   610 Lexington Avenue #814
   New York, NY 10022-1605
   212-644-1241
   800-838-0879

REFERENCES

Borden, W., & Berlin, S. (1990). Gender, coping and psychological well-being in spouses of older adults with chronic dementia. *American Journal of Orthopsychiatry, 60,* 603–610.

Hileman, J. W., Lackey, N. R., & Hassanein, R. S. (1992). Identifying the needs of home caregivers of patients with cancer. *Oncology Nurse Forum, 19*(5), 771–777.

Hirschfield, M. (1983). Homecare versus institutionalization: Family caregiving and se-

nile brain disease. *International Journal of Nursing Studies, 20*(1), 22.

Jed, J. (1989). Social support for caretakers and psychiatric rehospitalization. *Hospital and Community Psychiatry, 40*(12), 1297–1299.

Lawton, M. P. (1971). The functional assessment of elderly people. *Journal of the American Geriatric Society, 19,* 465–488.

Lawton, M., & Brody, E. (1969). Assessment of older people: Self-maintaining and instrumental activities of daily living. *The Gerontologist, 9,* 179–186.

Robinson, B. (1983). The caregiver strain questionnaire. *Journal of Gerontology, 38*(3), 334.

Smilkenstein, G. (1978). The family APGAR. *Journal of Family Practice, 6,* 1231–1239.

Wright L. M., & Leahey, M. (1984). *Nurses and families.* Philadelphia: Davis.

Zarit, S. H., Reever, K. E., & Bach-Peterson, J. (1980). Relatives of the impaired elderly: Correlates of feelings of burden. *The Gerontologist, 20,* 649.

G

Fear (See Anxiety)

Feeding Problems (See Activities of Daily Living Problems)

G

Grief and Loss Problems

PROBLEM DESCRIPTION

Loss is a change in the status of a significant person or object. It can be actual or threatened and reduces one's probability of achieving implicit or explicit goals. Loss requires that one give up something familiar, comfortable, and personal. Significant losses can cause strong emotional responses. Throughout life everyone experiences losses and the process of dealing with the loss is learned over time.

Reactions to loss are unique, individual, unpredictable, and dependent on several factors. The closer one is to the object the greater the loss. Loss can expose feelings of inadequacy, dependency, and insecurity. The more intense the involvement, the more profound the sense of loss. When the ultimate loss, the death of a loved one, occurs, a person has hopefully had some experience in dealing with the stages of grief. Attitudes and individual perceptions determine how individuals will react to or express grief; factors such as culture, guilt, financial issues, age, or developmental crises can compound the reaction. Individuals and families with adequate support systems will have fewer difficulties coping with loss and grief than those who face it alone. Those who have previously lost and coped successfully will more likely deal with the current loss.

Categories of Loss

1. Loss of a person through
   - Death, abortion, miscarriage, and stillbirth
   - Disease
   - Divorce
   - Separation
   - Moving
   - Changes (mental and physical)
   - Friendships
2. Loss of aspects of the self
   - Ideas
   - Dreams
   - Health
   - Body parts
   - Self-esteem
   - Identity
   - Innocence
   - Hospitalization
   - Role
3. Loss of external objects
   - Possessions
   - Pets
   - Natural disasters
   - Home
   - Thievery
4. Developmental losses
   - Breast-feeding to bottle to solids
   - Security objects
   - Change in daily activities (school, graduations, or work)
   - Love
   - Aging process
   - New baby or member in family

The reaction to loss is grief. Grief is a physical and emotional response to a loss. Bereavement is the actual grief process a person goes through after a major loss. Mourning is the psychological healing process through which the loss is made real and the grief is made manageable. Grief is not on a continuum but goes through stages over a period of time, becoming less intense, until the loss can be remembered without pain. A normal grief reaction usually lasts about a year, often with exaggerations or exacerbation around the time of holidays or anniversaries.

Factors That Influence or Contribute to the Grief Experience

1. Nature of the attachment
   - Who was the person who died?
   - Was the attachment strong? Weak?

- Was the deceased person's relationship vital to the bereaved's self-esteem or self-worth?
- Was the survivor highly dependent on the deceased?
- Was ambivalence present in the relationship?

2. Who the person was
   - Relationship—father, son, friend, distant cousin, etc
   - The deceased's age, gender, etc
3. Historical experiences
   - Past losses and coping mechanisms
   - Prior mental health
   - Prior physical health
   - Other life crises
   - Multiple losses
4. Mode of death
   - Expected
   - Unexpected
   - Accidental
   - Murder or suicide
   - Was the death near, distant, or far away?
5. Personality variables
   - Age
   - Gender
   - Ability to express feelings
   - Coping style
6. Social variables
   - Ethnic background
   - Religious background
   - Social background
   - Gains—primary and secondary

Grief may be anticipatory if the pt is expected to die or if a major loss is anticipated in the near future. All persons regardless of age or types of loss will work through four major tasks of grieving:

1. Accepting the reality of the loss
2. Experiencing the pain of the loss
3. Adjusting to life
4. Reinvesting energy into new relationships and experiences

Grief is a normal response to a loss, but if the grief is delayed, exaggerated, or absent it may lead to abnormal, complicated, or unresolved grief and depression.

Work in grief therapy flourished in the 1960s and 1970s. Dr. Elisabeth Kübler-Ross (1969) identified five stages that a dying person experiences

- Denial
- Anger
- Bargaining
- Depression
- Acceptance

Engel (1964) indicated three phases of grief

- Shock and disbelief
- Developing awareness
- Restitution

Westberg (1971) described 10 stages of grieving:

1. State of shock
2. Expressing emotion
3. Depression and loneliness
4. Physical symptoms of distress
5. Panic
6. Guilt feelings
7. Anger and resentment
8. Resistance
9. Hope
10. Affirming reality

According to Bowlby (1961) the three stages of bereavement are:

- Beginning stage—protest denial, crying, clinging to lost object, and hostility
- Middle stage—disorganization, despair, apathy, and aimlessness
- Termination stage—reorganization, with acceptance of lost object and acceptance of new object.

Grief therapy allows the pt to work through the feelings and come to acceptance. The goal in grief work is not to avoid or eliminate painful feelings but to review emotions and work toward integration of life minus the loss.

PROBLEM IDENTIFICATION

Characteristics and Observable Behaviors

- Absentminded
- Agitation
- Ambivalence
- Anger
- Anxiety
- Appetite decreased
- Blaming others and self
- Cognitive confusion and memory lapses
- Difficulty communicating
- Difficulty concentrating
- Crying
- Denial
- Disbelief
- Disinterest in ADLs
- Dreaming
- Emotional numbness or emotions out of control
- Emptiness
- Energy, lack of
- Exhaustion
- Fearful
- Forgetful
- Guilt
- Hallucinations, auditory and visual
- Hostility toward persons connected with the death
- Isolative and withdrawn
- Loneliness
- Relief
- Restlessness
- Rumination
- Sadness
- Searching for lost object
- Sense of unreality
- Shock
- Sighing, frequent
- Sleep disturbances
- Somatization
- Treasuring objects of the deceased

Factors Related to the Problem

- Social isolation
- Physical symptoms or illness
- Substance abuse
- Mood disorder
- Organic mental disorder
- Personality disorder
- Anxiety
- Perceived or actual loss
- Unexpected or sudden death of significant other
- Multiple overlapping losses with unresolved issues
- Inadequate social supports
- Stressful and prolonged anticipatory loss

Table II-9 presents Schneider's (1980) differential diagnosis between grief and depression.

G

Assessment Tools and Instruments (see Appendix I)

Consider administering the:

1. Beck Depression Inventory
2. Brief Psychiatric Rating Scale
3. Geriatric Depression Scale
4. Global Assessment of Functioning Scale
5. Mini-Mental State Examination
6. Social Dysfunction Rating Scale
7. Spiritual Perspective Clinical Scale
8. Suicide Risk Assessment Tool
9. TRIADS

PROBLEM LIST

- Comfort, Altered
- Communication, Impaired Verbal
- Grieving, Anticipatory or Dysfunctional
- Hopelessness
- Pain, Chronic
- Parenting, Altered
- Post-Trauma Response
- Powerlessness
- Sensory/Perceptual Alterations (specify)
- Sexual Dysfunction
- Sleep Pattern Disturbance
- Social Interaction, Impaired
- Social Isolation
- Spiritual Distress
- Thought Processes, Altered
- Violence, Risk for, self-directed or directed at others

Table II-9
Differences Between Grieving and Depression

Characteristic	Grieving Person	Person With Depression
Loss	Has suffered recognizable loss	Has suffered recognizable loss, or person may see loss as punishment
Mood state	Quickly shifts from sadness to more normal state in the same day	Has variability in mood; psychomotor activity level; verbal communication; appetite; and sexual interest, within the same day or week; sadness is mixed with anger
Energy level	Feels tension or absence of energy	Feels a consistent sense of depletion; psychomotor retardation; anorexia with weight loss; decreased interest in sex; decreased verbal communication; agitation; compulsive eating; and, sexuality or verbal output are diminished
Expression of anger	Shows open anger and hostility	Absence of externally directed anger and hostility
Expression of sadness	Weeps, can be managed	Has difficulty in weeping or in controlling weeping
Dreams, fantasies, and imagery	Vivid, clear dreams and fantasies; good capacity for imagery, particularly involving the loss	Relatively little access to dreams, low capacity for fantasy or imagery (except for self-punitive)
Sleep disturbance	Disturbing dreams and episodic difficulties in getting to sleep	Severe insomnia and early morning awakening
Self-concept	Sees self as being to blame for not providing adequately for lost object; has tendency to experience world as empty; has preoccupation with lost object or person	Sees self as bad; has tendency to experience self as worthless; preoccupation with self; has suicidal ideas and feelings
Responsiveness	Responds to warmth and reassurance	Responds to repeated promises, pressure, and urging or is unresponsive to most stimuli
Pleasure	Variable restrictions of pleasure	Persistent restrictions of pleasure
Reaction of others to affected person	Others show tendency to feel sympathy for person and to want to touch or hold person	Others show tendency to feel irritation toward person; others rarely feel like touching or reaching out to person

NURSING MANAGEMENT

Prevention, Maintenance, and Restorative Interventions

- Help the pt to accept the reality of the loss, to understand the normal process of grief and mourning, and to reorganize own life in a meaningful way without the significant other person.
- Talk about the loss with the pt and the circumstances surrounding the loss to make it more real and reduce anxiety.
- Talk about the loss to help the pt understand the significance of the loss because everyone experiences a loss in an individual way.
- Use broad opening statement to encourage pt to disclose.
- Reassure the pt that bereavement feelings are real.
- Encourage the pt to express anger and guilt feelings and their meanings.
- Repeat grief education as needed because the pt understands the dynamics in different ways at different times along the grief continuum.
- Allow time to gradually integrate the significance of the loss.
- Educate the pt that behavior resulting from anger and fear that is redirected or denied is misunderstood by others and has the potential for causing additional stress in families.
- Educate the pt that the anger felt is a normal process of grieving and is usually directed at someone who is close.
- Assist the pt to identify potential difficulties and plan for the "what if."
- Assist the pt and f/c in opening channels of communication.
- Educate pt that those who maintain hope will be better able to cope with death.
- Terminally ill pts experience anticipatory grief that results in depression and sadness and it is inappropriate to cheer them up because the losses they face are great and will necessitate eventual understanding and acceptance.
- Educate f/c that being around a terminally ill person is difficult and time consuming.
- Educate p/f/c to pace themselves and decide on how other responsibilities may be met.
- Provide grief information and educational support because sometimes fear of the unknown can cause the most anxiety.
- Assist the f/c to understand the role the dying person fills in the family, the person's value and equilibrium.
- Assist f/c in finding alternative members who can pick up some of those values, traits, and traditions.

Medication Management

Caution is recommended when sedative-hypnotic medications are prescribed for pts who are in a normal grieving state. Transient and judicious use of these medications should only be considered if the pt is having difficulty with sleeping, eating, irritability, and other stress-related disorders. If the pt requests prolonged use of sedative-hypnotics, unresolved grieving or depression should be considered.

Antidepressants may be indicated for pts with a previous history of depression or an identified history of poor coping skills in times of loss. Medications can have side effects dulling the senses, which does not allow the normal grief process to proceed. Close observation is necessary to balance the positive effects of medications within the grief process.

NURSING MANAGEMENT

Nursing Interventions and Rationales

☆ **Behavioral**

* Assist the pt to develop action plans to reach new goals. *Planning encourages responsibility and provides direction, goal achievement.*
* Encourage the pt to be tolerant of own ability to function at an optimum level during holiday seasons or anniversary dates. *This assists in the fatigue that feelings of loss will engender at that time.*
* Teach the pt to embrace the memory of the lost person or object. *Reminiscing assists in letting grief go but maintaining positive memories and feelings.*

♡ **Emotional**

* Use effective communication techniques and role playing. *These encourage awareness and expression of emotions associated with grief and loss.*
* Explore with the pt fears associated with the loss, especially regarding the loss of control. *This identifies potential coping mechanisms.*
* Encourage the pt to focus on assets and strengths. *Such focus promotes self-esteem and aids coping.*

△ **Cognitive**

* Encourage realistic goal setting. *This reduces distortions of reality associated with loss.*
* Assist the pt to identify goals that are unattainable because of the loss. *This reduces feelings of helplessness.*
* Assist the pt to find new ways to meet realistic goals. *Pts need to plan interventions and promote feelings of control.*
* Assist the pt to identify positive aspects of relationship with the person or object of loss that can be carried into the future. *Use positive aspects of relationship for coping with loss.*
* Reward and encourage the pt to make realistic statements about current situation that reflect acknowledgment of the loss. *This helps to face reality of loss.*

▢ **Physical**

* Educate the pt that stress related to a loss may increase a person's vulnerability to other physical and emotional problems. *This increases an awareness of the mind/body connection.*

◯ Social

- Explore with the p/f/c ways in which social support systems have changed as a result of loss. *Such exploration identifies changes and facilitates adaptation.*
- Refer the pt to self-help groups such as bereavement groups, Parents without Partners, Widowed Persons Service, Compassionate Friends, or other local groups. *Referrals promote support and prevent the complications of prolonged grief.*

✦ Spiritual

- Discuss ways to increase a sense of control over life situations. *This strengthens coping abilities and a sense of personal competence.*
- Explore with the p/f/c beliefs and attitudes that may be relevant to the pt's experience of loss. *This encourages grief work and adjustment to loss.*
- Assist the pt's awareness of options for creating meaning in life. *Such awareness reduces helplessness and despair.*
- Support and reinforce creative efforts. *This assists the pt to discover a new purpose in life.*

Nursing Goals

- To decrease secondary gain from dysfunctional grieving
- To facilitate progression through the stages of grieving
- To encourage the pt to consciously adapt their life-style to the loss
- To encourage the pt to make plans for the future
- To help the pt acknowledge terminal illness and assist in an anticipatory grievance process

Patient Goals

- The pt will acknowledge and verbalize acceptance of the loss.
- The pt will demonstrate integration of loss into life.
- The pt will verbalize changes in life-style and coping mechanisms that incorporate the fact of the loss.
- The pt will verbalize realistic future plans integrating the loss.
- The pt will demonstrate physical recuperation from the stress of loss and grieving.
- The pt. will progress through grieving process.
- The pt will demonstrate reestablished relationships or social support.
- The pt will participate in support groups.

Patient and Family/Caregiver Outcomes

The patient will:

- Express feelings of grief as demonstrated by _____ within _____ (weeks)
- Verbalize loss and its meaning by _____ (date)
- Verbalize knowledge of the grief process by _____ (specify)

- Express reduced feelings of guilt and blame to the provider by _____ (date)
- Make plans for the future as demonstrated by _____ within _____ (weeks)
- Make statements that reflect acceptance of own feelings (even though they may create discomfort and pain) within _____ (weeks)
- Describe physical manifestation of _____ (specify) by _____ (date)
- Recognize thoughts, feelings, or events that lead to _____ (specify) by _____ (date)
- Identify ways to increase sense of control over life as demonstrated by _____ within _____ (weeks)
- Examine and list _____ (specify number) needs that will be more difficult to meet as a result of the loss by _____ (date)
- Identify _____ (specify number) past losses and coping mechanisms previously used by _____ (date)
- Identify and verbalize thoughts, attitudes, and beliefs that contribute to feelings of guilt within _____ (weeks)
- Differentiate between concepts of responsibility and guilt as demonstrated by _____ by _____ (date)
- Identify (specify) personal strengths and assets within _____ (weeks)
- Practice new behaviors designed to facilitate goal attainment as demonstrated by _____ by _____ (date)
- Describe role changes resulting from the loss by _____ (specify)
- Express feelings associated with loss of old roles and creation of new ones within _____ (weeks)
- Discuss _____ (specify number of) life goals before the loss by _____ (date)
- Describe how loss has affected goal attainment by _____ (date)

The family/caregiver will:

- Discuss past experiences and beliefs associated with losses and anticipated course of illness and outcomes within _____ (weeks)
- Discuss preillness roles, rules, goals, and anticipated changes in roles, rules, and goals within _____ (weeks)
- Express feelings to _____ openly within _____ (weeks)
- Participate in pt's care within _____ (weeks)
- Adapt to changes in roles as demonstrated by _____ within _____ (weeks)
- Preserve cultural, ethnic, and religious practices as demonstrated by _____ within _____ (date)
- Resolve loss through grief and mourning as demonstrated by _____ within _____ (weeks)

RESOURCES AND INFORMATION

1. Alpo, Professional Relations (for copy of "Death of the Family Pet: Losing a Family Friend")
    PO Box 25200
    Lehigh Valley, PA 18002-5200
    610-398-4500

2. American Association of Retired Persons (AARP)
   601 E Street, NW
   Washington, DC 20049
   202-434-2277
3. American Cancer Society: 1-800-ACS-2345
4. Delta Society (video and written material on pet loss and bereavement)
   PO Box 1080
   Renton, WA 98057-1080
   206-226-7357
5. Hospice Education Institute
   190 Westbrook Rd.
   Essex, CT 06426-1518
   860-767-1620
6. National Hospice Organization (NHO)
   1901 North Moore Street
   Suite 901
   Arlington, VA 22209
   1-800-658-8898
7. National Institute for Jewish Hospice
   ASB/1 Building
   Suite 652
   8723 Alden Drive
   Los Angeles, CA 90045
   1-800-446-4448
8. In the white pages of the telephone book: bereavement groups, Parents without Partners, Widowed Persons Service, Compassionate Friends, or other local groups for grief work

REFERENCES

Bowlby, J. (1969). *Attachment and loss* (Vol. 1). New York: Basic Books.

Engel, G. (1964). Grief and grieving. *American Journal of Nursing, 64*(7), 93–96.

Kübler-Ross, E. (1969). *On death and dying.* New York: Macmillan.

Schneider, L. (1980, Fourth Quarter). Clinically significant differences between grief, pathological grief and depression. *Patient Counseling and Health Education,* 267–275.

Westberg, G. (1971). *Good grief.* Philadelphia: Fortress Press.

Grooming Problems (See Activities of Daily Living Problems)

H

Homicidal Behavior (See Suicidal and Homicidal Behaviors)

Hygiene Problems (See Activities of Daily Living Problems)

Hyperactivity (See Manic Behaviors)

I

Incontinence (See Activities of Daily Living Problems)

L

Loss Problems (See Grief and Loss Problems)

M

Manic Behaviors

PROBLEM DESCRIPTION

Mania is a state of excessive excitement or enthusiasm. Manic-depressive illness or bipolar affective disorder is a cyclic disorder characterized by recurrent fluctuations in mood between mania, depression, and normal periods. Manic episodes vary in intensity and time even within the same pt. Manic behaviors are characterized by at least three of the seven primary symptoms:

1. Inflated self-confidence or self-esteem, grandiosity, or excessive self-importance
2. Decreased sleep
3. More rapid speech, more talkative than usual, or feels pressure to keep talking
4. Flight of ideas, feels subjectively that thoughts are racing
5. Distractibility
6. Increased goal-directed activity, high energy level, or psychomotor agitation
7. Excessive involvement in pleasurable activities with unwanted consequences (eg, gambling, sex, driving fast)

Symptoms must be present during an episode of elevated mood that is present persistently for at least 1 week. The mood alteration must be of sufficient severity to cause marked impairment of functioning or to protect the person from harm to self or others, and not be secondary to an underlying medical condition or treatment.

Hypomanic behavior is less extreme than mania, but often with more lability and volatility. It is more likely that suicide will be attempted during the hypomanic phase. Often actions to initiate therapeutic interventions during hypomania are likely to be unsuccessful. Most pts like their hypomanic phases and their behavior is rarely disruptive enough for others to become involved in treatment. Hypomanic features include at least three primary symptoms (as discussed above) during an episode of elevated, expansive, or irritable mood present for at least 4 days, and is distinctly different from the nondepressed mood. The change is not severe enough to impair functioning or be apparent to others; it is not secondary to an underlying medical condition or treatment (American Psychiatric Association, 1994).

Secondary mania is a condition that develops subsequent to another medical disorder, such as substance abuse, multiple sclerosis, use of steroids, cerebral palsy, neurologic disorders, and endocrine disorders.

The onset of bipolar affective disorder is usually between ages 20 and 40. Mania can first occur as early as the late teens and early twenties. A few individuals can experience their first episode in their forties or fifties. About 90% of persons who experience manic episodes also experience severe episodes of depression.

PROBLEM IDENTIFICATION

Characteristics and Observable Behaviors

- Aggressive
- Ambitious
- Argumentative
- Delusional
- Denial of realistic danger
- Distractibility
- Elation or euphoria
- Emotional lability
- Excessive spending of money
- Expansiveness
- Flight of ideas
- Grandiosity
- Hostile, complaining
- Humor
- Hyperactivity
- Identification with religious leader
- Illusions
- Inadequate hydration, nutrition, hygiene, and inappropriate dress
- Increased creative activity
- Increased motor activity
- Inflated self-esteem
- Irresponsibility
- Irritability
- Lack of judgment
- Lack of shame or guilt
- Loose associations
- Need for little sleep
- Paranoid
- Pressured speech
- Provocative behaviors
- Sexual overactivity
- Short attention span and difficulty concentrating
- Increased social activity
- Substance use and abuse
- Unrealistic perception of self
- Unwarranted optimism
- Weight loss

Factors Related to the Problem

- Low self-esteem
- Bipolar affective disorder
- Psychotic process
- Sleep deprivation
- Psychiatric illness
- Altered thought process
- Sensory/perceptual alterations
- Hyperactivity
- Fatigue
- Cognitive impairment
- Substance abuse
- Endocrine disorders
- Multiple sclerosis
- Cerebral palsy
- Neurologic disorders

Drugs that can cause mania include steroids, antidepressants, isoniazid, L-dopa, marijuana, LSD, cocaine, mescaline, caffeine, dextroamphetamine (Dexedrine), methylphenidate (Ritalin), and pemoline (Cylert).

Assessment Tools and Instruments (see Appendix I)

Consider administering the:

1. Abnormal Involuntary Movement Scale
2. Brief Psychiatric Rating Scale
3. Global Assessment of Functioning Scale
4. Mini-Mental Status Examination

5. Modified Overt Aggression Scale
6. Social Dysfunction Rating Scale
7. Suicide Risk Assessment Tool

PROBLEM LIST

- Caregiver Role Strain
- Communication, Impaired Verbal
- Fatigue
- Noncompliance
- Nutrition, Altered: Less than Body Requirements
- Parental Role Conflict
- Parenting, Altered
- Personal Identity Disturbance
- Post-Trauma Response
- Self Care Deficit (specify)
- Self Mutilation, Risk for
- Sensory/Perceptual Alterations (specify)
- Sexual Dysfunction
- Sexuality Patterns, Altered
- Sleep Pattern Disturbance
- Social Interaction, Impaired
- Social Isolation
- Spiritual Distress
- Thought Processes, Altered
- Violence, Risk for, self-directed or directed at others

PROBLEM MANAGEMENT

Prevention, Maintenance, and Restorative Interventions

- The f/c needs to be involved in treatment and supervision.
- Educate the p/f/c about all aspects of bipolar affective disorder, manic behavior, medications, and adverse effects.
- Assist p/f/c to provide a consistent, structured environment to let the pt know what is expected.
- Ignore or withdraw attention from bizarre behaviors, appearances, or sexual acting out to minimize attention to unacceptable behaviors.
- Show acceptance of pt, use a firm, calm approach, and give simple and direct explanations.
- Do not make promises you cannot keep.
- Do not bargain or argue with the pt.

- Avoid highly competitive activities to decrease situations that could exacerbate hostile and aggressive feelings.
- Monitor drug therapeutic blood levels on a regular basis.

Medication Management

Antimanic medications are used to control the symptoms of bipolar disorder. Lithium has been the drug of first choice because it manages both the manic and depressive phases of bipolar affective disorder. Recently alternate antimanic medications have come into use: carbamazepine (Tegretol), clonazepam (Clonopin), valproic acid (Depakene), divalproex (Depakote), verapamil (Isoptin, Calan), clonidine (Catapres), and propranolol (Inderal). Research has shown that divalproex sodium (Depakote) is as effective as lithium, is often better tolerated, and may be more effective in certain forms of bipolar disorder (Carson, 1996). Monitoring therapeutic blood levels of antimanic medications is critical for maintaining a therapeutic dose level and avoiding toxicity.

ECT has been used successfully in treating mania in the earliest days of severely manic decompensations and it is a relatively safe and effective treatment for manic episodes during pregnancy.

Table II-10 presents guidelines for the commonly used antimanic medications.

M

Table II-10
Guidelines for Commonly Used Antimanic Medications

Medication	Dosage	Therapeutic Level	Adverse Reactions
Lithium	600–1200 mg po in divided doses daily	Acute therapy: 0.8–1.4 mEq/L Maintenance therapy: 0.4–1.0 mEq/L	Monitor blood levels to assess for toxicity above 1.5 mEq/L
Carbamazepine (Tegretol)	Initial: 200–400 mg/d po and may be increased up to 1.6–2.2 g/d po—use lower dosages when used in combination with other antimanic or antipsychotic drugs	4–12 µg/mL	Monitor blood levels to assess for blood dyscrasias
Valproic acid (Depakene/ Depakote)	Initial: 300–500 mg/d po and then gradually increased to 750–3000 mg/d po	50–125 µg/mL	Monitor blood levels to assess for elevated liver transaminase elevations or hepatic toxicity

NURSING MANAGEMENT

Nursing Interventions and Rationales

★ Behavioral

- Give simple, direct explanations for tasks. *Simple explanations assist the pt in completing tasks and state what is expected.*
- Avoid arguing with the pt. *Arguing interjects doubt and undermines the limits set.*
- Decrease stimuli before bedtime, turn down lights, turn down television, have pt take a warm bath to limit noise and other stimuli. *These measures encourage rest and sleep.*
- Limit excessive verbal activity by focusing on one topic at a time. *This encourages self-control.*
- Assist the pt to become aware of the effect of behavior on others and use feedback from others. *Feedback clarifies behaviors and reduces alienation and rejection.*
- Explore with the pt the consequences of manic behavior. *This encourages reality testing and shows how behavior interferes with health and safety.*

♡ Emotional

- Assist the pt to be aware that sadness is acceptable at times. *This helps pt understand that sadness is self-rewarding and that this state of mind may be difficult to give up.*

△ Cognitive

- Assist the pt to identify and express feelings. *This promotes self-awareness.*
- Interrupt when necessary to slow down stream of conversation. *Interruption increases pt awareness of behavior.*
- Assist the pt to stay with the subject being discussed. *This sets limits and increases attention span.*
- Provide the pt with paper or notebook to write or draw on as a way to express feelings. *Thoughts are mixed and this might help pt sort through feelings.*
- Limit flight of ideas by clarifying and validating the meaning of messages. *Such clarification focuses on logical thought processes and speech.*

▢ Physical

- Educate p/f/c about escalating manic behaviors and to observe for increasing s/s. *Early intervention prevents further complications.*
- Monitor medication blood levels. *Monitoring avoids toxic levels of antimania medications.*
- Educate p/f/c in ways to maintain salt, fluid, and electrolyte balance. *Proper balance decreases chance for toxic reaction.*
- Encourage p/f/c to limit caffeine and smoking. *These are often abused in a manic state and may increase manic behavior.*
- Assist the pt to identify inappropriate sexual behaviors. *This protects pt from embarrassment or potential diseases.*

⬭ Social

- Educate p/f/c on inappropriate behaviors, setting limits, and not encouraging inappropriate behaviors that may seem funny or playful. *This assists the pt from increasing behavior to extreme levels.*

✦ Spiritual

- Confront discrepancies in the pt's perception of self and real self once a therapeutic relationship is established. *Such action provides pt with a more realistic self-concept.*
- Discuss with the pt the ability to live a less disruptive, more satisfying life. *This discussion helps pt to accept the illness as one that can be relieved by medication.*
- Teach the pt that medication can maintain inappropriate behaviors at an acceptable level and release energy for more creative and productive efforts. *This encourages self-actualization and prevents future hospitalizations.*
- Discuss with the pt the fact that the euphoric feelings experienced are only a temporary release from the pain. *This promotes feelings and self-awareness.*

Nursing Goals

- To decrease hyperactivity, restlessness, and agitation
- To decrease bizarre appearance and behavior, sexual acting out, and other inappropriate behaviors
- To decrease disorientation, hallucinations, delusions, and other psychotic symptoms
- To promote safety and compliance with medication therapy

Patient Goals

- The pt will verbalize and comply with medication regimen, including periodic blood tests.
- The pt will state s/s of an approaching manic episode.
- The pt will have and state plans for asking for help when manic symptoms reappear.
- The pt will obtain help from supportive person(s) who can assist or listen to thoughts and feelings during stressful times.
- The pt will knowledgeably discuss factors contributing to manic behavior.
- The pt will control own behavior and participate in less stimulating activities that still provide satisfaction.

Patient and Family/Caregiver Outcomes

The patient will:

- Demonstrate decreased restlessness, hyperactivity, and agitation within _____ (weeks)
- Demonstrate decreased hostility as demonstrated by _____ within _____ (weeks)

- Demonstrate increased feelings of self-worth as demonstrated by _____ within _____ (weeks)
- Demonstrate more appropriate appearance as demonstrated by _____ within _____ (weeks)
- Demonstrate decreased hallucinations or delusions by _____ (date)
- Demonstrate an increased attention span as demonstrated by _____ within _____ (weeks)
- Demonstrate decreased pressured speech, tangentiality, and loose associations as demonstrated by _____ within _____ (weeks)
- Participate in learning about illness, treatment, and safe use of medications by _____ (date)
- Identify and verbalize painful feelings and distinguish between feelings of anger, anxiety, guilt, and sadness within _____ (weeks)
- Express realistic ideas without grandiose of exaggerated ideas of self-importance as demonstrated by _____ within _____ (weeks)
- Enhance self-concept by realistically appraising self for both _____ (specify number) strengths and specify number) limitations by _____ (date)
- Identify and list activities that provide satisfaction without producing stress by _____ (date)

M

The family/caregiver will:

- Establish clear lines of authority and boundaries for behavior as demonstrated by _____ within _____ (weeks)
- Describe role expectations that are realistic and promote individual growth and improved self-esteem by _____ (date)

RESOURCES AND INFORMATION

1. National Institute of Mental Health
   Information Resources and Inquiries Branch
   Office of Scientific Information, Room 15C
   5600 Fishers Lane
   Room 7-C02
   Rockville, MD 20857
   301-443-4513
2. National Depressive and Manic-Depressive Association
   53 West Jackson Boulevard
   Suite 505
   Chicago, IL 60604
   312-939-2442
   1-800-82-NDMDA
3. Helping Hands
   109 Chestnut Street
   Andover, MA 01810
   617-475-6888

REFERENCES

American Psychiatric Association. (1994). *Quick reference to the diagnostic criteria from DSM-IV.* Washington, DC: Author.

Carson, V. B., & Arnold, E. N. (1996). *Mental health nursing: The nurse-patient journey.* Philadelphia: Saunders.

Meaning and Purpose in Life Problems

PROBLEM DESCRIPTION

Meaning and purpose in life problems affect the pt's whole being. When the pt is unable to reconcile the illness with religious beliefs, spiritual convictions, cultural ties, or philosophy of life, the pt faces a threat to his or her belief or value system. Meaning and purpose in life improves the pt's capacity for recovery and healing; spiritual and religious beliefs assist with positive coping, and health potential is enhanced in the presence of meaning and purpose in life, the will to live, and faith in the self, God, and others (Ross, 1995). Various international organizations and the Joint Commission on the Accreditation of Healthcare Organizations mandate that meaning and purpose in life or spirituality be considered by those who provide care.

The interaction of many factors—personality, coping, environmental, relationships, finances, support system, and disease state—greatly affect meaning and purpose in life problems. Meaning and purpose in life are associated with personal growth, spiritual resources, and joy in living. Every age group, from child to elder, deals with this issue. Absence of meaning and purpose in life can lead to feelings of being unloved, depression, suicidality, poor use of coping skills, negative thought patterns, and difficulty in interpersonal relationships. Personal meaning and purpose in life beliefs that vary from those of family and friends may also stress relationships, especially if belief systems conflict.

PROBLEM IDENTIFICATION

Characteristics and Observable Behaviors

- Verbalizations and questions regarding meaning and purpose in life; suffering; death; self-blame; pessimism about the future; lack of control or power; morals and ethics; no fear of death; alienation and separation; forgiveness; fanaticism; belief in an afterlife
- Enhanced awareness of aging
- Direct or displaced anger or hate toward God or religious, or spiritual representatives
- Inability to participate in usual religious, spiritual, or cultural practices, sacraments, and customs
- Nightmares and other problems with sleep

- Ambivalent feelings about beliefs or abandoning usual beliefs, rituals, etc
- Inappropriate or gallows humor
- Emotional detachment from or emptiness toward others, self, community, nature, etc
- Alterations in behavior, thoughts, or mood (withdrawal, lack of eye contact, intrusiveness, decreased energy level, apathy, submissiveness, dependency, and estrangement)
- Lack of appetite or vomiting for no known reason
- Change in sexual activity
- Lack of participation and decision-making in self-care
- Expressed frustration and dissatisfaction over inability to perform previous activities and role performance
- Discouragement, despair, and crying
- Expressions of uncertainty or fatalism over outcomes and sense of abandonment
- Changes in personal hygiene
- Remorse and guilt that "bad" things are happening now because of mistakes earlier in life
- Pessimism and discouragement with a loss of hope and difficulty speaking about the future
- Expression of discomfort about not adhering to dietary traditions, usual rituals, etc
- Refusing to accept visits and solace from religious or spiritual advisor
- Feelings of distress for feeling angry at "higher power," church, temple, mosque etc for medical diagnosis and the symptoms of it
- Strong, overwhelming feelings regarding condition and degree of impaired functioning
- Social and occupational dysfunction or withdrawal
- Perception of the connection between religious faith and spiritual practices and current and past situations

Factors Related to the Problem

- Sense of meaning and purpose, inner strengths, interconnections, and forgiveness
- Age, ethnicity, gender, education, and income
- Loss of body part or function
- Abuse, rape, and other traumas
- Unknown or doubtful etiology of illness
- Terminal illness, debilitating disease, or pain
- Series of losses, grief, and changes (death, miscarriage, etc)
- Surgery and surgical procedures
- Medications and medical procedures
- Restriction of religious or spiritual practices
- Beliefs contrary to others in the home and those important to the pt
- Substance abuse
- Sexual drive and interest

- Energy level and motivation, appetite, and sleep pattern
- Medical and health status
- Coping repertoire and responses
- Impaired cognitive functioning
- Degree to which meaning and purpose in life needs are met
- Ability to pursue goals
- Meaning attached to medical diagnosis
- Sense of responsibility regarding illness
- Sense of self-esteem, self-worth, and adequacy
- Sense of control, dignity, pride, and autonomy

Questions for Assessment of Meaning and Purpose in Life Problems

1. Does the pt have strong, evident religious, spiritual, or cultural practices and ties?
2. Are there more subtle signs of religious, spiritual, or cultural commitment from the pt?
3. Does the pt have visits at home from family, friends, or religious, spiritual, or cultural representatives?
4. Does the pt express feelings of guilt, anger, or despair about own life?
5. How does the pt's illness affect life roles, goals, and degree of health?
6. Does the pt have positive self-esteem?
7. What does the pt consider the primary cause of spiritual distress?
8. Does the pt expect any conflicts between religious and spiritual approaches and medical treatment?
9. Does the pt have a sense of meaning and purpose in life? (Andrews & Boyle, 1995; Barry, 1996; Burkhardt & Nagai-Jacobson, 1989; Dossey, Keegan, Guzzetta, & Kolkmeier, 1995; Guzzetta & Dossey, 1992; Loxley & Cress 1983)

Assessment Tools and Instruments (see Appendix I)

Consider administering the:

1. Spiritual Perspective Clinical Scale
2. Suicide Risk Assessment Tool

Another assessment to consider is the Purpose-in-Life Test (Crumbaugh, 1968).

PROBLEM LIST

- Anger
- Decisional Conflict
- Grieving, Anticipatory or Dysfunctional
- Helplessness
- Hopelessness
- Pain (specify)

- Post-Trauma Response
- Powerlessness
- Self-Care Deficit (specify)
- Sensory/Perceptual Alterations (specify)
- Sexuality Patterns, Altered
- Sleep Pattern Disturbance
- Social Isolation
- Spiritual Distress
- Thought Processes, Altered

PROBLEM MANAGEMENT

Preventive, Maintenance, and Restorative Interventions

- Assess and educate self and peers about meaning and purpose in life, positive spirituality, and various religious, spiritual, and cultural beliefs, practices, and world views.
- Explore own religious beliefs and spiritual convictions to convey a nonjudgmental attitude toward the pt's religious beliefs and spiritual convictions, promote respect for and acceptance of the pt, to assist the pt to explore meaning and purpose in life issues, and promote a positive therapeutic relationship.
- Plan for activities that have a high likelihood of success, based on the pt's meaning and purpose and life experiences, strengths, and assets.
- Listen when the pt wants to share meaning and purpose in life and religious and spiritual concerns.
- Refrain from discussing, arguing about, or joking with the pt about the pt's belief and value systems that are directly related to problem behavior and meaning and purpose in life.
- Assist the p/f/c to make those life-style changes and required behavior changes that affect meaning and purpose in life issues.
- Reduce or eliminate those factors that are barriers to or reduce the pt's meaning and purpose in life and spiritual life, such as (but not limited to) disconnection from the natural world, lack of privacy, medals, articles, books, etc, which are unavailable to the pt due to small, print, sensory or literal loss, etc.
- As indicated, assist the pt to preserve those beliefs and practices that have a beneficial effect on health (Leininger, 1995).
- As indicated, assist the pt to adjust or adapt those beliefs and practices that are neutral or indifferent in terms of the pt's health status (Leininger, 1995).
- As indicated, assist the pt to readjust or repattern those beliefs and practices that have a potential or actual harmful effect in terms of the pt's health status (Leininger, 1995).

Medication Management

No specific medications are indicated for this behavior, except for the medications indicated for the physical and psychological problems associated with this problem.

NURSING MANAGEMENT
Nursing Interventions and Rationales
☆ Behavioral

- Plan and assist the pt to engage in activities that assist the pt in coping with the diagnosis. *Activity enhances pts coping skills and sense of self-sufficiency.*
- Assist the pt to complete a life satisfaction chart, journal, or values clarification exercise. *This determines the pt's present fulfillment of and future goals for meaning and purpose in life.*
- If appropriate and acceptable, pat the pt's hand or hug the pt. *Touch conveys support and strengthens the relationship.*

♡ Emotional

- Assist the pt to express any feelings of anger or negativity toward God, etc. *This relieves tension and enhance meaning and purpose in the pt's life.*
- Facilitate the pt celebrating, mourning, or acknowledging events that influence the pt's feelings about meaning and purpose in life and spirituality. *Acknowledging milestones can enhance personal growth and resolution.*

⊿ Cognitive

- Identify life-affirming ideas, values, and beliefs through values clarification exercises. *These assist the pt to understand the impact of his or her world view on meaning and purpose in life, health, and illness.*
- If indicated, teach the pt how to affirm, change, or eliminate beliefs that are life-denying. *This helps pt to move beyond mental blocks and negativity.*
- Teach the pt to use mental imagery techniques. *Imagery helps the pt to heal old memories, forgive others, and envision a meaningful and purposeful future.*
- Refer the pt for psychotherapy (cognitive or existential). *Psychotherapy helps pt to deal with personal growth and self-investigation regarding meaning and purpose in life.*

⊓ Physical

- Adapt the therapeutic regimen and routine to adhere to the pt's beliefs. *This maintains pt preferences and meaning and purpose in life during the course of home care.*
- Obtain referrals to make adaptations to diet, activity, etc. *Referrals may provide for the coexistence of the pt's preferences and therapeutic regimen.*
- Assess for adequate nutritional intake. *The pt with meaning and purpose in life problems may not have a desire to eat or may have stress-related digestive problems.*

◯ Social

- Share, when appropriate, prayer and personal experiences with meaning and purpose in life problems. *Sharing offers support to the pt as pt adapts to a new life circumstance.*
- Refer and provide access to or transportation of a religious or spiritual person. *This permits clarification of beliefs and use of available religious and spiritual care resources.*

M

- Assist the p/f/c to contact spiritual or religious advisors and community groups. *Such contact provides for meaning and purpose in life and spiritual and social support.*
- Assist the pt to participate in formal or informal religious system through large-print books, television programs, radio shows, visits from clergy, etc, as appropriate. *Such involvement decreases the pt's sense of social isolation.*

✳ Spiritual

- Assess the pt's beliefs about health and illness and meaning and purpose in life. *This reduces the pt's sense of aloneness and abandonment.*
- Involve the pt in meaningful, purposeful personal activities. *Helps pt to maintain identity, role relationships, and positive memories.*
- Intentionally be present and "in touch" with the pt. *This provides reliability and basis for trust by displaying care.*
- Assess the pt's beliefs and convictions regarding the illness as it affects meaning and purpose in life and family functioning. *Pt needs to examine which beliefs are useful at this time.*
- Assess the religious affiliation or spiritual identification of the p/f/c and the degree of congruence among family members. *The assessment allows the provider to determine the need for referrals.*
- Listen to the pt and assist the pt to discuss and explore religious or spiritual beliefs. *Listening validates the importance of religious and spiritual matters and conveys respect to the pt.*
- Teach the terminally ill pt about the stages of death and dying (Kübler-Ross, 1969). *This helps pt to feel control and to acknowledge goals.*
- Assist the f/c to arrange for the pt to have significant symbols, engage in preferred rituals, and have visits from identified religious or spiritual representatives as needed. *These measures provide comfort for the pt, reduce anxiety, and enhance meaning and purpose in life.*
- Encourage hope in nonjudgmental and respectful ways. *Directing positive energy and respect toward the pt improves self-esteem and provides basis for patient hope.*

Nursing Goals

- To assist the pt to meet spiritual needs, according to the pt
- To demonstrate a respect and caring attitude toward the pt's religious and spiritual beliefs and practices
- To plan for the pt's spiritual care based on pt's religious views, etc
- To advocate for the pt's individual religious and spiritual needs
- To honor the pt's own religious, spiritual, ethical, and other beliefs and values
- To assist the pt to identify any conflicts between beliefs and practices or convictions and medical diagnosis
- To assist the pt to identify ways to adapt to anticipated loss or death
- To consider the various cultural ways the pt may express own spirituality and find meaning and purpose in life

Patient Goals

* The pt will continue to develop spiritually.
* The pt will ascribe meaning and purpose to current life circumstances.
* The pt will attach meaning to unmet suffering and life circumstances.
* The pt will identify and use appropriate resources to continue to explore how religion and spirituality can provide meaning and purpose for the experience of _____ illness and life.
* The pt will practice religious and spiritual activities after discharge.
* The pt will express a sense of spiritual peace and physical comfort.
* The pt will understand and accept own death.

Patient and Family/Caregiver Outcomes

The patient will:

* State an understanding of the differences and similarities between spiritual health and physical health by _____ (date)
* Verbalize thoughts and feelings about meaning and purpose in life, death, and loss within _____ (weeks)
* Identify _____ (specify) positive aspects of using faith and convictions to give meaning and purpose to the experience of the _____ illness by _____ (date)
* Identify _____ (specify) negative aspects of using faith and convictions that detract from meaning and purpose to the experience of the _____ illness by _____ (date)
* Identify _____ events and _____ feelings that contributed to a loss or lack of meaning and purpose in the pt's life within _____ (weeks)
* Engage in life-affirming activities as demonstrated by _____ by _____ (date)
* Verbalize how current illness and treatment interferes with meaning and purpose in life by _____ (date)
* Define meaning and purpose in life and list spiritual needs within _____ (weeks)
* Identify _____ feelings related to condition and list _____ (specify) support systems to use when meaning and purpose in life problems arise by _____ (date)
* Share perceptions of how death will affect the f/c functioning within _____ (weeks)

The family/caregiver will:

* Discuss their perceptions of how the pt's death will affect the f/c functioning within _____ (weeks)
* Identify and provide _____ (specify) predictable activities that increase the pt's sense of control and meaning and purpose in life by _____ (date)
* Assist the pt to use faith and conviction to cope with the pt's _____ illness within _____ (weeks)
* Discuss thoughts and feelings about the situation with _____ (specify), a religious or spiritual leader, within _____ (weeks)

RESOURCES AND INFORMATION

1. Center for Attitudinal Healing
   19 Main Street
   Tiburon, CA 94920
   415-435-5022
2. Spirituality and Healing in Medicine and Healing Words, Healing Practices (videos)
   Harvard Medical School
   Harvard MED-CME
   PO Box 825
   Boston, MA 02117-0825
   Phone: 617-432-1525
   Fax: 617-432-1562
3. National Institutes of Health
   Office of Alternative Medicine
   6120 Executive Boulevard
   Executive Plaza South
   Room 450
   Rockville, MD 20892-9904
   301-496-4000

REFERENCES

Andrews, M. M., & Boyle, J. S. (1995). *Transcultural concepts in nursing care* (2nd ed.). Philadelphia: Lippincott.

Barry, P. D. (1996). *Psychosocial nursing care of physically ill patients & their families* (3rd ed.). Philadelphia: Lippincott-Raven.

Burkhardt, M., & Nagai-Jacobson, M. G. (1989). Spirituality: The cornerstone of holistic nursing practice. *Holistic Nursing Practice, 3*(3), 18–26.

Crumbaugh, J. C. (1968). Cross validation of the Purpose in Life Test based on Frankl's concepts. *Journal of Individual Psychology, 24,* 74–81.

Dossey, B. M., Keegan, L., Guzzetta, C. E., & Kolkmeier, L. G. (1995). *Holistic nursing: A handbook for practice* (2nd ed.). Gaithersburg, MD: Aspen Publishers.

Guzzetta, C. E.. & Dossey, B. M. (1992). *Cardiovascular nursing: Holistic practice*. St. Louis: Mosby-Yearbook.

Kübler-Ross, E. (1969). *On death and dying*. New York: Macmillan.

Leininger, M. (1995). *Transcultural nursing concepts, theories, research, and practice*. New York: McGraw-Hill.

Loxley, C. M., & Cress, S. S. (1983). *The pocket guide to clinical nursing process for the adult medical-surgical client*. New York: Miller Press.

Ross, L. (1995). The spiritual dimension: Its importance to patients' health, well-being and quality of life and its implications for nursing practice. *International Journal of Nursing Studies, 32,* 457–468.

Medication Reactions
(See Adverse Reactions)

Memory Problems (See Delirium, Dementias, and Depression and Depressive Behaviors)

N

Neglect and Exploitation

PROBLEM DESCRIPTION

On the part of the pcg or the f/c, neglect is:

1. The refusal or failure to attend to the necessary care and needed treatment, including preventive care, of a pt, including deliberate refusal to implement the individualized treatment plan designed for the pt by the treatment team
2. The inaction or action that denies the prescribed care and treatment to which the pt is entitled
3. Action(s) contrary to the prescribed treatment or regimen
4. Unauthorized removal or denial of a pt's personal possessions or normal comforts (eg, bed, heat, light), including failure to secure proper clothing and see that the pt is properly clothed
5. Unauthorized denial of a pt's scheduled meals or snacks
6. Failure to intervene or protect a pt from abusive behaviors, mistreatment, neglect, and exploitation by another family member or provider

On the part of the pcg or f/c, exploitation is:

1. The unauthorized denial, misuse, or theft of the pt's money, property, or other resources
2. A direct or indirect act or process that uses or removes the resources of the pt for monetary or personal gain

PROBLEM IDENTIFICATION

Characteristics and Observable Behaviors

Neglect

Patient. Poor hygiene; poor nutrition with weight loss and anemia; dehydration; poor skin integrity; contractures; urine burns or excoriation; pressure ulcers; and impaction (Fulmer & Ashley, 1989); lethargy, passivity, withdrawal, overcompliance, or indifference; inappropriate dress; anemia; repeated CHF; infections; excessive reminiscing and subtle changes in cognition (especially confusion, disorientation, and forgetfulness) or personality (particularly anger and hostility); and expressed frustration about receiving care

Primary Caregiver and Family/Caregiver. Inadequate concern, privacy, attention, respect, socialization, interest, and supervision (when needed); changes in cognition or personality; expressed frustration about caregiving; emotional, mental, physical, social, or spiritual abandonment; omission of care

Home. High weeds in yard with garbage strewn about; lack of routine and needed repairs to home; evidence of animal infestation; presence of rotted food in or about the home; evidence of fire hazards; cold or wet home; utilities and services cut off; overcrowded home; house lacks minimum equipment and supplies; and house has architectural barriers

Exploitation

Patient. Lack of belongings, food, assistive devices, clothing, medications, etc, particularly when finances are available; extreme expressions of interest in the pt's finances and other assets by the pt; pt isolated from others; failure or reluctance to discuss financial plans or arrangements; verbalizations about offers of financial assistance or requests for help from others; changes in bank accounts; unexplained overdrafts and charges for insufficient funds; missing property, belongings, assets, etc; noticeable difference in the appearance between the pt and the pcg or f/c; oversedation; confusion regarding paying bills or inability to afford transportation; inconsistency in accounts or contradictions regarding the pt's money, property, or other resources; pt "forced" out of their home for economic pressures; deprived of rights (civil, legal, personal, and sexual) by force or duplicity; verbally coerced or threatened to engage in activity against the pt's wishes or best interest; participates in or prevented from participating in medical, scientific, or other activity without informed consent; unnecessarily hospitalized or otherwise institutionalized by the f/c; bribed through the deceit of another, to give something away unwittingly; forced to relinquish money, assets, or other resources to the pcg or f/c for their benefit and advantage rather than the pt's

Primary Caregiver and Family/Caregiver. Evasive about pt's finances; has detailed information about pt's finances; urges pt "not to worry" and says that is taking care of pt by supervising financial matters; acquires pt's property; provides extensive or fantastic rationalizations for unnecessary pt hospitalization, institutionalization, or removal from home; keeps pt in physical or social isolation; unwilling to spend money for health and medical care, especially when resources are available; provides story regarding financial arrangements that is inconsistent or contradictory to pt's statements; professes belief that because pt is incapacitated they "don't need" certain objects, money, bank accounts, or property

Factors Related to the Problem

The pt at risk for neglect and exploitation:

- Female and over age 75
- History of previous violence, abuse, neglect, or exploitation

- Increasingly complex needs that meet or exceed the f/c's ability to meet them
- Physical impairment, especially severe difficulty with vision, hearing, speech, or ambulation
- Behavior problems, especially anxious and withdrawn ones
- Mental and emotional impairments
- Low self-esteem
- Social isolation
- Substance abuse
- Resistance to or anger about receiving care

The pcg or f/c at risk for committing neglect and exploitation:

- Difficulty providing for physical care and safety of the pt and others
- Resentful of caring for the pt
- Difficulty providing emotional nurturance
- Financial and resource limitations
- History of previous violence, abuse, neglect, or exploitation
- Low self-esteem
- Severe external stress
- Social isolation and lack of support systems
- Lack of knowledge or skills
- Conflicting or multiple responsibilities
- Compromised health history and status
- Substance abuse
- Inadequate developmental level

Communities at risk for neglect and exploitation:

- Migrant or transient population
- Over- or underpopulated with older and other vulnerable adults

Assessment Tools and Instruments (see Appendix I)

Administer the:

1. Mini-Mental State Examination
2. TRIADS

PROBLEM LIST

- Apathy
- Constipation
- Diversional Activity Deficit
- Family or Caregiver Role Strain
- Family or Caregiver Role Stress
- Fluid Volume Deficit
- Helplessness
- Hopelessness

- Nutrition, Altered
- Pain (specify)
- Parenting, Altered
- Personal Identity Disturbance
- Post-Trauma Response
- Powerlessness
- Self-Care Deficit (specify)
- Sensory/Perceptual Alterations (specify)
- Sleep Pattern Disturbance
- Social Interaction, Impaired
- Social Isolation
- Spiritual Distress
- Thought Processes, Altered

PROBLEM MANAGEMENT

Prevention, Maintenance, and Restorative Interventions

- Be knowledgeable with the agency's policy and procedure regarding neglect and exploitation.
- Intervene immediately if the pt or anyone else in the home setting is in imminent danger of neglect and exploitation.
- Assess for s/s of neglect and exploitation.
- Interview the pt initially to collect baseline information and build trust with the pt.
- Compare the information obtained from the pt to that provided by the pcg, f/c, or others.
- In a nonjudgmental manner and in private, listen to the pt first and then listen to the pcg and f/c after regarding potential neglect and exploitation.
- If needed, use a translator from the home care agency; do not use a f/c, friend, or neighbor as a translator to obtain information regarding neglect and exploitation.
- Assess the p/f/c and home environment for the risk and signs of neglect and exploitation.
- Educate yourself, peers, public, and the p/f/c about establishing methods of alleviating social conditions that influence neglect and exploitation and ways to reduce opportunities for neglect and exploitation.
- Support the development and maintenance of services and legal and legislative efforts to eliminate or prevent neglect and exploitation.
- Intervene when neglect and exploitation occur; if necessary, arrange for separation of the parties, and for the parties to connect with their families of origin.
- Identify and develop a plan to deal with the identifiable, associated risk factors for neglect and exploitation.
- Make plans in advance for providing care (neglect and exploitation prevention planning) well in advance of a pcg or f/c becoming at risk for neglecting or exploiting a pt.
- Develop plans, which include cultivation of personal resources; early recognition of neglect and exploitation; referrals for counseling, personal assistance, respite

care for the pcg and f/c, emergency shelters, hospitals, and foster homes, other community services, mental health programs, or crisis intervention; and for minimizing stressors and preventing further neglect and exploitation, if they have occurred.

- Assist the pt to anticipate difficult circumstances and make preparations, such as writing a will and preparing powers of attorney.
- Assist the pcg and f/c to identify sources of support and how to ask for understanding and emotional support before caregiving responsibilities contribute to neglect and exploitation.
- Teach that neglect and exploitation are spiritual problems and create spiritual pain.

Medication Management

No specific medications are indicated for this behavior, except for the medications indicated for the physical and psychological problems associated with this problem.

NURSING MANAGEMENT

Nursing Interventions and Rationales

☆ Behavioral

- Continually monitor the home care setting. *Monitoring prevents or confirms allegations of neglect and exploitation.*
- Monitor for factors that are associated with neglect and exploitation to provide baseline data. *Early recognition and intervention promote the integrity of the p/f/c relationships.*
- Document suspected neglect and exploitation accurately and objectively. *Comprehensive documentation is necessary for diagnosis and possible legal or social intervention.*
- Provide or refer to individual, couple, group, or family therapy to focus on skills used to prevent or change neglectful and exploitative behavior. *Therapy facilitates and supports changes in f/c roles and behaviors, as well as decrease isolation or shame.*
- Provide or refer to appropriate support groups for information, effective use of existing resources, and long-term support. *This focuses on skills used to prevent or change cycle of neglect and exploitation.*

♡ Emotional

- Provide reassurance to the pt regarding suspected or validated neglect and exploitation. *Such reassurance minimizes anxiety.*
- Use a nonjudgmental approach to talk about feelings with the pt and then pcg and f/c. *Pt and pcg may not have had a chance to talk about the situation previously and may welcome the opportunity to receive help instead of blame.*
- Encourage the pt, if willing, to talk about experiences with neglect and exploitation. *Recalling experiences provides pt validation, promotes the grieving process, and provides basis for trust with provider.*

△ Cognitive

- Obtain a neuropsychological or other evaluations. *Evaluation prevents dismissal of allegations of neglect and exploitation based on pt's cognitive status.*
- Educate the pcg and f/c regarding pt care, the aging process, and support services. *This provides options and improves the coping skills of the pcg and f/c.*
- Provide or refer for cognitive and other types of therapy. *Therapy assists the p/f/c to prevent or change their own part in the neglect and exploitation pattern or cycle.*
- Obtain an understanding of the pt's perception of the threat or reality of neglect and exploitation. *This facilitates the development of interventions that directly address the pt's concerns.*
- Teach the p/f/c about neglect and exploitation. *This creates a framework to identify and express feelings and face the reality of the situation.*

☐ Physical

- Teach the pcg and f/c to provide for the pt's personal and medical needs. *This provides for appropriate physical care and nurturing.*
- Assess for evidence of neglect and exploitation. *Assessment allows nurse to prevent or intervene early in such situations.*
- Observe the pt and home setting (including the yard). *This allows nurse to document and treat injuries, correct conditions, and minimize or prevent injury and complications.*
- Determine risk for physical harm and report to the appropriate authorities if the risk is probable. *P/f/c safety is paramount.*

◯ Social

- Explore alternative living and caregiving situations if there is actual or potential pt neglect and exploitation. *This preserves the rights and dignity of the pt.*
- Provide referrals, as indicated, to the police, social services, protective services, ombuds program, advocacy group, etc. *Such action protects the pt legally and financially.*
- Discuss options and provide referrals for services such as respite, transportation, companion, volunteer, or other forms of assistance. *This action prevents or minimizes neglect and exploitation.*
- Contact previous health care providers, health care settings, bank officials, and f/c outside of the home (with the requisite permission). *This helps the provider, legal authorities, and f/c to determine if the information presented is congruent and complete regarding the neglect and exploitation.*
- Institute measures to include the pt in social or business activities. *This prevents neglect and exploitation.*
- Intervene when criminal damage to a person or property is involved, when there is the potential for serious injury or death, and when there is a likelihood of damage to public health and safety. *Such intervention preserves life and is caring, accountable, and lawful.*
- Provide the p/f/c with information regarding legal considerations and options. *Such knowledge allows them to obtain legal protection or prosecution or have information for future use.*

- Provide or arrange for legal assistance for the p/f/c. *This helps p/f/c to cope with the legal ramifications of neglect and exploitation.*
- Assist the pt to explore having neighbors call the police when they hear or see anything that may indicate neglect and exploitation are pending or are in progress. *This provides additional support for pt.*

✴ Spiritual

- Teach the p/f/c about the connection between neglect and exploitation and spiritual pain. *This validates pt's pain and distress and opens issues for discussion.*
- Ensure that the pt has access to a telephone, personal items, belongings, etc. *This increases pt's ability to take and maintain control over own life and aspects of care.*
- Institute measures to include the pt in spiritual or religious activities. *This enhances spiritual well-being and prevents neglect and exploitation.*

Nursing Goals

- To intervene appropriately when there is suspected neglect and exploitation
- To eliminate or reduce the factors for neglect and exploitation
- To promote the prevention of, recognition of, and intervention in situations of neglect and exploitation
- To accurately assess the potential for neglect and exploitation of the pt and others, institute measures to prevent it, and connect the parties with their families of origin
- To assist the p/f/c to identify choices and make future plans to develop alternative ways of dealing with unhealthy interaction patterns
- To teach about the connection between neglect and exploitation and spiritual pain

Patient Goals

- The pt will be or remain free from neglect and exploitation.
- The pt will consider the provider(s) as a valuable contact if or when problems involving neglect and exploitation occur.
- The pt will state that the precipitating factors for neglect and exploitation have been reduced or eliminated.
- The pt will state that he or she feels safe in own home.
- The pt will state that incidents of neglect and exploitation have not occurred or have stopped.
- The pt will understand the connection between neglect and exploitation and spiritual pain.

Patient and Family/Caregiver Outcomes

The patient will:

- Provide baseline information to the provider on admission or _____ (specify) regarding suspected or actual neglect and exploitation
- Identify passive and active neglect and exploitation from the pcg and f/c as demonstrated by _____ within _____ (weeks)
- Identify exploitation as demonstrated by _____ within _____ (weeks)

- State that incidents of neglect and exploitation have not occurred within _____ (weeks)
- Demonstrate decreased behavioral, emotional, cognitive, physical, social, and spiritual effects of neglect and exploitation by _____ within _____ (weeks)
- Express an understanding of the right to be free from any form of neglect or exploitation by _____ (date)
- Verbalize identification and acceptance of losses and changes associated with the neglectful and exploitative relationship(s) by _____ (date)
- Make future plans based on an awareness of relationship(s) characterized by neglect and exploitation as demonstrated by _____ by _____ (date)
- Make alternative plans for the future in the event that the caregiving situation changes by discharge
- Express an understanding of the right to remain free of and protected from all forms of neglect and exploitation within _____ weeks
- Have a written plan for preventing or managing neglect and exploitation by discharge
- Understand the relationship between neglect and exploitation and spirituality as demonstrated by _____ within _____ (specify)

The family/caregiver will:

- Contact and attend a respite service, support group, social service, or self-help group (specify) by _____ (date)
- Report an increased ability to cope with the responsibilities and activities involved in caring for the pt as demonstrated by _____ within _____ (specify)
- Identify the provider as a person to contact when problems arise by verbalizing _____ within _____ (specify)
- Understand the relationship between neglect and exploitation and spirituality as demonstrated by _____ within _____ (specify)
- Provide baseline information to the provider on admission or _____ (specify) regarding suspected or actual neglect and exploitation
- Consistently provide for the pt's emotional, cognitive, physical, social, and spiritual needs as demonstrated by _____ and _____ within _____ (weeks)

RESOURCES AND INFORMATION

1. Local, state, and federal health and human services, adult protective services, and police
2. American Medical Association Council on Scientific Affairs (1987). High risk profile for elder abuse and neglect. *Journal of the American Medical Association, 257,* 966–971.

REFERENCES

Fulmer, T. T., & Ashley, J. (1989). Clinical indicators of elder neglect. *Applied Nursing Research,* 2(4), 161–167

Noncompliance (See Apathy)

O

Obsessive-Compulsive Disorders

PROBLEM DESCRIPTION

Obsessive-compulsive disorder is described in the *DSM IV* (American Psychiatric Association, 1994) as a form of anxiety. It can occur at any age, but often begins in childhood, and is one of the more common anxiety disorders in older adults. Obsessive thoughts are persistent, repeated, intrusive, and unwanted thoughts that cause distressing emotions. Compulsive behaviors are ritualistic behaviors, usually repetitive in nature, and may be attempts to control or diminish obsessive thoughts. Rituals are the behaviors that a person engages in as a response to compulsions. An individual with OCD can often identify the obsessions and compulsions and knows they are irrational; the person feels ashamed of these actions and hides them from others. OCD can trap a person in a vicious cycle that is excessive but seems like the only way available to lessen discomfort. An individual often enters therapy only when the thoughts or behaviors inhibit the overall ability to function.

The OCDs can be associated with other diagnoses, such as depression, schizophrenia, dementia, or psychosis. Obsessions can exist without compulsions, but this is rare. Phobias are also related to obsessions. Phobias are persistent, irrational fears of an object, anxiety, or situation. Compulsions can range from mild (normal and healthy) to total incapacitation of the ability to function.

Obsessive Thoughts

Obsessive thoughts are designed to minimize anxiety and maintain interpersonal security. Obsessions do not satisfy the anxiety-producing situation, leading to guilt and feelings of self-punishment, which leads to dread and countermeasures to reduce the feelings. Obsessions are learned responses that are repeated to reduce anxiety, and they can lead to perfectionist tendencies in the self and others. Obsessions substitute for relationships and social interactions and can cause communication problems. Obsessions do not allow for differences of opinions because prejudices are firmly fixed and religious beliefs are often rigid. The obsessive individual may become depressed, hopeless, and disillusioned when high standards for self and other are not met.

Compulsive Behaviors

Compulsive behaviors can cause serious physical problems when the behaviors are exhausting or excessive. Transient relief for the anxiety-provoking situation is achieved with compulsive behaviors. Rituals and acts prevent, control, and undo the forbidden thoughts and impulses associated with the anxiety. Inhibiting or controlling behavior may result in terror. Compulsive behaviors are often a substitute for verbal expression of fears. The behavior is recognized as irrational but is difficult to stop. Compulsions are self-perpetuating due to their usefulness in reducing anxiety and so become learned behavior patterns. These patterns block learning of new adaptive behaviors. The person with compulsive behaviors has little option for change or growth. Security and relief from anxiety are the primary goals, which prevent risk taking or involvement in new experiences.

PROBLEM IDENTIFICATION

Characteristics and Observable Behaviors

- Ambivalence and indecision
- Anxiety
- Changes frightening
- Communication problems
- Compulsive, ritualistic behaviors such as repeated handwashing
- Controlling of others and self
- Denial
- Detail oriented
- Distress and despair
- Disturbances in normal function due to obsessive thoughts or compulsive behaviors
- Emotionally distant
- Excessive devotion to work and productivity
- Fearfulness
- Guilt feelings
- Hoarding behaviors
- Impaired judgment and insight
- Inability to tolerate deviations from the norms
- Irrational, bizarre thoughts of violence, contamination, or doubts
- Isolative
- Judgmental
- Limited ability to express emotions
- Low self-esteem
- Obsessive thoughts that may be destructive or delusional
- Obstinate or stubborn
- Overemphasis on cleanliness and neatness
- Perfectionistic
- Physical problems
- Slowness or difficulty completing activities of daily living
- Rationalization and symbolization
- Relationship problems
- Rigid and inflexible
- Ruminations
- Self-mutilation

Factors Related to the Problem

- Aggression toward others
- Alcohol ingestion
- Depression
- Financial, relationship, or employment problems
- Fire setting
- Gambling
- Lack of control over events
- Organic mental disorders
- Over- or undereating
- Phobias
- Rigidity
- Schizophrenia
- Self-destructive behaviors
- Stealing
- Substance abuse
- Inadequate support systems
- Unanticipated life or role changes
- Unmet needs

Assessment Tools and Instruments (see Appendix I)

Consider administering the:

1. Beck Depression Inventory
2. Brief Psychiatric Rating Scale
3. Brief Psychiatric Schizophrenia Rating Scale
4. Geriatric Depression Scale
5. Global Assessment of Functioning Scale
6. Mini-Mental State Examination
7. Obsessive-Compulsive Disorder Screening Checklist
8. Social Dysfunction Rating Scale
9. Spiritual Perspective Clinical Scale

PROBLEM LIST

- Activity Intolerance
- Body Image Disturbance
- Caregiver Role Strain
- Communication, Impaired Verbal
- Decisional Conflict
- Diversional Activity Deficit
- Fatigue
- Grieving, Dysfunctional
- Growth and Development, Altered
- Hopelessness

- Infection, Risk for
- Noncompliance
- Nutrition, Altered
- Parental Role Conflict
- Parenting, Altered
- Personal Identity Disturbance
- Post-Trauma Response
- Powerlessness
- Relocation Stress Syndrome
- Self-Care Deficit (specify)
- Self Mutilation
- Sensory/Perceptual Alterations (specify)
- Sexual Dysfunction
- Sexuality Patterns, Altered
- Skin Integrity, Impaired
- Sleep Pattern Disturbance
- Social Interaction, Impaired
- Social Isolation
- Spiritual Distress
- Therapeutic Regimen, Ineffective Management of
- Thought Processes, Altered

PROBLEM MANAGEMENT

Prevention, Maintenance, and Restorative Interventions

- Instruct the p/f/c that a contract will outline a plan to lessen the compulsive or ritualistic behavior.
- Provide low-stress, secure environment to prevent exacerbation of obsessions and associated compulsive behavior.

Medication Management

Clomipramine (Anafranil), fluoxetine (Prozac), and fluvoxamine (Luvox) are the medications of choice for treating OCDs. Psychosurgery is reserved for severely ill pt who are unresponsive to medications or behavior therapy.

NURSING MANAGEMENT

Nursing Interventions and Rationales

✫ Behavioral

- Avoid arguing or persuading about fears and anxieties. *This prevents the pt from holding onto obsessions even more tightly.*

- Give verbal support to the pt for attempts to lessen obsessive thinking and decrease frequency of compulsive behaviors. *Support reinforces appropriate behavior.*
- Assist the pt to say directly what is needed. *Such honesty eliminates nonessential details and clarifies communication.*
- Identify baseline frequency of obsessive thinking and compulsive behaviors and keep a record of time and frequency. *A baseline and a subsequent record measure progress.*

Emotional

- Observe the pt for increasing anxiety and when possible intervene before the compulsive behavior begins. *Observation and intervention prevent the need for compulsive behavior and increase awareness of the connection between anxious feelings and OCD.*
- Ask pt to describe feelings about own OCD and what pt thinks motivates these behaviors. *Empathy and supportive listening help to remove stigmatization and silence and move toward healing.*
- Assist the pt to use humor and laughter and to have fun. *This decreases the pt's serious, unemotional nature.*

Cognitive

- Use thought-stopping and thought-switching techniques. *These help the pt change to a positive way of thinking.*
- Explore differences between thoughts and actions. *This allows the pt to see that thinking and acting are not the same.*
- Be conscious of time and consistent when making visits. *Consistency sets limits on behavior and decreases OC behavior.*

Physical

- Observe pt for signs of infection or tissue breakdown if common compulsive behaviors of handwashing, showering, nail biting, or other excessive self-care tasks are present. *This maintains skin integrity.*
- Ask pt if obsessions or compulsions interfere with eating, sleeping, and other self-care. *Pt needs basic physical needs met.*
- Observe pt for compliance with medication regimen and avoidance of any side effects; inquire as to reasons if medication is not being taken. *This encourages compliance with medication regimen and monitors for adverse effects.*

Social

- Explore with the pt the prejudices and stereotypes that hinder self-growth. *Such exploration allows pt to be aware that stereotypes of mental illness do not reflect realilty.*
- Consider other ways of perceiving the environment and be more accepting of others. *This helps pt to establish relationships without imposing OC thought patterns or letting these behaviors interfere.*
- Discuss OCD facts with p/f/c, answer questions, and listen to their concerns. *P/f/c support can remove fears and help f/c provide more support and presence to pt.*

✴ Spiritual

- Assist the pt to question rigid beliefs and personal standards. *This helps the pt be open and accept other ways of believing and thinking without being threatened.*
- Encourage the pt to be curious about new information and knowledge. *Such encouragement motivates consideration of new experiences with less anxiety.*

Nursing Goals

- To decrease or eliminate obsessive thoughts
- To decrease or eliminate compulsive behaviors
- To facilitate therapy for OCDs

Patient Goals

- The pt will experience decreased obsessive thoughts.
- The pt will experience decreased compulsive behaviors.

Patient and Family/Caregiver Outcomes

The patient will:

- Demonstrate decreased anxiety, fears, guilt, rumination, or aggressive behaviors by _____ (date)
- Identify anxiety underlying compulsive behaviors as demonstrated by _____ within _____ (weeks)
- Describe and explore causes of obsessive thinking within _____ (weeks)
- Decrease or eliminate obsessive thinking as demonstrated by _____ within _____ (weeks)
- Become less controlling of self and others as demonstrated by _____ within _____ (weeks)
- Show more flexibility in thinking as demonstrated by _____ within _____ (weeks)

The family/caregiver will:

- Communicate feedback to the pt when they see obsessive-compulsive behaviors that are out of control and reinforce learned coping skills to help pt to decrease behaviors within _____ (weeks)

RESOURCES AND INFORMATION

1. Obsessive-Compulsive Information Center
   Dean Foundation for Health Research and Education
   2711 Allen Boulevard
   Middleton, WI 53562
   608-827-2390

2. Anxiety Disorders Association of America
    6000 Executive Boulevard
    Suite 513
    Rockville, MD 20852-3801
    301-231-9350
3. National Self-Help Clearinghouse
    25 West 43rd Street
    New York, NY 10036
    212-354-8525
4. National Mental Health Association
    1021 Prince Street
    Alexandria, VA 22314-2971
    703-684-7722
5. National Institute of Mental Health
    Information Resources and Inquiries Branch
    Room 7C-02
    5600 Fishers Lane
    Rockville, MD 20857
    301-443-4513
6. National Alliance for the Mentally Ill
    200 N. Glebe Road
    Suite 1015
    Arlington, VA 22203
    703-524-7600

REFERENCES

American Psychiatric Association. (1994). *Quick reference to the diagnostic criteria from DSM-IV*. Washington, DC: Author.

Overdose (See Adverse Medication Reactions, Substance Abuse Behaviors, and Suicidal and Homicidal Behaviors)

P

Pain

PROBLEM DESCRIPTION

Pain is medically defined in terms of actual or potential tissue damage, with associated psychological factors, or as a general medical condition with psychological factors. Pain, a discomfort or sensation that is uncomfortable, is dynamic and is also defined by the person experiencing pain (Meinhart & McCaffery, 1983). Ninety to 98% of the time, pain can be managed (Dossey, Keegan, Guzzetta, & Kolkmeier, 1995). Fear and anxiety related to physical pain can exacerbate physical pain, cause mental stress, and make pain management more difficult.

The experience of pain is highly individual and subjective. An individual's definition of the severity of pain is important. The pt's past experience with pain and psychological factors will influence the current pain and coping skills. Unacknowledged, unrecognized, and underrated pain diminishes the quality of life of the p/f/c.

Classification of Pain

- Acute pain: warns of injury; usually localized; is a sudden surprise; causes fear and anxiety; can be objectively noted (eg, by changes in heart rate, respiration, pupil dilation, blood pressure, nausea, and diaphoresis); can be intense and of short duration; pt usually complains of pain or discomfort and requests relief from pain.
- Chronic pain: may begin as acute, but does not lessen or resolve 1 to 6 months after healing is expected to occur; poorly localized; can be limited, intermittent, persistent, or intractable; usually little to no change in vital signs; contributes to and is highly correlated with depression; contributes to social isolation and changes in sleep pattern and appetite, muscle spasms, and changes in reflexes; fear of reinjury is present.

Severity of Pain
The following words represent the continuum of pain intensity: mild, discomforting, distressing, horrible, and excruciating.

Time Patterns of Pain
Pain can follow one of these three time patterns:

1. Continuous, steady, or constant
2. Rhythmic, periodic, or intermittent
3. Brief, momentary, or transient (Barker, 1994)

Table II-11
Types of Pain

	Source	Location
Somatic pain	Nociceptor stimulation	Skin and subcutaneous tissues; deep somatic tissues (ie, blood vessels, connective tissues, muscle)
Visceral pain	Stretching, inflammation, or ischemia	Organs
Referred pain	Accompanies visceral pain	Distal from the original source or cause
Afferentation pain	Injury	Peripheral or CNS

From Newman & Smith (1991)

Types of Pain

The recognized types of pain and their sources and locations are presented in Table II-11.

PROBLEM IDENTIFICATION

Characteristics and Observable Behaviors

The pt may exhibit pain either verbally or nonverbally. Nonverbal expression of pain are facial grimacing or crying; moaning, sighing, gasping, whimpering, and screaming; anorexia; fatigue; guarding movements; decreased social interaction; changes in sleep pattern; anxiety; changes in behavior (especially pacing and restlessness or withdrawal) and mood (especially irritability and hostility).

Words Commonly Used to Describe Pain

- aching
- annoying
- attack
- bearable
- beating
- boring
- burning
- cold
- cool
- cramping
- cruel
- crushing
- cutting
- deep
- dreadful
- drawing
- drilling
- dull
- exhausting
- fearful
- flashing
- freezing
- frightening
- gnawing
- gripping
- grueling
- heavy
- hot
- jumping
- intense
- itchy
- killing
- lancing
- nagging
- nauseating
- numb
- piercing
- pinching
- pounding

- pressing
- pricking
- pulling
- pulsing
- punishing
- radiating
- scalding
- sensations
- sharp
- shooting
- sickening

- smarting
- sore
- spasm
- splitting
- spreading
- stabbing
- squeezing
- stinging
- suffocating
- tearing
- tender

- terrifying
- throbbing
- tingly
- torturing
- tugging
- unbearable
- unrelenting
- vicious
- violent
- wrenching

Factors Related to the Problem

- Chemical agents
- Aging
- Attitude of pt and f/c
- Past experiences with pain
- Coping styles previously used
- Personality style
- Nationality and cultural influences
- Guilt
- Depression
- Anxiety and fear
- Somatoform disorders
- Psychosis
- Acute illnesses, infections, and contagious diseases (eg, herpes zoster and postherpetic neuralgia)
- Chronic illnesses (eg, diabetes, CAD, and depression)
- Degenerative conditions (eg, osteoarthritis and osteoporosis)
- Stress and recent loss or other precipitating event
- Vascular conditions (eg, peripheral vascular disease and dependent edema)
- Trauma and injuries
- Treatments and procedures
- Over- and underactivity
- Pregnancy
- Allergic responses
- Stress
- Constipation, intestinal spasms and disorders
- Secondary gain
- Hemiplegia and amputations
- Cancers
- Unknown causes (idiopathic pain)

Assessment Tools and Instruments (see Appendix I)

Consider administering the:

1. Beck Depression Inventory
2. Brief Psychiatric Rating Scale
3. Falls Risk Assessment
4. Geriatric Depression Scale
5. Mini-Mental State Examination
6. Suicide Risk Assessment Tool

Other Assessments

1. Ask the pt to use one word to describe the current pain and a word to describe the worst pain ever to gauge the pain being experienced (Jacox, 1977).
2. Use a Visual Analog Scale (VAS) in which the pt marks on a 100-mm line the status of current pain (no pain to worst possible pain) and current pain relief (0% pain relief to 100% pain relief). (Barker, 1994)
3. Administer the McGill Pain Questionnaire (Melzack, 1975).
4. Have pt use a pain drawing, with the figures commonly seen on the initial assessment form.

PROBLEM LIST

- Activity Intolerance
- Anxiety
- Breathing Pattern, Ineffective
- Caregiver Role Strain
- Communication, Impaired Verbal
- Constipation
- Diversional Activity Deficit
- Fatigue
- Fluid Volume Deficit
- Helplessness
- Hopelessness
- Infection, Risk for
- Mobility, Impaired
- Nutrition, Altered
- Pain (specify)
- Personal Identify Disturbance
- Powerlessness
- Role Performance, Altered
- Self Care Deficit (specify)
- Self Concept Disturbance
- Sensory/Perceptual Alterations (specify)
- Skin Integrity, Impaired
- Sleep Pattern Disturbance
- Social Isolation

- Spiritual Distress
- Thought Processes, Altered
- Violence, Risk for, Self-directed or Directed at Others

PROBLEM MANAGEMENT

Prevention, Maintenance, and Restorative Interventions

- Assess for depression because there is a high correlation between chronic pain and depression.
- Teach all those present in the home about pain phenomena and management.
- Instruct that depending on the disease state, pain and symptom management are particular to each pt's illness.
- Provide reassurance that nonmedical interventions (eg, breathing exercises, music, imagery, distraction, relaxation, yoga, Tai Chi, etc) and medications produce the best results.
- Administer, and teach the f/c to administer, medications for pain before pain increases, at regular intervals, to prevent pain from becoming intolerable.
- When possible, facilitate pt control and administration of pain medication.
- Assess the pt's pain: onset; nature; location, severity; intensity; duration; relief measures; quality; precipitating factors; aggravating factors; associated s/s; radiation, numbness, or paresthesia; response to pain control measures; and impact on daily life.
- Pay careful attention to the nonverbal expressions of pain because some pts, especially older ones, either do not feel pain fully or deny that they are experiencing pain.
- Consult with the p/f/c and providers to determine the pt's response to all interventions and pain management to determine if a regular pattern has developed.
- Evaluate pain medication on each home visit and remind the pt that the pain medication is in the pt's body and working (ie, teach about the half-life of medications).
- Monitor the pt for the potential side effects and adverse effects of pain medications and consider alternatives if side effects persist or adverse effects are manifest.
- Teach preventive approaches to pain.

Nonpharmacologic Interventions

Simple relaxation (eg, progressive muscle relaxation or music) and complex relaxation (eg, biofeedback and imagery) are effective in reducing mild to moderate pain and as adjuncts to pain medications for severe pain; pt and f/c education and instruction regarding pain management is effective in reducing pain (Agency for Health Care Policy and Research, 1992). Other nonpharmacologic approaches for pain control include (but are not limited to): cryotherapy, superficial heat, massage, therapeutic and healing trough, acupressure, TENS, cognitive-behavioral psychotherapy, distraction, and positive suggestion.

Medication Management

Various types of medications are used to control pain. Specific medications are used to control the pain associated with particular conditions, such as nitroglycerin for angina and indomethacin for gout, or H_2-receptor inhibitors for gastroesophageal reflux.

For the pt with a terminal condition and pain, the goal is to provide comfort—physical, emotional, psychological, and spiritual. Full and effective doses of pain control medications to achieve adequate pain control are necessary and just because a pt is sedated does not mean that pain is tolerable. "The increasing titration of medication to achieve symptom control, even at the expense of life, thus hastening death secondarily, is ethically justified" (American Nurses Association, 1992).

Drugs that potentiate the effects of narcotics, such as promethazine (Phenergan), are often used. Antidepressants, antihistamines, anxiolytics, neuroleptics, corticosteroids, anticonvulsants, and psychostimulants are used as adjuncts in pain management. Antidepressant medications decrease depression (often associated with chronic pain), enhance pain relief, promote sleep, reduce anxiety, and potentiate other medications used for analgesia. Monitor the pt's blood level of antidepressant medication used for pain control. (See Depression and Depressive Behaviors.)

Anticonvulsants are used to control the burning or tingling associated with nerve injury. Anticonvulsants can damage the liver and lower the number of white and red blood cells in the blood. Steroids help to relieve pain caused by brain and spinal cord tumors, bone pain, and the pain caused by inflammation. Steroids can cause gastric bleeding and irritation. They increase appetite and may cause fluid to accumulate in the body. Some pts who take steroids become confused.

Often combinations of nonnarcotic and narcotic medications are administered as alternatives to narcotic agents when nonnarcotic analgesics alone are not effective in alleviating pain. Pain that is not relieved by pain medication can be treated with radiation therapy, nerve blocks, neurosurgery, and surgery.

Nonnarcotic Pain Control Medications

The NSAIDs and aspirin decrease inflammation. NSAIDs, such as acetaminophen, ibuprofen, naproxen, and ketoprofen, effective for mild to moderate pain, may mask a fever. Some are available in oral suspension. Acetaminophen 1000 mg po given every 4 hours can cause liver toxicity, as can ingesting large amounts of alcohol with acetaminophen. Aspirin has anticoagulant properties and is to be avoided in pt's with a low platelet count, bleeding tendencies, and a history of gastric or duodenal ulcers. NSAIDs can interfere with blood clotting and cause gastric irritation, ulceration, stomach bleeding, renal problems, dizziness, anxiety, drowsiness, tinnitus, and confusion.

Narcotic Pain Medications

Narcotic pain medications stimulate opiate receptors and help to manage severe pain. The preferred route of administration is oral. However, long-acting transdermal patches are available. Other routes of administration include sublingual and buccal preparations; rectal and vaginal suppositories; subdermal, intramuscular, epidural, and intrathecal injections and infusions; continuous intravenous infusions; subcutaneous injections; catheters; implanted devices; and interpleural analgesia delivery systems. Codeine, hydrocodone, hydromorphone, levorphanol, meperidine, methadone, morphine, oxycodone, and oxymorphone are the common opioid agonists.

The common side effects and adverse effects of narcotic medications are allergy, nausea, vomiting, constipation, hypotension, dry mouth, grogginess, dizziness, itching, urinary retention, respiratory depression, increased intracranial pressure and CNS depression, physical tolerance, and dependence. Most pts with severe pain are not adequately treated for their pain due to lack of knowledge, underestimation of the needed amount of analgesic, overestimation of the duration of action, and fears of addiction (Wise & Rundell, 1994).

There is an enormous difference between psychological addiction and physical tolerance or dependence. Prescribers, providers, p/f/c, and the public often confuse *physical* tolerance and dependence with *psychological* addiction. It is extremely rare for a pt treated for pain to become psychologically addicted; the incidence is probably between 0.0003% and 0.1% in pts with no prior history of substance abuse or untreated psychiatric disorder (Angel, 1982; Jaffe & Martin, 1990).

Physical tolerance and dependence is easily managed and can develop in the first few weeks of opiate use, which means that the dosage requirements will increase (tolerance), and if the drug is discontinued suddenly, withdrawal symptoms will surface (dependence), which can be prevented if the dosage is tapered off gradually.

Psychological addiction is a behavioral disorder (see Substance Abuse Behaviors) characterized by compulsive use, overwhelming involvement with the drug, extreme efforts to secure a supply of it, and relapse after withdrawal.

NURSING MANAGEMENT

Nursing Interventions and Rationales

⭐ **Behavioral**

- Teach behavior modification techniques to the p/f/c. *These techniques alleviate or prevent pain experiences and reduce secondary gain.*
- Teach the p/f/c to allow the pt to take as much time as needed to complete activities and tasks and assist only when necessary. *A pt in pain will take longer to accomplish tasks.*
- Reinforce, and teach the f/c to reinforce, the pt's "well" behavior and not the "pain behavior" with praise and attention. *Such reinforcement prevents the pt from developing a pain syndrome.*
- Teach the pt to use distraction and other behavioral techniques. *This decreases the objective and subjective experience of chronic and acute pain.*
- Assist the p/f/c to develop an individualized pain control plan. *Planning helps p/f/c to anticipate pain control activities and evaluate pain control measures.*

♡ **Emotional**

- Assist the pt to express feelings associated with the experience of pain. *This assists the pt to tolerate the pain.*
- Listen to and allay the p/f/c's fears and concerns about addictions, tolerance, and side effects of medications for pain. *Such behavior enhances treatment and comfort.*

△ Cognitive

- Teach the p/f/c to record and graph progress regarding pain management. *Recording assists with coping.*
- Assist the pt to confront thoughts and fears regarding pain. *This helps the p/f/c to accurately appraise the situation.*
- Teach the p/f/c about the theories and dynamics of the experience of pain. *This information enhances treatment effectiveness.*
- Teach the p/f/c about the facts regarding physical tolerance and dependence versus psychological addiction. *This ensures that the pt will take the medication for pain on a regular basis at the prescribed dosage.*
- Refer to a pain specialist if the pt's pain experience becomes the focus of life or is unresponsive to management. *In this situation, specialized assistance is needed* (McCaffery & Beebe, 1989).
- Teach the pt to use imagery and other cognitive techniques. *This helps to decrease chronic and acute pain.*

⊔ Physical

- Assess the pt for skin breakdown, constipation, shortness of breath, nausea and vomiting, fatigue, vascular insufficiency, contractures, muscle spasms, mobility numbness, neuropathy, etc. *Assessment for these conditions reduces or prevents complications from pain.*
- Teach the pt to exercise, stretch, and perform other physical maneuvers and techniques. *Such activity increases comfort, decreases pain, and enhances physical conditioning.*
- Before and after the pt takes pain medication, instruct the pt to use techniques to relax. *Relaxation provides relief from pain.*
- Refer the pt for a PT, OT, social work, or other evaluation. *Such assessments may determine the pt's need for assistive devices, energy conservation, safe ambulation, lifestyle and home adaptation, exercise tolerance, prevention of the hazards of immobility, for structural support, and diversional activity guidance.*
- Refer the pt for acupressure, biofeedback, home TENS, etc to be used singly or in combination with pain medication. *These measures will improve the pain experience.*
- Instruct the p/f/c to ensure that the pt receives sufficient rest and sleep. *This helps pt to better tolerate the pain and conserve energy for activities and ambulation.*
- Provide and teach the f/c noninvasive techniques, such as hot or cold packs, bedtime backrubs, or massage. *These measures relieve pain and improve comfort.*
- Instruct the p/f/c to administer the pain medication regularly, rather than on a prn basis. *This prevents pain, decreases anxiety, and releases muscle tension.*

◯ Social

- Assess the effects of pain on the p/f/c. *The pain experience can affect role performance, social interaction, finances, daily life, ADLs, cognition, and the responses of others in the pt's life.*
- Discuss with the p/f/c the social problems of pain. *Such discussion diminishes the pt's feeling of stigma, powerlessness, and learned helplessness.*

- Encourage the pt to maintain social contact. *Contact with others counters the socially debilitating effects of pain.*
- Monitor the p/f/c for role changes and adjustment to role changes during the pt's pain experience. *This prevents or minimizes relationship problems.*
- Assess the most effective (in terms of cost, complexity, precautions, and convenience) method of pain control in the home setting. *Assessment avoids duplication of services and inappropriate referrals.*
- Teach the f/c to keep a daily diary of the pt's pain experiences. *A diary helps to identify factors or social stressors that may contribute to or alleviate the pt's pain level and may be useful in planning interventions* (Haley & Dolce, 1986).
- Assess and intervene, if indicated, regarding the pt's loneliness. *Loneliness will exacerbate the pt's pain level.*
- Refer for social services. *Financial factors and other social considerations may interfere with the pt's pain regimen.*

✦ Spiritual

- Explore the pt's beliefs about pain, suffering, and concerns about being a "good" pt. *This ensures effective planning and intervention.*
- Inform the pt that he or she is the expert regarding the pain being experienced. *The pt is credible, and pain is whatever the pt says it is whenever it is* (McCaffery and Beebe, 1989).
- Ask the pt to make decisions regarding pain management. *This enhances the pt's sense of control.*
- Obtain devices that allow the pt to safely self-administer pain medications. *This promotes self-confidence, control, and pain relief.*
- Encourage the pt to pray, read inspirational material, meditate, listen to music, etc. *These measures assist with the management and acceptance of pain and decrease boredom.*
- Explore with the pt the meaning of pain in life. *Discussion helps to find meaning and purpose in the pt's life.*

Nursing Goals

- To be accountable and responsible for effective pain management
- To promote optimal mobility
- To teach and assist the pt to use techniques to reduce pain
- To evaluate the pt for a decrease in pain
- To teach the p/f/c about the treatment for pain, the side effects of pain treatments, and preventive and safety measures to be taken

Patient Goals

- The pt will identify factors that trigger pain.
- The pt will not be preoccupied with pain.
- The pt will demonstrate a decrease or elimination of pain through the use of nonpharmaceutical methods of pain control.

- The pt will demonstrate a decrease or elimination of pain through the use of pharmaceutical methods of pain control.
- The pt will report a stabilization, decrease, or elimination of the use of pain medications.
- The pt will increase mobility and activities formerly limited by pain.
- The pt will relate that others in the home validate that the pain exists.
- The pt will experience control or relief from physical, psychological, emotional, and spiritual pain.

Patient and Family/Caregiver Outcomes

The patient will:

- Use distraction or _____ and _____ to decrease pain _____ (specify) a day, beginning _____ (specify)
- Demonstrate decreased _____ (specify) and other manifestations of the pain experience within _____ (specify)
- Plan and engage in one activity, when comfortable, _____ a day within _____ (weeks)
- State that pain has improved _____% and increase daily activities as evidenced by _____ within _____ (weeks)

The family/caregiver will:

- Believe and accept that the pt is in pain as demonstrated by _____ by _____ (date)
- Provide the pt with attention when the pt is not in pain _____ (specify) a day within _____ (weeks)
- Take measures to protect the safety of the pt as demonstrated by _____ within _____ (specify)

P

RESOURCES AND INFORMATION

1. American Pain Society
   Book: *Principles of Analgesic Use in the Treatment of Acute Pain and Chronic Cancer Pain* (1993)
   4700 W. Lake Avenue
   Glenview, IL 60025-1485
   847-375-4715
2. U.S. Department of Health and Human Services
   Agency for Health Care Policy and Research (AHCPR)
   2101 East Jefferson Street
   Suite 501
   Rockville, MD 20852
   To receive copies of the clinical guidelines:

Center for Research Dissemination and Liaison
AHCPR Publications Clearinghouse
PO Box 8547
Silver Spring, MD 20907
1-800-358-9295
301-495-3453
Fax: 301-594-2800
Clinical Practice Guidelines
   a. Acute Pain Management: Operative or Medical Procedures and Trauma Clinical Practice Guideline (AHCPR 92-0032)
   b. Management of Cancer Pain (AHCPR 94-0592)
   c. Management of Chronic Low Back Pain (AHCPR 1994)
   d. Pain Control After Surgery—A Patient's Guide (AHCPR 92-0021)
3. Oncology Nursing Society (ONS)
   501 Holiday Drive
   Pittsburgh, PA 15220
   412-921-7373
   ONS Position Paper on Cancer Pain Assessment and Management Monograph
4. Arthritis Foundation Information Line (literature and referrals to local chapters, exercise groups, and self-help groups)
   1330 W. Peachtree Street
   Atlanta, GA 30309
   1-800-283-7800
   404-872-7100
5. American Council for Headache Education (ACHE)
   875 Kings Highway
   Suite 200
   Woodbury, NJ 08096
   1-800-255-2243
   609-845-0322
6. American Chronic Pain Association (for information on coping skills, support groups, printed materials, videos, audiotapes, and chapters)
   PO Box 850
   Rocklin, CA 95677
   916-632-0922
7. National Chronic Pain Outreach Association (for information about any type of chronic pain and support groups)
   540-997-5004
8. National Cancer Institute (booklet: "Questions and Answers About Pain Control")
   1-800-ACS-2345
9. Pain Management in the Home (videotape)
   Judith A. Paice
   Lippincott
   PO Box 1600
   Hagerstown, MD 21741-9910
   1-800-777-2295
   Fax: 301-824-7390
   e-mail: lrorders@phl.lrpub.com

REFERENCES

Agency for Health Care Policy and Research. (1992). *Guideline report. Acute pain management: Operative or medical procedures and trauma* (AHCPR Publication No. 92-0001). Rockville, MD: Author.

American Nurses Association. (1992). *Position statement on promotion of comfort and relief of pain in dying patients*. Washington, DC: Author.

Angel, M. (1982). The quality of mercy. *New England Journal of Medicine, 306,* 98–99.

Barker, E. (1994). *Neuroscience nursing*. St. Louis: Mosby-Yearbook.

Dossey, B. M., Keegan, L., Guzzetta, C. E., & Kolkmeier, L. G. (1995). *Holistic nursing: A handbook for practice* (2nd ed.) Gaithersburg, MD: Aspen.

Haley, W. E. & Dolce, J. J. (1986). Assessment and management of chronic pain in the elderly. *Clinical Gerontologist, 5,* 435–455.

Jacox, A. (1977). *Pain: A sourcebook for nurses and other health professionals*. Boston: Little, Brown.

Jaffe, J. H. & Martin, W. R. (1990). Opioid analgesics and antagonists. In A. G. Gilman, T. W. Rall, A. S. Nies, et al. (Eds.), *The pharmacological basis of therapeutics* (8th ed.). New York: Pergamon.

McCaffery, M., & Beebe, A. (1989). *Pain: Clinical manual for nursing practice*. St. Louis: Mosby.

Meinhart, N., & McCaffery, M. (1983). *Pain: A nursing approach assessment and analysis*. East Norwalk, CT: Appleton-Century-Crofts.

Melzack, R. (1975). The McGill Pain Questionnaire: Major properties and scoring methods. *Pain, 1,* 277–299.

Newman, D. K., & Smith, D. A. J. (1991). *Geriatric care plans*. Springhouse, PA: Springhouse.

Wise, M. G. & Rundell, J. R. (1994). *Concise guide to consultation psychiatry* (2nd ed.) Washington, D.C.: American Psychiatric Press.

Panic

PROBLEM DESCRIPTION

Panic disorder is a diagnostic subtype of anxiety disorder. It is characterized by a spontaneous panic attack, usually lasting 5 to 30 minutes, with intense fear or discomfort that does not occur in association with a specific anxiety-provoking beginning and end, and is accompanied by distressing physical sensations. Panic is anxiety to the extreme and often occurs in pts with restricted movement or access to help. The sense of terror can be so severe that individuals can become disorganized, disoriented, and depersonalized. These fears can lead to extreme behaviors to avoid the panic situation. In most situations, panic attacks are experienced while engaging in routine activities. They can occur as frequently as several times a day or as rarely as once or twice a year. If experienced at night, the panic is referred to as night terrors. Being tired or under stress is more likely to cause panic attacks in a variety of apparently normal situations. Panic attacks are unpleasant, but not physically critical and can occur in up to 5% of the population, primarily affecting the CV and respiratory systems. Without any apparent reason, the person experiences a sudden sense of overwhelming apprehension, fear, terror, and doom. This starts an upward spiral and a vicious cycle of thoughts and physical symptoms. Individuals with panic disorder have been reported to have more suicidal ideation and suicide attempts (Busch, 1996).

The *DSM-IV* refined the disorders to include panic disorder with or without agoraphobia and agoraphobia without history of panic attack. Studies now validate the pharmacologic and behavioral interventions used in panic situations and their effectiveness (Stuart & Laraia, 1996).

The etiology of panic disorder is complex and controversial. Theories propose that relationships exist among the environment, heredity, psychology, and biology. It is thought that a severe environmental stressor might trigger a panic attack. Studies indicate that a high incidence of negative life events precedes the first panic attack. The psychological model considers that panic is a response to bodily sensations with an alarm reaction that has either been conditioned from prior experience or is the result of cognitive processing errors or an appraisal of loss of safety. The person becomes preoccupied with stopping these physiologic sensations (behavioral) or searching for their meaning (cognitive appraisal) (Stuart & Laraia, 1996). The neurobiologic theory proposes that panic attacks are biochemically provoked and have their origin in the CNS. Carbon dioxide, isoproterenol, and high doses of caffeine also can induce acute panic anxiety.

Panic symptoms are similar to many medical illnesses and must be differentiated before any therapeutic intervention is initiated. Pain complaints, chest pain, epigastric distress, and headaches were the presenting symptoms in 80% of primary care patients who met criteria for panic disorder (Katon, 1988). Panic disorder is differentiated from generalized anxiety disorder by the lack of focus on an object of concern. It is also differentiated from PTSD by the lack of a traumatic event. Panic attacks usually begin between late adolescence and mid-thirties. If untreated, persons with panic attacks risk increased chances for alcohol and substance abuse, strained relationships, and suicide.

PROBLEM IDENTIFICATION

Characteristics and Observable Behaviors

- Chest pain or discomfort
- Chills or hot flushes
- Dizzy or lightheaded
- Fear of dying
- Fear of losing control or going crazy
- Feeling of choking
- Feelings of unreality
- Feelings or being detached from body
- Nausea or abdominal distress
- Numbness
- Palpitations
- Shortness of breath or smothering
- Sweating
- Trembling or shaking

Factors Related to the Problem

- Alcohol abuse
- Alcohol withdrawal
- Substance abuse
- Caffeinism (consuming more than 250 mg/d)
- Hypoglycemia
- Hyperthyroidism
- Mitral valve prolapse
- Temporal lobe epilepsy
- Depression
- Suicide

Assessment Tools and Instruments (see Appendix I)

Consider administering the:

1. Suicide Risk Assessment Tool

For additional assessment consider administering:

1. Panic Attack Questionnaire, a 23-item clinician-rated inventory (Norton, Dorward, & Cox, 1986)
2. Panic Attack and Homework Diary, the pt's ongoing record of panic parameters and real-life exposure activities (Thyer, 1987)

PROBLEM LIST

- Breathing Pattern, Ineffective
- Coping, Ineffective Individual
- Diarrhea
- Fatigue
- Hopelessness
- Pain
- Powerlessness
- Sensory/Perceptual Alterations
- Sleep Pattern Disturbance
- Social Isolation
- Spiritual Distress
- Swallowing, Impaired
- Thought Processes, Altered
- Urinary Elimination, Altered
- Violence, Risk for, Self-Directed or Directed at Others

PROBLEM MANAGEMENT
Prevention, Maintenance, and Restorative Interventions

- Instruct p/f/c that panic attacks may aggravate existing physical conditions.
- Assess for panic disorder when physical symptoms are present and combined with fear of leaving home.
- Use measurement tools as baseline on initiation of treatment and throughout course of treatment to document effect and alter strategy when necessary.
- Encourage pts to share beliefs about illness, ask them to specify what they believe is wrong, what treatment is expected, and what they would like to gain from care.
- Assess pt's level of commitment and motivation or discover any intervening issues that might cause secondary gain, before beginning cognitive therapies.
- Teach p/f/c that the most effective cognitive behavioral techniques include exposure therapy, cognitive restructuring, breathing control, and relaxation.
- Teach p/f/c that exposure therapy is a systematic confrontation by the pt, in imagination or in reality, accompanied or alone, of the feared objects or events; it stops the expectation of panic, reduces the avoidance behavior, produces habituation or

extinction, and enhances development of self-efficacy or confidence (Craske, Street, & Barlow, 1989).

- Instruct the pt to keep a diary of activities to document progress.
- Teach the pt that interoceptive exposure (exposure to internal cues) are somatic sensations, are not harmful, and can be experienced without fear.
- Teach p/f/c that cognitive restructuring emphasizes the discrepancy between the pt's catastrophic predictions, the reality of events, experiences, and outcomes.
- Help the pt monitor thoughts, assess consistent erroneous predictions, place doubts on predictions, determine alternative explanations for symptoms, and desensitize worst fears.
- Instruct pt to keep 3 × 5-inch file cards with positive, reality-based statements on them that can be used at times when negative thoughts are overwhelming.
- Teach pt that cue cards are tangible tools to gain better control of panic.
- Teach the pt breathing control exercises to decrease the frequency of panic attacks and reset the pCO_2 levels back to normal.
- Teach the p/f/c that combining cognitive techniques and breathing control assists the pt to identify mental and physical sensations to gain control over condition.
- Teach diaphragmatic breathing to control hyperventilation.
- Teach pt to consciously control slow, deep, even, abdominal breaths, rather than shallow, rapid, thoracic breaths.
- Do not have the pt breath into a paper bag for hyperventilation because this will cause the pt to rebreathe the exhaled carbon dioxide and may make the panic attack worse (Stuart & Laraia, 1996).

Symptom Management, Categories, and Techniques

Table II-12 lists the psychotherapeutic strategies for panic.

Medication Management

The goal for treating panic attacks with medications is to block spontaneous and situational panic attacks. The medications best suited for this are tricyclic antidepressants, MAOIs, benzodiazepines, and SSRIs.

The tricyclic antidepressants might require 4 to 24 weeks to show significant effectiveness. Seventy to 90% of pts who comply with the medication regimen show moderate to marked improvements. Imipramine (Tofranil) is the tricyclic antidepressant of choice (Shader, 1994).

The MAOIs are also useful for treating panic disorders. Phenelzine (Nardil) is the drug of choice. The pt must be given special dietary instructions for MAOIs.

Benzodiazepines are effective in treatment of panic disorders and are used primarily for rapid action and intervention. The disadvantage of benzodiazepines is that they can cause physiologic dependence or seizures with abrupt discontinuation. Alprazolam (Xanax), clonazepam (Klonopin), and lorazepam (Ativan) are the usual drugs of choice for treatment.

The SSRIs are effective in the treatment of panic disorders, with fewer side effects than tricyclic antidepressants or MAOIs. Fluoxetine (Prozac) and sertraline (Zoloft) are a few of the SSRIs used to treat panic.

Table II-12
Psychotherapeutic Strategies for Panic

Presenting Problems	Treatment Strategies
Knowledge deficits	Patient education
	Reading materials
	Self-help support groups
Panic attacks	Breathing control
	Cognitive restructuring
	Interoceptive exposure
	Psychopharmacology
Agoraphobic avoidance	Exposure
	Cognitive restructuring
	Breathing control
	Relaxation training
Negative cognitions	Cognitive restructuring
Anticipatory anxiety	Relaxation training
	Cognitive restructuring
	Exposure techniques
Sensitivity to body sensations	Interoceptive exposure
	Cognitive restructuring
Numbness and tingling	Breathing control
Shortness of breath	Breathing control
Psychosocial problems	Psychotherapy
Marital discord	Marital therapy
Skills deficit	Skills training
Lack of treatment efficacy	Reevaluation of treatment plan
	Compliance counseling

From Stuart & Laraia (1996)

P

NURSING MANAGEMENT

Nursing Interventions and Rationales

☆ **Behavioral**

- Instruct the pt in cognitive behavioral strategies such as exposure therapy, cognitive restructuring, breathing control, and relaxation. *These measures diminish physiologic sensations, restructure cognitions, and change avoidance behaviors.*

♡ **Emotional**

- Assess and instruct the pt in ways to deal with feelings of low self-esteem, difficulty expressing anger, lack of assertiveness, or prolonged feelings of rejections and unhappiness. *This provides the pt with more adaptive coping mechanisms and decreases the tendency for relapse.*

△ Cognitive

- Instruct pt in keeping a daily diary of activities that cause panic situations; what precipitated the attack; how long the attack lasted; what methods were used to decrease the situation; and the feelings that were experienced during the time. *This assists the pt in documenting progress, increasing the level of involvement and commitment, and providing new ways to deal with situations.*
- Instruct the pt in use of cue cards. *These help pt to gain better control over the panic disorder.*

◻ Physical

- Instruct the pt in foods, medications, and caffeine products that will cause panic attacks. *This creates awareness of stimulants and that avoidance will decrease physical symptoms in panic attacks.*

◯ Social

- Assess the pt for stressful life events by exploring previous family experiences and coping mechanisms. *This assists p/f/c in learning source of panic disorder.*
- Instruct the pt that life stressors or chronic daily problems place them at increased risk for panic attack. *Such information decreases social and psychological distress and enhances self-esteem.*

✦ Spiritual

- Educate pt about panic disorders. *Information may help pt to feel empowered to deal with the panic.*
- Instruct the pt in medication and therapeutic interventions. *The pt is able to facilitate a holistic and comprehensive biopsychosocial-spiritual approach to treatment.*

Nursing Goals

- To assist the pt in learning cognitive behavioral strategies
- To collaborate with pt in assessing strengths and determine best therapeutic approach for treatment of panic

Patient Goals

- The pt will demonstrate a significant decrease in symptoms of panic.
- The pt will actively use cognitive behavioral measures to control panic situations.
- The pt will demonstrate marked reduction in avoidance behavior when confronted by feared or stressful situations.
- The pt will express hopeful and futuristic plans.

Patient and Family/Caregiver Outcomes

The patient will:

- Demonstrate a significant decrease in symptoms of anxiety related to panic as demonstrated by _____ within _____ (weeks)

- Actively use measures to control panic attacks as demonstrated by _____ within _____ (weeks)
- Demonstrate a marked reduction in avoidance behavior when confronted with panic situations within _____ (weeks)
- Verbalize understanding of medication, behavioral, and cognitive methods of treatment for panic disorders as demonstrated by _____ within _____ (weeks)
- Limit intake (specify how much) of caffeine, nicotine, or other CNS stimulants that exacerbate panic situations by _____ (date)
- Participate in program to desensitize panic and phobic responses as demonstrated by _____ within _____ (weeks)
- Demonstrate sense of control over behavior and management of own care by _____ (date)

The family/caregiver will:

- Recognize stages of panic and provide assistance in accordance with limitations as specified within _____ (weeks)

RESOURCES AND INFORMATION

1. National Institutes of Health (NIH)
   Office of Clinical Center Communications
   Building 10, Room 1C255
   Bethesda, MD 20892
   301-496-2563
2. Anxiety Disorders Association of America
   6000 Executive Boulevard
   Suite 513
   Rockville, MD 20852
   301-231-9350
   Fax: 301-231-7392
3. American Psychiatric Association
   Division of Public Affairs/Code P-H
   1400 K Street, NW
   Washington, DC 20005
   202-682-6220

P

REFERENCES

American Psychiatric Association. (1994). *Quick reference to the diagnostic criteria from DSM-IV.* Washington, DC: Author.

Busch, P. E. (1996). Panic disorder the overlooked problem. *Home Healthcare Nurse,* 14(2), 111–116.

Craske, M. G., Street, L., & Barlow, D.H. (1989). Instructions to focus upon or distract from internal cues during exposure treatment of agoraphobic avoidance. *Behavior Research and Therapy,* 27(6), 663–672.

Katon, W., Sheehan, T., & Uhde, T. (1988, March). Panic disorder: A treatable problem. *Patient Care, 30,* 149–154.

Norton, G. R., Dorward, J., & Cox, B. J. (1986). Factors associated with panic attacks in non-clinical subjects. *Behavior Therapy, 17,* 239–252.

Shader, R. I. (1994). *Manual of psychiatric therapeutics* (2nd ed.) Boston: Little, Brown and Co.

Stuart, G. W., & Laraia, M. T. (1996). Panic disorders with agoraphobia. In A. B.

McBride & J. K. Austin (Eds.), *Psychiatric-mental health nursing: Integrating the behavioral and biological sciences* (pp. 297-314). Philadelphia: Saunders.

Paranoia

PROBLEM DESCRIPTION

Paranoid behaviors can best be described on a continuum, from mild suspicion to paranoid personality disorder. Paranoid behaviors are characterized by a lack of trust, suspiciousness, grandiose or persecutory delusions, hallucinations, and hostility. Paranoid ideation or behaviors may be rooted in earlier experiences and are related to issues of trust, which are formed in the first 2 years of life. Paranoid traits emerge during adolescence or early adulthood and have a gradual onset.

Paranoid individuals believe that everything is linked to them. They interpret the actions of others as deliberately demeaning or threatening. Paranoid persons are usually sensitive to other people's motives and feelings but externalize their own emotions. They often reject or avoid responsibility and blame others. Their fault-finding behavior is a reflection of their own internal anxieties and self-dislike. They feel vulnerable, state they are being treated unfairly, and can be argumentative even if what they perceive is not true. If confronted, they can respond with anger and aggression and easily lose control.

To cope with these feelings, the paranoid person often uses defense mechanisms such as denial and projection. The ego needs to protect itself and uses these defenses to compensate with delusions to bolster self-esteem and decrease the feelings of powerlessness. The delusions may be grandiose, destructive, or conspiratorial and involve ideas of reference.

To be considered a paranoid personality disorder, individuals must exhibit at least four of the following:

- Suspicion that others are exploiting, harming, or deceiving them
- Preoccupation with doubts about loyalty or trust in significant others
- Reluctance to confide in others for fear that the information could be used against them
- Perception of hidden demeaning or threatening meanings from simple remarks made by others
- Holding grudges against others who they perceive might have previously insulted or injured them
- Perception of attacks on character or reputation with quick angry reactions
- Recurrent suspicions, without justifications, regarding fidelity of spouse or sexual partner

Paranoid disorders occur frequently in older individuals and may be chronic or transient. Earlier relationship problems, social isolation, and illness become more aggravated with age. When older paranoid persons live alone, they often include their neighbors and caregivers in their delusional system and can cause disruptions and problems with and for them. Deafness, stress, illness, medications, depression, and organic brain disorders also contribute to additional paranoid behaviors in adults and older adults.

PROBLEM IDENTIFICATION

Characteristics and Observable Behaviors

- Affect guarded or flat
- Alterations in perceptions
- Anger and hostility
- Anxiety
- Avoidance of others
- Belief in conspiracy
- Communication problems, misinterpretations
- Delusions, especially grandiose and persecutory
- Denial
- Disorganized, illogical thoughts
- Fears
- Feelings of persecution
- Feelings of powerlessness, inferiority
- Hypersensitive to criticism
- Ideas of delusions of reference or feelings of persecution
- Impaired judgment
- Impaired problem-solving
- Inability to perform ADLs
- Insecurities
- Isolative, withdrawn
- Lack of trust, mistrust
- Low self-esteem
- Nonreality-based thinking
- Projection of blame on others
- Rationalization
- Refusal or reluctance to take medications
- Sexual problems
- Superior attitude toward others
- Suspiciousness

Factors Related to the Problem

- Aggression
- Altered thought processes
- Anxiety
- Crisis, maturational and situational
- Delusions

- Dementia
- Depression
- Fear or loss of autonomy or self-control
- Hearing loss in the elderly
- Hostility, aggression or homicidal ideation
- Ineffective interpersonal relationships
- Manic behaviors
- Psychoactive substance disorder
- Schizophrenia
- Sensory deprivation or overload
- Suicidal ideation
- Thought disorders
- Vision problems

Assessment Tools and Instruments (see Appendix I)

Consider administering the:

1. Brief Psychiatric Rating Scale
2. Brief Psychiatric Schizophrenia Rating Scale
3. Global Assessment of Functioning Scale
4. Mini-Mental State Examination
5. Modified Overt Aggression Scale
6. Social Dysfunction Rating Scale
7. Spiritual Perspective Clinical Scale
8. Suicide Risk Assessment Tool

P PROBLEM LIST

- Activity Intolerance
- Caregiver Role Strain
- Fatigue
- Noncompliance
- Nutrition, Altered: Less than Body Requirements
- Parental Role Conflict
- Parenting, Altered
- Personal Identity Disturbance
- Post-Trauma Response
- Powerlessness
- Relocation Stress Syndrome
- Self-Care Deficit, ADLs
- Sensory/Perceptual Alterations
- Sexual Dysfunction
- Sexual Patterns, Altered
- Sleep Pattern Disturbance
- Social Interaction, Impaired

- Social Isolation
- Spiritual Distress
- Thought Processes, Altered
- Violence, Risk for, Self-Directed or Directed at Other(s)

PROBLEM MANAGEMENT

Prevention, Maintenance, and Restorative Interventions

(See Section 1 for common general interventions.)

- Do not argue with paranoid persons that their beliefs are not true; gently respond to the feelings instead.
- Do not placate paranoid persons because it only increases their anxiety and lack of trust.
- Do not agree with paranoid beliefs; this can add credibility to paranoid statements.
- Acknowledge beliefs but do not offer an opinion about them.
- Be cautious in use of touch and be aware of pt's personal boundaries and space and honor them.
- Ask for permission or clearly explain that you will be touching or performing a procedure, so pt is not caught unaware.
- All movement should be purposeful rather than rushed because haste triggers fear.
- Determine if there is a relationship between expression of suspiciousness and potential for aggression.
- Do not place pt in confrontational situation; pt may react aggressively.
- Once the dynamics of suspiciousness are understood, do not encourage repetitive talk but focus on underlying feelings or process.
- Make short, frequent contacts initially to establish trust and relationship.
- Interest, tolerance, and impartiality help establish an initial connection.
- Limit the number of providers and caregivers to establish consistency and decrease suspicious behaviors.
- Help pts to understand that they are overinterpreting experiences because they are feeling isolated.

Teach p/f/c that:

- Emotional tension (anxiety) may interfere with rational thinking and behavior
- Cognitive functioning is influenced by physiologic status, environmental status, and emotional status, and that it becomes distorted in persons who do not develop trust
- The cognitive process of perception is influenced by the individual's current needs, interests, and fund of knowledge, which can result in vigilance and suspiciousness
- A disruption in the quality and quantity of incoming stimuli can affect an individual's thought process and result in suspiciousness
- Lack of security and trust may contribute to the development of suspiciousness and paranoia

- Failure of parent–child bonding may result in mistrust about relationships
- Persons feeling threatened in interpersonal situations are unable to feel secure and satisfied until the fear is reduced
- Suspicious and paranoid behaviors result from an inability to check the validity of observations, to look at the situation from another viewpoint, or question conclusions

Medication Management

Pimozide (Orap), an antipsychotic, is an effective medication in treatment of paranoid disorders in conjunction with psychotherapy. It may be used alone or in combination with an antidepressant. Other antipsychotics have not been as consistently effective, as shown by individual case studies (Shader, 1994). When paranoia is a part of a mood disorder, lithium or carbamazepine (Tegretol) may be useful. Pimozide shows less incidence of tardive dyskinesia than other antipsychotics, except for clozapine (Clozaril) (Yudofsky, Hales, & Ferguson, 1991).

Medications That Can Cause Paranoia

- Albuterol (Proventil, Ventolin)
- Amphetamines
- Atropine
- Baclofen
- Bromocriptine
- Cimetidine
- Clonazepam
- Cocaine
- Corticosteroids
- Digitalis
- Disulfiram
- Ephedrine
- Indomethacin
- Levodopa
- Methylphenidate
- Propranolol
- Pseudoephedrine

P

NURSING MANAGEMENT

Nursing Interventions and Rationales

✰ Behavioral

- Instruct pt on acceptable and unacceptable behaviors and their consequences. *Instruction provides clear communication and decreases anxiety.*
- Assess pt for harmful behaviors to self or others and develop steps to maintain control. *This exerts self-control over situation.*
- Teach coping skills that help pt maintain individuality to provide new skills. *This reduces anxiety and increases self-esteem and fosters trust.*
- Instruct f/c to approach the pt in nonthreatening way, be consistent in interactions, use a calm and steady voice, and not surprise the pt. *These steps decrease situations the pt may interpret as threatening.*
- Instruct f/c to recognize paranoid behaviors that may escalate due to overstimulation and to decrease stimuli in the environment before pt escalates and loses control. *These measures help f/c to assist the pt in controlling paranoid behaviors.*

♡ Emotional

- Establish a working and therapeutic relationship. *This creates trust to accomplish goals.*
- Understand that self-disclosure is uncomfortable and self-awareness is difficult for the pt with paranoia. *Such awareness prevents pressuring or pushing pt and losing trust.*
- Assist pt to gain experience in sharing feelings. *Sharing promotes an alternative way to validate thoughts and feelings and receive feedback.*
- Give positive feedback when pt demonstrates trust of another. *This reinforces trust of others.*

△ Cognitive

- Assist the pt in developing communication skills. *These skills enable pt to validate reality with others.*
- Help pt to clarify thoughts. *This avoids misinterpretation.*
- Teach pt to become consciously aware of feelings of suspiciousness. *Such awareness helps pt to make an effort to check feelings out objectively or to act appropriately despite the fear.*
- Teach pt steps in formation of trusting relationship. *This allows pt to build and recognize such relationships.*
- Teach pt to recognize consequences of paranoid behavior on life and how it affects ADLs. *This motivates pt to reduce paranoid behavior.*

⊐ Physical

- Provide medications in well marked containers and assist the pt to be involved in medication setup. *This decreases suspiciousness or paranoia about medications and their safety.*
- Assist p/f/c to understand effect of caffeine on paranoid behaviors. *This decreases anxiety and paranoid feelings from overstimulation.*
- Assist p/f/c in obtaining better eyeglasses, hearing aids, or lighting. *These help to decrease misinterpretation.*

◯ Social

- Encourage involvement in activities the pt is able to tolerate and participate in. *Activity increases interactions and promotes trust.*
- Give feedback on behaviors that are insulting, threatening, or rejecting. *Feedback helps pt recognize behavior and its impact on others.*

✴ Spiritual

- Assist the pt to recognize worth and relatedness to others. *This enables pt to value self and promote a positive self-concept.*

Nursing Goals

- To decrease paranoid behaviors and suspicions
- To promote expression of feelings and behaviors
- To promote social interaction and improved interpersonal relationships

Patient Goals

- The pt will make appropriate appraisals of situations and people.
- The pt will identify situations in which distrust occurs.
- The pt will demonstrate increased levels of trust.
- The pt will learn ways of socially validating perception.

Patient and Family/Caregiver Outcomes

The patient will:

- Demonstrate decreased paranoid behaviors (specify) _____ by _____ (date)
- Demonstrate reality-based thinking as evidenced by _____ within _____ (weeks)
- Demonstrate decreased suspicious behaviors as evidenced by _____ within _____ (weeks)
- Identify and list trusting characteristics in self and others within _____ (weeks)
- Verbalize practical options for changing life situations and becoming more trusting as demonstrated by _____ within _____ (weeks)

The family/caregiver will:

- Verbalize understanding of pt's personal boundaries (specify) _____ within _____ (weeks)
- Verbalize understanding of personal behaviors (specify) that could potentiate aggressive acts by pt within _____ (weeks)

RESOURCES AND INFORMATION

1. National Alliance for the Mentally Ill (NAMI)
    2101 Wilson Boulevard
    Suite 302
    Arlington, VA 22201
    703-524-7600
    Fax: 703-524-9094
2. National Mental Health Association (NMHA)
    1021 Prince Street
    Alexandria, VA 22314-2971
    703-684-7722
    1-800-969-NMHA
    Fax: 703-684-5968

REFERENCES

Shader, R. I. (1994). *Manual of psychiatric therapeutics* (2nd ed.). Boston: Little, Brown.

Yudofsky, S. C., Hales, R. E., & Ferguson, T. (1991). *What you need to know about psychiatric drugs*. New York: Ballantine.

Perceptual Problems

PROBLEM DESCRIPTION

Perception is the individual experience of sensing, interpreting, and comprehending the environment. Perception is derived from the five senses: vision, hearing, taste, touch, and smell. When inner reality is congruent with external reality, the person is grounded in reality or reality oriented. When internal and external reality are incongruous, the individual has a distorted sense or perception of reality. The distortion is limited to the individual and can affect all aspects of thinking and behavior, as in hallucinations and delusions.

Perceptual development begins at birth and the relationship with parents. Infants who develop a broad and positive array of interpersonal experiences with parents, including visual and language stimuli, are better equipped to develop their own skills and self-understandings as they grow. The relationships with parents, significant others, and life experiences continue to be incorporated and developed as individuals mature. Absence of perceptual acuity can lead to problems at any stage of development; for example, a child who needs glasses may not do well in school, or a retiree who is losing hearing may develop paranoid and panic behaviors.

Perceptual dimensions continue to develop over time and increase in complexity. Individuals who develop healthy perceptual abilities are able to view situations in broad terms, using sensory and cognitive skills. They are able to maintain a congruency between internal and external reality. Illness, physical problems, psychological issues, spiritual suffering, aging, and drugs can affect perceptual abilities and cause significant distortions. In determining whether a person's perception is normal, certain behaviors show a person is experiencing a distorted reality. The behaviors related to perceptual problems include hallucinations, illusions, sensory integration problems, poor visceral pain recognition, problems with stereogenesis (recognition of objects by touch), problems with graphesthesia (recognition of letters "drawn" on the skin), and misidentification of faces (including self).

Perceptual Distortions

Hallucinations

Hallucinations are false sensory perceptions that do not exist in external reality. The types of hallucinations include:

- Visual—seeing objects that are nonexistent. Visual hallucinations are rare in people with schizophrenia.

- Tactile—feeling objects or sensations that are nonexistent. This is common in cognitive or other toxic-induced psychosis.
- Auditory—hearing voices, bells, or other sounds that are nonexistent. Auditory hallucinations signify that there is no physical or toxic cause to the dysfunction; they are most commonly found in schizophrenia.
- Olfactory—smelling putrid, foul, and rancid odors that are repulsive. Olfactory hallucinations are typically associated with stroke, tumor, seizures, and dementias.
- Gustatory—tasting putrid, foul, and rancid tastes that are repulsive.

Illusions
Illusions are distortions or misinterpretations of actual stimulus. The pt distorts an image into another meaning.

Depersonalization
Depersonalization is a loss of sense of control over self and a feeling of detachment from the surroundings.

Derealization
Derealization is a sense of unreality, a distortion or a loss of reality about the environment.

PROBLEM IDENTIFICATION

Characteristics and Observable Behaviors

- Aggressive behaviors
- Agitation
- Apathy and altered posture
- Bizarre behavior
- Decreased problem-solving ability
- Depersonalization
- Derealization
- Difficulty with communication
- Disorganized, illogical thinking
- Disorientation
- Fatigue
- Feelings of anxiety, fear, or agitation

- Hallucinations
- Illusions
- Impaired ability to conceptualize
- Isolative
- Loss of ego boundaries
- Low self-esteem
- Misperceptions, false perceptions
- Poor interpersonal relationships
- Poor personal hygiene
- Regressive behavior
- Restlessness

Factors Related to the Problem

- AIDS
- Auditory nerve damage
- Blindness
- Brain tumor
- Cerebral vascular accident
- Confusional states
- Decreased sensory stimulation

- Delirium
- Delusions
- Dementia
- Developmental delays
- Encephalopathy
- Hallucinogen-induced disorders
- Head injury

- Impaired cognition
- Intoxication
- Mood disorders
- Multiple sclerosis
- Neurobiochemical changes in the brain
- Organic brain syndrome
- Paranoia
- Parkinson's disease
- Personality disorders

- Physical illness
- Post-traumatic stress disorder
- Psychosis
- Schizophrenia
- Stress
- Substance abuse
- Temporal lobe epilepsy
- Transient ischemic attacks
- Withdrawal

Assessment Tools and Instruments (see Appendix I)
Consider administering the:

1. Brief Psychiatric Rating Scale
2. Brief Psychiatric Schizophrenia Scale
3. Clinical Inventory Withdrawal Assessment
4. Global Assessment of Functioning Scale
5. Mini-Mental State Examination
6. Modified Overt Aggression Scale
7. Social Dysfunction Rating Scale
8. Suicide Risk Assessment Tool

PROBLEM LIST

- Body Image Disturbance
- Caregiver Role Strain
- Communication, Impaired Verbal
- Fatigue
- Growth and Development, Altered
- Noncompliance
- Pain
- Parental Role Conflict
- Post-Trauma Response
- Relocation Stress Syndrome
- Sensory/Perceptual Alterations
- Sexual Dysfunction
- Sleep Patterns, Altered
- Social Interaction, Impaired
- Social Isolation
- Spiritual Distress
- Thought Processes, Altered
- Violence, Risk for, Directed at Self or Others

PROBLEM MANAGEMENT

Prevention, Maintenance, and Restorative Interventions

- Assess pt's description of type, frequency, and intensity of hallucinations or illusions.
- Assess need for adaptive devices (glasses, hearing aids), or appropriate use.
- Assess whether medical evaluation of pt might be needed to determine extent or nature of perceptual disturbance.
- Observe pt for orientation to reality, level of anxiety, and sleep patterns.
- Do not attempt to reason with pt or challenge hallucinations because attempts to reason with pt increase anxiety and exacerbate hallucinations.
- Remember that delirious pts have limited ability to accurately interpret and respond to environmental, physical, or emotional stimuli because of biochemical changes in the brain.
- Repeat explanations and orientation to the setting to provide calm reassurances.

Medication Management

Medications for perceptual disturbances are necessary if the behavioral symptoms are out of control. Careful observation of s/s will determine the types of medications used. Medications used might include antianxiety drugs, neuroleptics, or antidepressants.

NURSING MANAGEMENT

Nursing Interventions and Rationales

☆ Behavioral

- Encourage the pt to identify and initiate anxiety-reducing measures. *This gives the pt a sense of control.*
- Use directive statements when speaking to the pt; have the pt pay attention to what is being said and not listen to voices. *This helps the pt focus on external and not internal stimuli.*
- Schedule regular times for physical activity that require concentration and exertion. *Activity distracts the pt from internal stimuli.*
- When the pt is out of control, approach in a calm, confident manner. *Calmness helps de-escalate.*
- Assist and encourage the pt to use adaptive devices. *This increases appropriate sensory stimulation.*
- Assist the pt to maintain reality orientation by calling by name, providing clock and calendar, using large signs and visual cues, using pictures of family and past, and providing access to television, newspapers, or radio. *These measures provide additional stimuli and orient pt to reality.*

- Instruct the pt to turn off the television or decrease other stimulating situations. *This controls and limits sensory overload.*
- Instruct the pt that establishing regular sleep patterns and receiving sufficient rest will improve tolerance to stimuli. *Sufficient rest helps the pt deal with perceptual distortions.*

Emotional

- Encourage the pt to express feelings related to experiencing hallucination. *Such expression promotes understanding of the experience and emotions to decrease anxiety.*

Cognitive

- Explain that hallucinations result from organic causes and can be effectively treated. *This reduces stress and anxiety.*
- Assist the pt to identify situations that evoke hallucinatory experiences. *This increases self-awareness and builds coping skills to avoid hallucinations.*
- Teach the pt ways to intervene during hallucinations, such as telling the voices they are not real and to go away. *Such interventions maintain a sense of control and reduce frequency and duration of hallucinations.*
- Instruct the pt to check with others about reality of perception. *This improves orientation to reality.*

Physical

- Arrange the pt's environment to provide familiar surroundings. *Familiarity decreases sensory deprivation, ensures safety, and promotes a sense of identity.*

Social

- Encourage social systems to maintain consistent contact with pt. *Social contact improves orientation to reality.*

Spiritual

- Teach the pt that perceptual processes and self-concept can be changed through healthy interpersonal relationships and exploration of the misperception. *This establishes control over situation.*

Nursing Goals

- To orient the pt to reality
- To assist the pt to recognize cause of perceptual or sensory disturbance
- To promote appropriate medical interventions in response to physical causes of perceptual disturbance

Patient Goals

- The pt will demonstrate improved orientation to reality.
- The pt will describe perceptual disturbance reactions and feelings related to them.
- The pt will identify situations that increase perceptual distortions.
- The pt will demonstrate improved social skills.
- The pt will demonstrate ability to avoid sensory overload situations.

Patient and Family/Caregiver Outcomes

(See Section 1 for common outcomes)
The patient will:

- Remain oriented to surroundings as demonstrated by _____ within _____ (weeks)
- Demonstrate awareness that hallucinations are caused by internal stimuli within _____ (weeks)
- Describe and practice methods of reality testing at onset of hallucination as demonstrated by _____ within _____ (weeks)
- Use adaptive devices, such as glasses or hearing aids (specify) by _____ (date)
- Reestablish usual sleep cycle by _____ (date)
- State measures to reduce sensory overload as demonstrated by _____ within _____ (weeks)

The family/caregiver will:

- Orient pt to reality during times of perceptual disturbances as demonstrated by _____ within _____ (weeks)
- Express understanding of measures to reduce sensory overload (specify) _____ by _____ (date)

RESOURCES AND INFORMATION

1. National Alliance for the Mentally Ill (NAMI)
   2101 Wilson Boulevard
   Suite 302
   Arlington, VA 22201
   703-524-7600
2. National Mental Health Association
   1021 Prince Street
   Alexandria, VA 22314-2971
   1-800-969-NMHA
3. National Institute of Mental Health (NIMH)
   Information Resources and Inquiries Branch Office of Scientific Information,
   5600 Fishers Lane
   Room 7C02
   Rockville, MD 20857
   301-443-4513

Personality Disorder Problems

PROBLEM DESCRIPTION

Personality disorders are so designated to note maladaptive personality characteristics and defense mechanisms (American Psychiatric Association [APA], 1994). A personality disorder is defined as an enduring pattern of inner experience and behavior that deviates markedly from the expectations of the individual's culture. This pattern is manifested in two or more of the following areas:

1. Cognition (ways of perceiving and interpreting self)
2. Affectivity (emotional response)
3. Interpersonal functioning
4. Impulse control

It is an inflexible enduring pattern across a broad range of personal and social situations. The enduring pattern leads to clinically significant distress or impairment in important areas of functioning. The pattern is stable and of long duration; the onset is traced back to adolescence and early adulthood. A personality disorder is not a manifestation of another mental disorder or directly related to substance use or a general medical condition (APA, 1994).

Clusters of the Personality Disorders

Personality disorders are grouped in clusters, with each cluster having distinctive patterns and profiles (APA, 1994).

Cluster A

The common trait in cluster A is that these disorders often appear odd or eccentric and begin in early adulthood.

*   Paranoid personality disorder: pervasive distrust and suspiciousness of others
*   Schizoid personality disorder: pervasive pattern of detachment from social relationships and restricted range of expressions of emotions in interpersonal settings
*   Schizotypal personality disorder: pervasive pattern of social and interpersonal deficits marked by acute discomfort with and reduced capacity for close relationships

Cluster B

The common trait among these personality disorders is that they typically exhibit dramatic, emotional, or erratic behaviors, and they begin in early adulthood.

*   Antisocial personality disorder: pervasive pattern of disregard for and violation of the rights of others occurring since the age of 15 years. An antisocial personality disorder does not exhibit any sense of guilt or remorse and is often manipulative.
*   Borderline personality disorder: pervasive pattern of unstable interpersonal relationships, difficulty defining self and determining self-image, labile affects, and

marked impulsivity. Those with a borderline personality disorder often engage in manipulation or "splitting," which means that they tend to view people as all good or all bad, and become angry when others fail to be perfect.

- Histrionic personality disorder: pervasive pattern of excessive emotionality and attention-seeking behaviors. Persons with a histrionic personality disorder tend to feel uncomfortable or unappreciated when they are not the center of attention.
- Narcissistic personality disorder: pervasive pattern of grandiosity, need for admiration, and lack of empathy toward others.

Cluster C

These disorders typically display anxious or fearful behaviors.

- Avoidant personality disorder: pervasive pattern of social inhibitions, feelings of inadequacy, and hypersensitivity to negative evaluation from others
- Dependent personality disorder: pervasive and excessive need to be taken care of that leads to submissive, clinging behavior, and fears of separation
- Obsessive-compulsive personality disorder: pervasive pattern of preoccupation with orderliness, perfectionism, and mental and interpersonal control, at the expense of flexibility, openness, and efficiency

Personality disorders affect 5% to 10% of the adult general population; most individuals are not aware of their disorder and seek no treatment. Antisocial personality disorder affects approximately 3% of American men and 1% of American women. Borderline personality disorders are more pervasive in women than in men (Carson, 1996). People with personality disorders have a tendency to sustain chronic impairment in social and occupational functioning, have an increased incidence of substance use, and are frequently involved in legal complications. Pts with a personality disorder are among the most difficult of all groups to treat and they challenge even the most seasoned therapist. It is imperative that providers working with pts with a personality disorder receive close clinical supervision, to avoid the manipulative, splitting, demeaning, and demoralizing reactions that treating them can engender.

In treating pts with personality behavior disorders it is often helpful to understand where the behavior pattern originated. Scientists and researchers have debated the cause and have determined at least three sources of personality disorders.

1. Developmental: Described by Margaret Mahler (1971, 1972), the object relations theory suggests that during the rapprochement subphase of the separation–individuation phase of development that the "mother" is either too emotionally distant from the child or excessively clinging to a child who needs to explore the environment. This traditionally happens between 16 and 25 months of age. The child who works through the conflicts of going away from the "mother" but knows that the "mother" will still be there for emotional support is able to deal with love and trusting parents and has realistic relationships with others (Mahler, 1971, 1972).
2. Biologic: Correlations have been noted between genetics and family traits schizotypal personality disorder.
3. Neurotransmitters: Studies show that there is a link with 5-hydroxyindoleacetic acid, a major metabolite of serotonin, and aggressive and suicidal behaviors (Brown et al., 1982; Brown & Linnoila, 1990).

Personality disorders are evidenced by the pt demonstrating maladaptive coping mechanisms. Behaviors that demonstrate this concept include manipulation, passive-aggressive behaviors, dependency or inadequacy, antisocial behaviors, borderline personality behaviors, histrionic behaviors, delusional disorder behaviors, and schizoid or schizotypal personality behaviors.

PROBLEM IDENTIFICATION

Characteristics and Observable Behaviors

- Alcohol or drug use
- Alternate clinging and avoidance behavior in relationships
- Anger or hostility
- Anxiety
- Apathy and forgetfulness
- Attention-seeking behaviors
- Calculating, demanding, manipulative, and intimidating behaviors
- Conflict with authority and difficulty following rules and obeying laws
- Dependency on others and feelings of victimization
- Dishonesty, lying, and withholding of information
- Dissatisfaction with life
- Doubt of role performance
- Exaggeration of emotions
- Feelings of boredom, emptiness, inadequacy, and worthlessness
- Impulsive behaviors and physically self-damaging acts, including suicidal threats or gestures
- Inability or refusal to express emotions directly and superficial relationships with others
- Inability to delay gratification
- Inability to tolerate stress or deal with conflict
- Inadequate skills for daily living to meet changes and crises
- Inconsistent behaviors and mood swings
- Poor interpersonal relationships
- Intolerance of being alone
- Lack of consideration for others
- Perceived lack of control
- Lack of feelings of guilt or remorse
- Lack of insight and poor judgment
- Low frustration tolerance
- Low self-esteem
- Noncompliant
- Pessimistic
- Poor impulse control
- Seductive behavior or sexual acting out
- Socially unacceptable behaviors
- Somatic complaints
- Splitting

P

Factors Related to the Problem

- Denial of problems of feelings
- Dependency
- Depression
- Failure to accept or handle responsibility
- Helplessness
- History of abuse
- History of frequent hospitalizations or therapy
- Ineffective interpersonal relationships
- Intellectualization or rationalization of problems
- Lack of insight
- Low self-esteem
- Manipulative behaviors
- Resistance to therapy
- Self-mutilating and self-destructive behaviors
- Sense of entitlement
- Substance abuse
- Suicidal threats or gestures

Assessment Tools and Instruments (see Appendix I)

Consider administering the:

1. Brief Psychiatric Rating Scale
2. Brief Psychiatric Schizophrenic Rating Scale
3. Global Assessment of Functioning Scale
4. Mini-Mental State Examination
5. Modified Overt Aggression Scale
6. Obsessive-Compulsive Disorder Screening Checklist
7. Social Dysfunction Rating Scale
8. Suicide Risk Assessment Tool

PROBLEM LIST

- Activity Intolerance
- Body Image Disturbance
- Caregiver Role Strain
- Communication, Impaired Verbal
- Fatigue
- Growth and Development, Altered
- Hopelessness
- Noncompliance
- Parental Role Conflict
- Post-Trauma Response
- Self Mutilation, Risk for
- Sensory/Perceptual Alterations

- Sexual Dysfunction
- Sexuality Patterns, Altered
- Sleep Pattern Disturbance
- Social Interaction, Impaired
- Social Isolation
- Spiritual Distress
- Thought Process, Altered
- Violence, Risk for, Self-Directed or Directed at Others

PROBLEM MANAGEMENT
Prevention, Maintenance, and Restorative Interventions

- Teach the p/f/c that anxiety results from the fear that the inhibited anger will be discovered.
- Teach the p/f/c that limit setting is important because passive-aggressive behaviors are active and reactive and are reinforced, both positively and negatively.
- Teach the p/f/c that the family or cultural milieu may encourage the indirect expression of negative feelings or acting-out behaviors.
- Teach the p/f/c that the person who behaves passively or aggressively sees the self as a victim and uses this to control others.
- Instruct the f/c that the pt uses manipulation as a controlling behavior to gain power over others and to protect self from a sense of failure or frustration.
- Instruct the f/c that when the pt uses manipulative behaviors the f/c will often feel angry, rejected, and punished, which in turn causes the pt to increase anxiety and continue using manipulation.
- Teach the p/f/c that power struggles result when the unconscious needs of both the manipulator and the person being manipulated are in conflict.
- Teach the f/c that inconsistent parental love may have caused the pt as a child confusion and insecurity, so that now the pt may use manipulative behavior to obtain love and resolve confusion.
- Teach the p/f/c that lack of self-respect, self-esteem, and a strong need to manipulate leaves the pt with little capacity to care about others.
- Instruct the f/c that manipulation prevents the pt from valuing the self and achieving a sense of self-worth.
- Be aware that the pt who uses manipulative behavior has little motivation to change unless pt needs to get out of a crisis or situation.
- As a provider, remember that it is not necessary or even desirable for the pt to like you personally.
- Be aware that the pt with a borderline personality disorder is frequently demanding, pessimistic, contrary, and self-destructive.
- Know that in interpersonal relationships a pt who has a borderline personality disorder will alternate between periods of clinging dependency and hostile rejection.

P

- Teach the p/f/c that relationships may be intense and that the pt with a borderline personality disorder may go to extremes to avoid feeling lonely, bored, or abandoned.
- Know that the pt with a borderline personality disorder may have an identity disturbance involving sexual orientation, value or belief system, and future goals.
- Know that the pt with a borderline personality disorder may be extremely labile, going from highs to lows, seeking attention, reacting emotionally, threatening aggressive or self-destructive behaviors, acting impulsively, and that short-term, brief, crisis- oriented therapy is often the choice for treatment.
- Teach the p/f/c that histrionic behavior is often used when an audience is present during an unpleasant situation.
- Know that histrionic behavior is often exhibited in sexual or seductive dress, advances, or improper comments, so the provider must take caution to avoid being accused of improper sexual behaviors.
- Teach the p/f/c that the pt with a schizoid or schizotypal personality disorder is frequently isolated by own choice, and pt does not have close relationships or want to establish any to achieve accurate expectations.
- Teach the p/f/c that the pt with a personality disorder interacts primarily within the home or with the family, and if pt encounters social situations with unfamiliar people anxiety will increase.
- Know that the symptoms of personality disorder are not severe enough to support a diagnosis of schizophrenia, but under extreme stress the pt could experience a psychotic episode.
- Realize that exploration of the cause of the pt's behavior is essential for successful intervention with demanding and manipulative behaviors, but realize that confronting demanding and manipulative behaviors increases anxiety and anger.
- To decrease excessive demands use a proactive approach by talking about plans and sources of anxiety, acknowledge stressors, and explain information about changes ahead of time to work on solutions.
- Establish limit setting early in the therapeutic relationship using signed contracts or agreements to establish parameters.
- Encourage participation by the f/c to reinforce the limits set to maintain consistency and communications with all persons involved in care.
- Understand that setting personal boundaries requires discipline and practice, and encouragement is needed because the pt who is not used to setting boundaries tends to be rigid initially, and may need encouragement to set achievable limits.
- Establish personal boundaries with clear limits on crossing them, and model appropriate behaviors, interrelations, and communications.
- Use clinical supervision to deal with personal feelings toward pt to understand that working with a pt who has a personality disorder requires patience, persistence, consistency, flexibility, and trust.
- Use a direct and matter-of-fact approach in confronting behaviors.

Medication Management

Pharmacotherapy for the personality disorders has generated much research, but questions about the cause of the disorders has led more to symptom treatment rather than treatment of the diagnosis.

- Aggressive or impulsive behaviors have been treated successfully with carbamazepine (Tegretol), fluoxetine (Prozac), sertraline (Zoloft), antipsychotics, lithium, and MAOIs.
- Haloperidol (Haldol) is effective to enhance the pt's global functioning.
- The unstable responds to amitriptyline (Elavil) for hostility and lack of impulse control.
- Out-of-control or violent behavior can be treated with an anxiolytic or sedative-hypnotic medication.
- Psychotic behaviors respond to neuroleptic medications.

NURSING MANAGEMENT

NURSING INTERVENTIONS AND RATIONALES

☆ Behavioral

- Set limits early at the beginning of the therapeutic relationship, clarify reasons for setting limits, and describe consequences for breaking limits. *This models direct, open communication and avoids miscommunication.*
- Use a calm, matter-of-fact attitude. *This demeanor conveys acceptance and consistency.*
- Teach the p/f/c to maintain consistency in following specified limits. *This avoids inconsistency and manipulation.*
- Convey expectations in a clear, direct manner and request clarification from pt of understanding. *Such communication decreases use of manipulation through misunderstanding.*
- Continuously direct attention to pt's behavior and provide immediate feedback. *Feedback increases pt's awareness of own behaviors.*
- Assist the pt to focus on own behavior and not that of others. *This allows the pt to examine own behavior.*
- Assist the pt to learn alternative techniques to control impulsive actions. *These techniques teach the pt to control his or her own behavior.*
- Explore with the pt the consequences of inappropriate behavior. *Such exploration helps the pt to understand the effect on others.*
- Understand that pt may attempt to have the provider do therapeutic work and will find ways to withdraw from contract while blaming provider. *This increases awareness of the pt's ability to manipulate.*
- Understand the pt's need to test interpersonal limit. *This helps the pt learn to control his or her own behavior.*
- Hold the pt accountable for being at home for visits and completing assignments as required. *This promotes pt accountability.*
- Assist the pt to clarify what is wanted. *This lets f/c discover what needs the pt is trying to fill through manipulation.*
- Reframe and model the pt's statements. *This assists the pt to more directly express the self.*
- Ask the pt to verbalize when anger is an advantage and a disadvantage. *The pt needs to consider the best options for handling anger..*

- Review the pt's way of expressing anger and appropriate expression that will not hurt others. *Review helps the pt to accept responsibility for angry feelings.*
- Review with the pt the motivations associated with expressing anger or resentment. *Review helps p/f/c to determine underlying reasons for anger or resentment.*
- Role play or rehearse behaviors that the pt will use. *Practice develops effective coping and communication skills.*
- Assist the pt to identify situations that are upsetting and cause negative feelings, and identify thoughts associated with them. *This assists the pt in gaining insight into negative feelings and connecting them to specific situations.*
- Teach the pt to substitute thoughts that are more objective and realistic. *This promotes realistic thinking.*
- Provide positive feedback to the p/f/c for successful expression of anger. *Feedback reinforces appropriate behavior.*
- Ignore pt communications when the pt is argumentative, complaining, or sarcastic. *Lack of attention extinguishes undesirable behaviors.*
- Provide positive reinforcement when the pt makes effort to compromise. *This acknowledges appropriate behavior.*
- Call attention to the pt's tone of voice and the syntax of the words when pt complains or whines. *This promotes awareness of communication patterns and how to alter them.*
- Interrupt blaming behaviors or using the past as justification for present behavior. *This helps the pt examine behaviors and own responsibility.*
- Develop specific consequences for unacceptable behaviors. *Such consequences help to decrease or eliminate unacceptable behaviors.*
- Assist the pt to recognize situations in which pt feels bored and identify appropriate activities to diminish boredom. *This helps the pt see that boredom is the problem and the pt is responsible for resolution.*

Emotional

- Suggest that the pt may be hurt, irritated, or upset rather than angry. *This allows the pt to accept negative feelings.*
- Use self-disclosure appropriately to share experiences that cause irritation and anger. *This assists the pt in recognizing normal ways of handling these feelings and to model self-disclosure.*
- Demonstrate a willingness to admit mistakes. *The pt may be quick to recognize mistakes and use them as a measure to gain control of interpersonal situation.*
- Give positive feedback for honesty. *Feedback assists the pt in recognizing that truth is more appropriate than dishonesty.*
- Discuss with the pt that feelings of guilt do not indicate that the person has done something bad. *This helps the pt understand feelings of guilt in relation to behavior.*

Cognitive

- Instruct the pt to note thoughts and feelings that occur before self-mutilation. *This increases awareness of feelings and actions related to self-mutilation and decreases incidence of self-abuse.*
- Instruct the pt to express feelings rather than using intellectualization. *Such teaching assists in dealing with feelings and emotions and not rationalizing behavior.*

- Promote a realistic perception of self by identifying discrepancies. *This assists the pt to recognize immature behavior and responses by others.*
- Encourage the pt to use independent thinking, problem-solving, and reframing of questions from "What should I do?" to "What do I want to do?" *This decreases dependency and passivity and increases self-reliance.*
- Assess the pt's response to subtleties or cues. *The pt may lack the ability or desire to interpret concepts or abstract ideas.*

⊔ Physical

- Provide sexual counseling. *This assists the pt in understanding disturbances in sexual activity and prevents physical and emotional complications.*
- Encourage physical activities. *Activity decreases restlessness associated with anxiety and anger.*
- Assist the pt in identifying physical manifestations of anger. *This promotes awareness of bodily sensations of anger and allows planning of interventions.*

◑ Social

- Explore with the pt problems in interpersonal relationships and alternative ways to relate without seduction or intimidation. *Pt gains awareness of behavior and impact on others.*
- Assess the pt's response to subtleties or social cues. *Pt may lack social awareness and comfort.*
- Instruct the pt in social skills, describing and demonstrating specific skills such as eye contact, attentive listening, nodding, and social conversation. *This models and teaches social interaction skills.*

✦ Spiritual

- Encourage and guide the pt to discuss feelings. *This promotes pt introspection and motivates change.*
- Assist the pt to identify and clarify personal values and beliefs. *Such clarification helps pt to gain a direction in life.*

P

Nursing Goals

- To decrease the following behaviors: manipulative; attention-seeking; seductive; dishonest; and other socially unacceptable activities
- To promote satisfying interpersonal communications
- To facilitate the pt's taking responsibility for self, problems, and behaviors
- To alleviate the pt's boredom
- To promote behavior containment within acceptable limits with the p/f/c
- To assist in decreasing the pt's acting-out behaviors
- To assist the pt in improving impulse control
- To decrease secondary gains the pt receives from physical complaints
- To terminate the therapeutic relationship effectively
- To facilitate development of healthy interpersonal relationships

Patient Goals

- The pt will remain safe from self-abusive behaviors.
- The pt will develop efficient, direct, and effective means of expressing feelings such as hostility, anger, retribution, and hurt.
- The pt will become more adept in interpersonal relations demonstrating less resistance and more self-determination.
- The pt will express needs and wants in a clear, direct manner that does not harm others and demonstrates responsibility for own actions.
- The pt will terminate the therapeutic relationship effectively.
- The pt will develop appropriate sexual contacts in healthy interpersonal relationships.

Patient and Family/Caregiver Outcomes

The patient will:

- Verbalize and demonstrate increased self-responsibility for behavior as demonstrated by _____ within _____ (weeks)
- Verbalize fewer somatic complaints as demonstrated by _____ within _____ (weeks)
- Demonstrate decreased manipulative, attention-seeking, passive-aggressive, or _____ (specify) behaviors by _____ (date)
- Express feelings, especially anger, directly and in a nondestructive manner (specify) _____ within _____ (weeks)
- Demonstrate mature interactions with _____ (specify) as demonstrated by _____ within _____ (weeks)
- Discuss the relationship of physical complaints, legal difficulties, or substance use to ineffective coping skills as demonstrated by _____ within _____ (weeks)
- Acknowledge the need to work through memories of childhood abuse to assist in decreasing repressed memories as demonstrated by _____ within _____ (weeks)
- Verbalize and demonstrate adequate skills to deal with changes or crises (specify) _____ within _____ (weeks)
- Identify ways to meet own needs that do not infringe on rights of others as demonstrated by _____ within _____ (weeks)
- Achieve or maintain satisfactory work performance as demonstrated by _____ within _____ (weeks)
- Eliminate acting-out behaviors as demonstrated by _____ within _____ (weeks)
- Ask for what is needed in an acceptable manner _____ (specify) within _____ (weeks)
- Demonstrate impulse control as evidenced by _____ by _____ (date)
- Delay gratification of needs and requests without acting out as demonstrated by _____ within _____ (weeks)
- Verbalize and list plans for moderation of life-style by _____ (date)
- Participate in relationships without excessive clinging, avoidance, or _____ (specify) by _____ (date)

- Meet dependency needs in a socially acceptable manner as demonstrated by _____ within _____ (weeks)
- Express an intensity of emotion that is appropriate to the situation (specify) _____ by _____ (date)
- Communicate effectively, both listening and speaking as demonstrated by _____ within _____ (weeks)
- Express genuine care and concern for others as demonstrated by _____ within _____ (weeks)
- Become more adept in relating to others in an effort to understand them as demonstrated by _____ within _____ (weeks)
- Exhibit less resistance to and more cooperation with others as demonstrated by _____ within _____ (weeks)
- Refrain from inappropriate sexual activity within _____ (weeks)
- State needs without using manipulation by _____ (date)
- Expresses feelings of frustration, powerlessness, and inadequacy appropriately within _____ (weeks)
- Verbalize an understanding of the connection to self-mutilate with escalating anxiety levels as demonstrated by _____ within _____ (weeks)
- Discuss events, behaviors, or situations that indicate manipulative behaviors as demonstrated by _____ within _____ (weeks)
- Discuss ways their behavior affects the self and others (specify) _____ by _____ (date)
- Distinguish needs and wants to learn to delay immediate gratification as demonstrated by _____ by _____ (date)
- Accept responsibility for their own actions, not blame others, tell lies or rationalize behavior (specify) by _____ (date)
- Respect and value the self, make realistic statements about the self, and act independently and autonomously (specify) _____ by _____ (date)

The family/caregiver will:

- Listen and communicate honestly when the pt is asking for feedback on behavior and interactions as demonstrated by _____ within _____ (weeks)
- Provide a safe, supportive environment for the pt to explore firm limits and boundaries on acceptable interpersonal relations (specify) _____ by _____ (date)

RESOURCES AND INFORMATION

1. American Psychiatric Association (APA)
    Division of Public Affairs/Code P-H
    1400 K Street, NW
    Washington, DC 20005
    202-682-6220
2. American Psychological Association (APA)
    750 First Street, NE
    Washington, DC 20001
    202-336-5500
    1-800-296-0272

3. Parents Anonymous
   520 South Lafayette Park
   Room 316
   Los Angeles, CA 80057
   213-388-6685 (Administration)
   1-800-421-0353 (24-hour Parent Stress Line)
4. National AIDS Hotline: 1-800-342-AIDS

REFERENCES

American Psychiatric Association. (1994). *Quick reference guide to the diagnostic criteria from DSM-IV.* Washington, DC: Author.

Brown, G. L., Ebert, M. H. M., Goyer, P. F., et al. (1982). Aggression, suicide and serotonin relationships to CSF amine metabolites. *American Journal of Psychiatry, 139,* 741–745.

Brown, G. L., & Linnoila, M. I. (1990, April). CSF serotonin metabolite (5-HIAA) studies in depression, impulsivity, and violence. *Journal of Clinical Psychiatry, 51* (Suppl), 31–43.

Carson, V. B. & Arnold, E. N., eds. (1996). *Mental health nursing: The nurse-patient journey.* Philadelphia: Saunders.

Mahler, M. S. (1971). A study of the separation-individuation process and its possible application to borderline phenomena in the psychoanalytic situation. *Psychoanalytic Study of the Child, 26,* 403–424.

Mahler, M. S. (1972). Rapprochement subphase of the separation-individuation process. *Psychoanalytic Quarterly, 41,* 487–506.

Phobias and Phobic Anxiety (See Anxiety)

Post-Traumatic Stress Disorder (PTSD)

P

PROBLEM DESCRIPTION

A type of anxiety disorder, at the extreme end of the stress reaction continuum, PTSD is a dramatic reexperiencing of a traumatic event, such as combat experience, a natural disaster, assault, rape, and other catastrophes (eg, abuse, torture, or an epidemic). A catastrophe is one extraordinary event or series of events that is overwhelming, sudden, and often dangerous to the pt or significant others (Figley, 1985). PTSD, an emotional state of discomfort and memories, is associated with intense fear, helplessness, or horror related to the exposure to or experience with trauma; a person's sense of invulnerability to harm is shattered (Figley, 1985). PTSD can develop quickly, within 6 months or less, be delayed (occurring more than 6 months after the trauma), or chronic (the stress reaction symptoms last longer than 6 months). Long-term self-medication with alcohol or drugs can delay PTSD up to 30 years. A severe illness or stress can dramatically induce a delayed episode of PTSD. Many people with PTSD who were engaged in wars have been improperly diagnosed as having an anxiety reaction, schizophrenia, or a personality disorder problem. Of those pts with PTSD, about 30% recover, 40% have mild symptoms, 20% have more moderate symptoms, and the remaining 10% remain unchanged or become worse (Kaplan & Sadock, 1988).

PROBLEM IDENTIFICATION

Characteristics and Observable Behaviors

- Reexperiencing of the trauma (called "flashbacks," a sudden feeling or acting as if the traumatic or catastrophic event were happening all over again) and other recollections of the trauma
- Recurrent or intrusive dreams, sleep disturbance(s), especially nightmares, or sleep phobia (avoiding sleep at night)
- Emotional "numbness," a feeling of detachment, and constricted affect
- Dysphoria (depressed and withdrawn), apathy, diminished involvement and interest in one's life and in others or overinvolvement with others
- Rage, explosiveness, and irritability
- Fear reaction, startle response, and increased emotional arousal
- Demandingness, suspiciousness, hyperalertness, hypervigilance, and paranoia
- Inflated concerns regarding one's safety
- Crying, active grieving, and sadness
- Issues regarding personal responsibility
- Fear of death or repeated trauma
- Shame and self-blame for the trauma
- Alienation from others and difficulty with relationships
- Difficulty expressing love and compassion
- Difficulty with social or occupational relationships and activities
- Legal problems and criminal activity
- Underachievement or OCD
- Repeated and excessive verbalizations about the traumatic event
- Survivor guilt
- Substance abuse and other forms of self-destructiveness and thrill seeking
- Difficulty concentrating
- Loss of meaning and purpose in life with vagueness regarding values
- Avoidance of reminders of the trauma and increased symptoms in the presence of reminders of the trauma
- Passiveness, submissiveness, stereotyped behavior
- Somatic complaints and body memories
- Difficulty adjusting to the home care milieu

Factors Related to the Problem

- Medical and psychiatric illness
- Actual, potential, or perceived loss of control
- Individual vulnerability: younger age, physical injury, perceived threat, biologic integrity, underlying psychiatric disorder, or family history of psychotic disorder (Marshall, 1995; Yehuda & McFarlane, 1995)

- Risk of exposure to traumatic events (eg, a high-risk neighborhood)
- Severe burns
- Emotional dependence
- Reminders, conditions, or environmental stimuli that resemble the original traumatic event or catastrophe
- Substance abuse
- Depression

Assessment Tools (see Appendix I)

Consider administering the:

1. Beck Depression Inventory
2. Brief Psychiatric Rating Scale
3. Geriatric Depression Scale
4. Mini-Mental Status Examination
5. Suicide Risk Assessment Tool

PROBLEM LIST

(See Section 1 for common problems.)

- Adjustment, Impaired
- Body Image Disturbance
- Communication, Impaired Verbal
- Diversional Activity Deficit
- Family Processes, Altered
- Grieving, Anticipatory
- Grieving, Dysfunctional
- Growth and Development, Altered
- Helplessness
- Hopelessness
- Parenting, Altered
- Personal Identity Disturbance
- Post-Trauma Response
- Powerlessness
- Rape-Trauma Syndrome
- Role Performance Alteration
- Self-Care Deficit (specify)
- Self-Concept Disturbance
- Sensory/Perceptual Alterations (specify)
- Sexual Pattern Disturbance
- Sleep Pattern Disturbance
- Social Isolation
- Spiritual Distress

- Thought Processes, Altered
- Violence, Risk for, Self-Directed or Directed at Others

PROBLEM MANAGEMENT

Prevention, Maintenance, and Restorative Interventions

- Observe the pt's behavior for s/s of post-trauma distress, especially when the pt is hesitant to reveal or discuss a traumatic or catastrophic event.
- Seek professional consultation to assist in the provider's own responses to the pt's experience of or expression of thoughts and feelings related to the pt's PTSD.
- Evaluate the severity of the pt's responses to the traumatic event and the extent to which current function is affected.
- Refer the pt for alcohol or drug treatment, as indicated.

Medication Management

No specific medications are indicated for this behavior, except for those prescribed for the physical and psychological problems associated with PTSD, usually short-term treatment for the core symptoms of anxiety, depression, panic, and sleep disturbance. Some antihypertensives (ie, propranolol and clonidine) and some anticonvulsants (eg, carbamazepine) are effective in treating the symptoms of PTSD. If the pt is extremely agitated, benzodiazepines or antipsychotic medications may be used briefly.

NURSING MANAGEMENT

Nursing Interventions and Rationales

☆ Behavioral

- Observe the pt in a structured activity to assess ability to complete tasks and concentrate. *Observation allows the provider to plan effective care based on the extent to which current function is affected.*
- If necessary, assist the pt to identify and avoid situations and stimuli that precipitate distress. *This encourages going through the phases of recovery from PTSD toward adaptive, healthy coping behavior.*
- Teach the pt how to stay "in the present." *This avoids or minimizes becoming overwhelmed by memories of the traumatic experience.*
- Assist the p/f/c to make changes and take action (eg, change locks). *This fosters a sense of personal safety and control and decreases vulnerability* (Taylor, 1983).
- Assist the pt to draw or use movement. *This readjusts and reappraises the traumatic experience.*

♡ Emotional

- Provide emotional support to the pt. *Support promotes the pt's expression of feelings connected with the PTSD to facilitate the healing process.*
- Observe the pt for signs of emotional withdrawal from others. *Such observation detects and eliminates or reduces the factors or reminders in the pt's home environment that may be associated with the traumatic experience.*
- Teach the p/f/c that the feelings and symptoms related to PTSD the pt is having are often experienced by others who have undergone traumatic events. *This provides reassurance.*

△ Cognitive

- Observe the pt for signs of difficulty concentrating, preoccupation, or disinterest. *This determines if factors or reminders are present in the pt's home environment that may be associated with the traumatic experience to help reduce or eliminate such factors or reminders.*
- Provide or arrange for time-limited psychotherapy for the pt with PTSD. *This is an effective form of treatment to resolve the conflicts associated with the traumatic event.*
- When the pt initiates the topic, discuss the content of dreams and nightmares. *Such discussion reduces or manages anxiety and fears associated with the PTSD.*
- Teach the p/f/c that there are four phases (recovery, avoidance, reconsideration, and adjustment) to long-term adjustment. *This gives pt understanding of the process of healing from PTSD.*

☐ Physical

- Teach the pt to use relaxation skills in anxiety-arousing situations and after experiencing the startle response. *This reduces the overall intensity of the anxiety and startle response as well as facilitating recovery and healing from PTSD.*
- Teach the f/c to arouse the pt according to the pt's desires. *The pt with PTSD may startle easily even when asleep so this intervention prevents injury, lessens anxiety, and avoids embarrassment.*
- Keep abreast of and teach the p/f/c about research studies suggesting a relationship between trauma and changes in brain structure and function. *This allows all to understand the relationship between biology and the environment* (Glod & McEnany, 1995).
- Instruct the pt regarding the need for physical exercise or to substitute safe physical activities. *Activity releases tension in a nondestructive manner.*

◯ Social

- Observe the pt for signs of social withdrawal or detachment when others are present. *This determines the extent to which the pt with PTSD is socially affected.*
- Remain, and teach to f/c to remain, with the pt to listen to pt "tell the story." *This prevents the triggering of severe anxiety or panic.*
- Refer the pt for an occupational, vocational, recreational, social, or other evaluation. *Evaluation facilitates the reintegration of the pt's life with social skills, diversional activities, and leisure time counseling because the pt with PTSD is often socially isolated and may have little interest in recreational activities.*

- Refer the p/f/c to sources of self-help, professional organizations, or groups specifically for people affected by PTSD. *Referral facilitates the p/f/c's understanding of the event and symptom resolution and prevents compromised family functioning.*
- Keep abreast of and teach the p/f/c about research studies suggesting a relationship between trauma and changes in brain structure and function. *This helps p/f/c to understand how interpersonal relationships may have been affected* (Glod & McEnany, 1995).

✦ Spiritual

- Identify cultural, religious, and spiritual values that help and hinder pt's recovery from the traumatic experience. *Such interventions will assist the pt to work through the trauma and heal.*
- Assist the pt to identify personal strengths and resources that can be used to avoid or cope with triggering situations. *This gives pt an overall sense of self-worth and confidence.*
- Explore the possible meaning and purpose of the traumatic event with the pt. *Exploration helps the pt make sense of the event(s).*
- Assist the pt to determine actual or symbolic activities that will make amends for other actual or potential people at risk for PTSD. *This gives the pt a sense of contribution, solace, and meaning.*
- Refer the pt for psychotherapy. *This alleviates underlying guilt and sense of inadequacy associated with the PTSD and enhances self-esteem as well as security and safety.*
- Encourage the pt to use techniques such as drawings or movement. *This assigns appropriate responsibility regarding the traumatic experience and achieves inner peace.*
- Assist the p/f/c to make changes and take action (eg, get more fire extinguishers). *Action fosters a sense of control and self-efficacy* (Taylor, 1983).
- Obtain support, preferably in a group setting, to deal with the provider's own feelings and reactions regarding the pt's responses to traumatic experience(s). *Support provides trust, competence, authenticity, and relatedness.*

P

Nursing Goals

- To identify the s/s of PTSD and educate the p/f/c regarding the phenomenon
- To identify the s/s of PTSD and refer the pt for specialized treatment (eg, critical incident debriefing, hypnosis, or substance abuse treatment)

Patient Goals

- The pt will acknowledge that the traumatic event occurred.
- The pt will report that reexperiencing of the trauma has diminished.

Patient and Family/Caregiver Outcomes

The patient will:

- Identify the experience with or exposure to _____ traumatic situations by _____ (date)

- State _____ (specify number) reminders, conditions, or environmental stimuli that are similar to the initial traumatic event(s) in the home care milieu
- Identify _____ (specify number and type) stimuli in the home environment that will elicit the fear or startle response by _____ (date)
- Participate in a social activity in the home by _____ (date)
- Become involved with others related to a support group or specific organization connected to the traumatic event by _____ (date)

The family/caregiver will:

- Assist with identifying the pt's experience with or exposure to a traumatic event(s) within _____ (weeks)
- Verbalize an understanding that the pt is having difficulty completing _____ (specify tasks or activity) due to the difficulty concentrating associated with PTSD by _____ (date)
- Assist with managing the pt's behavior related to the traumatic experience by setting limits on _____ behavior, allowing the pt to ventilate feelings, or _____ within _____ (weeks)
- Become involved in a support group for or specific organization connected to the traumatic event by _____ (date)

RESOURCES AND INFORMATION

1. In the telephone book: Veteran's organizations, rape crisis centers, and victim and witness assistance programs through the district attorney's office
2. National Victim Center (for local support groups): 1-800-FYI-CALL
3. National Organization for Victim Assistance: 202-232-6682
4. National Association of Crime Victim Compensation Boards: 703-370-2996
5. Epstein, M. & Hosking, S. (1992). *Falling apart (avoiding, coping with, & recovering from stress breakdown)*. Sebastopol, CA: CRCR Publications.

REFERENCES

Figley, C. (1985). *Trauma and its wake*. New York: Brunner/Mazel.

Glod, C. A., & McEnany, G. (1995). The neurobiology of posttraumatic stress disorder. *Journal of the American Nurses Association, 1*, 196–199.

Kaplan, H. I., & Sadock, B. J. (1988). *Clinical psychiatry from the synopsis of psychiatry*. Baltimore: Williams & Wilkins.

Marshall, R. D. (1995). Pharmacotherapy in the treatment of posttraumatic stress disorder. *Psychiatric Annals, 25*, 588–597.

Taylor, S. (1983). Adjustment to threatening life events: A theory of cognitive adaptation. *American Psychologist, 38*, 1161–1173.

Yehuda, R., & McFarlane, A. C. (1995). Conflict between current knowledge about posttraumatic stress disorder, and its original conceptual basis. *American Journal of Psychiatry, 152*, 1705–1713.

Psychosis

PROBLEM DESCRIPTION

Psychotic behaviors include many different symptoms resulting from disturbed thought processes, distorted perceptions, brain damage, or chemical toxicity. A person who is psychotic has difficulty telling reality from unreality. A person whose reality testing is impaired is said to be in a psychotic state. Psychosis is frequently seen in schizophrenia, but it can also be a part of other mental and physical illnesses. Hallucinations, delusions, or thought disorders can impair a person's ability to adequately test reality.

Causes of Psychosis

Psychosis can be caused by a variety of factors, including schizophrenia, mania, depression, stroke, tumor, head injury, seizures, fever, infections, alcohol, medications, legal or illegal drugs, and toxic substances.

Functional Psychosis

Functional psychosis is a psychotic disorder that has no active physical abnormality related to it. Functional psychotic disorders consist of brief reactive psychosis, delusional disorder, substance-induced psychotic disorder, major depressive episode with psychotic features, manic episode with psychotic features, schizoaffective disorder, schizophrenia, and schizophreniform disorder.

Cognitive Mental Disorder Psychosis

This psychosis is caused by specific, measurable deterioration in the physical structures or chemical functioning of the CNS. Causes of CMD psychosis include:

1. Metabolic: changes in the endocrine glands and deficiencies in the electrolyte blood levels, including:
    *   Addison's disease (hypoadrenalism)
    *   Cushing's syndrome (hyperadrenalism)
    *   Hyperthyroidism
    *   Hypothyroidism (myxedema)
    *   Hyperparathyroidism
    *   Hypoparathyroidism
    *   Hyperinsulinism
    *   Pituitary problems
    *   Calcium: hypercalcemia and hypocalcemia
    *   Sodium: hypernatremia and hyponatremia
    *   Phosphorus: hypohosphatemia

- Potassium: hyperkalemia and hypokalemia
- Base bicarbonate: alkalosis and acidosis

2. Convulsive disorders: electrical disturbances and disorders caused by partial and generalized seizures

3. Neoplastic diseases (cancers), benign or malignant, can cause psychotic behaviors depending on the location, size, and type of tumor. The major cause for change in psychiatric function is related to the increase in intracranial pressure, agnosia (loss of ability to interpret sensory perceptions such as vision and hearing), or apraxia (loss of ability to perform complex tasks or loss of motor control).

4. Degenerative causes
   - Multiple sclerosis
   - Systemic lupus erythematosus
   - Alzheimer's disease
   - Huntington's chorea
   - Creutzfeldt-Jakob disease

5. Arterial diseases
   - Cerebrovascular accidents
   - Cerebral arteriosclerosis
   - Multiple infarct dementias

6. Mechanical causes
   - Head injuries
   - Subdural hematoma
   - Normal pressure hydrocephalus

7. Infections
   - AIDS dementia complex
   - Encephalitis
   - Meningitis
   - Cerebral abscess
   - Syphilis

8. Nutritional causes due to lack of
   - Vitamin B_{12}
   - Folic acid
   - Nicotinic acid
   - Thiamine

9. Drugs
   - Alcohol
   - Hallucinogens
   - Heavy metals
   - Prescribed medications (at least 75 medications cause psychosis)

Understanding the etiology of psychosis will determine the treatment approach. Some types of psychosis have a good prognosis and the pt returns to premorbid functioning. In schizophrenia or dementias the pt will not return to premorbid functioning. Managing symptoms, treating underlying problems, providing reality orientation, preventing injury, building self-esteem, and expressing feelings are the main focuses of treatment.

PROBLEM IDENTIFICATION

Characteristics and Observable Behaviors

- Flat, blunted, or inappropriate affect
- Clenched teeth or fists, hostile or threatening behavior, and other forms of aggression
- Anxiety, fear, and feelings of insecurity
- Short attention span, attention deficits, and distractibility
- Bizarre behaviors, such as holding the body rigidly
- Cognitive deficits, impaired memory, and confusion
- Impaired concentration, judgment, and decision-making ability
- Illusions, delusions, hallucinations, and other distorted perceptions and nonreality-based thinking
- Disorganized, illogical thinking
- Disturbance of self-initiated, goal-directed activity, including poor personal hygiene
- Poor ego boundaries and emotional impairment
- Feelings of frustration
- Inability to perceive harmful stimuli or situations
- Irritability, labile affect, and mood swings
- Lack of awareness of physical or cognitive impairment
- Loss of personal control
- Mistrust, suspicion, and negativism
- Rambling and incoherent speech
- Sensory or motor defects
- Inappropriate social interactions
- Withdrawn behavior

Factors Related to the Problem

- Alcohol or drug withdrawal
- Alteration in mental status
- Anxiety
- Attention deficit disorders
- Cognitive and perceptual impairment
- Delusions, hallucinations, and illusions
- Depression and bipolar disorder (manic-depressive disorder)
- Medication noncompliance
- Metabolic disorders
- Low levels of antipsychotic medications
- Perceptual and cognitive impairment
- Physical problems related to immobility
- Psychomotor retardation
- Schizophrenia
- Seizure disorders
- Sensorimotor deficits
- Sensory deprivation or overload
- Sexual conflicts
- Sleep disturbances

P

Assessment Tools and Instruments (see Appendix I)

Consider administering the:

1. Abnormal Involuntary Movement Scale
2. Beck Depression Inventory
3. Brief Psychiatric Rating Scale
4. Brief Psychiatric Schizophrenic Rating Scale
5. Clinical Inventory Withdrawal Assessment
6. Falls Risk Assessment
7. Geriatric Depression Scale
8. Global Assessment of Functioning Scale
9. Mini-Mental State Examination
10. Modified Overt Aggression Scale
11. Obsessive-Compulsive Disorder Screening Checklist
12. Social Dysfunction Rating Scale
13. Suicide Risk Assessment Tool
14. TRIADS

PROBLEM LIST

- Activity Intolerance
- Body Image Disturbance
- Caregiver Role Strain
- Communication, Impaired Verbal
- Fatigue
- Growth and Development, Altered
- Mobility, Impaired
- Noncompliance
- Pain
- Parental Role Conflict
- Parenting, Altered
- Personal Identity Disturbance
- Post-Trauma Response
- Powerlessness
- Relocation Stress Syndrome
- Self Care Deficit (specify)
- Self Mutilation, Risk for
- Sensory/Perceptual Alterations
- Sexual Dysfunction
- Sexuality Patterns, Altered
- Sleep Pattern Disturbance
- Social Interaction, Impaired
- Social Isolation
- Spiritual Distress
- Therapeutic Regimen, Ineffective Management of
- Thought Processes, Altered
- Violence, Risk for, Self-Directed or Directed at Others

PROBLEM MANAGEMENT

Prevention, Maintenance, and Restorative Interventions

- Establishing a trusting relationship is the first step in treatment so that the pt trusts what the provider says is true.
- Obtain active involvement of the f/c to educate them on the disease process and problems and assist them in providing support to keep pt in the family setting as long as possible.
- Teach the f/c signs of psychosis that are harmful or unsafe and in need of immediate intervention.
- Support and encourage pts with psychotic behavior in a concrete, literal manner and avoid intense confrontation or emotionalism.
- Give directions simply and a few steps at a time.
- Teach the f/c to spend time with the pt, even when pt is not able to respond verbally or coherently, and to reorient the pt to reality as necessary.
- Carefully assess the pt who exhibits a psychosis to determine causes and plan for appropriate intervention and outcome.

Medication Management

The primary medications used to treat psychosis are antipsychotic or neuroleptic drugs. They reduce and assist to organize chaotic, disorganized, and psychotic thinking and reduce or remove delusions and hallucinations. Antipsychotic or neuroleptic medications are classified into three groups: low potency, high potency, and intermediate potency. Potency is not related to effectiveness but to the dosages necessary to produce a therapeutic effect. Antipsychotics work on dopamine and serotonin in the brain. Before starting neuroleptics the pt should have a complete history and physical examination to rule out medical problems. Noncompliance with medications is one of the greatest challenges for pts with a psychotic disorder. Denial, side effects, and f/c opposition to medications are major contributors to noncompliance. New antipsychotic medications such as clozapine (Clozaril) and risperidone (Risperdal) show success for compliance because of their decreased side effects. With both agents, appropriate laboratory and physical evaluation must be maintained to reduce adverse reactions.

In older adults, the use of antipsychotics must be assessed even more carefully. Conditions such as glaucoma, benign prostatic hypertrophy, metabolic disorders, and cardiac problems could be worsened by the use of antipsychotics.

P

NURSING MANAGEMENT

Nursing Interventions and Rationales

✯ Behavioral

- Set nonpunitive, clear, easy to understand limits on the pt's behavior. *Limits establish external controls when the pt is not able to exert self-control.*

- Reorient the pt to person, place, time, and situation. *Reorientation reinforces repeated presentation of concrete reality.*
- Limit the pt's environment. *Such limits enhance feelings of security because unknown boundaries or a perceived lack of limits can foster insecurity.*
- Establish and maintain a daily pattern to provide a safe, known routine. *The therapeutic regimen will have a greater likelihood of being followed.*
- Encourage new tasks or behaviors at a time of the day when the pt will be most able to concentrate and participate. *This maximizes the pt's ability to participate successfully.*

♡ Emotional

- Approach the pt with a calm, positive attitude that conveys the idea that pt will succeed in a new activity. *This attitude enhances the pt's confidence.*
- Redirect the treatment approach when the pt becomes agitated to a more neutral approach and re-engage the pt in a more calming or pleasurable activity. *This allows the pt to express self without becoming overwhelmed.*

△ Cognitive

- Approach the pt in a directive manner and state what needs to be done, rather than giving choices. *The pt's ability to make decisions is impaired and making decisions is frustrating.*
- Allow the pt more responsibility for making decisions when the more intense portion of the psychosis passes. *This encourages the pt to accept responsibility and regain independence.*

⊓ Physical

- Protect the pt from self-destructive activities by maintaining a safe environment and removing items that could be used in self-destructive behavior. *This maintains pt safety.*

◯ Social

- Teach specific social skills that the pt is lacking. *Such teaching increases knowledge and usage of appropriate skills.*
- Assist the p/f/c to provide an adequate amount of stimulations and not isolate. *This maintains contact with reality and decrease hallucinations when pt is alone.*
- Assess the pt's current capability of engaging in former hobbies or activities and make them available as much as possible. *It is best for pt to continue or resume previous interests rather than develop new ones.*

✦ Spiritual

- Encourage the p/f/c to discuss the pt's losses in terms of what is no longer possible and what can still be done to assist the p/f/c to discuss realistic changes. *Discussion enhances patient coping.*
- Do not falsely reassure the pt and answer all questions honestly and directly. *False reassurances can be condescending and a barrier to healthy adaptation.*

Nursing Goals

- To provide reality orientation and contact
- To decrease fears, anxiety, agitation, and mistrust
- To facilitate compliance with medications
- To interrupt the pattern of hallucinations or delusions
- To encourage pt contact with real people, interactions, and activities
- To anticipate ways to deal with possible recurrence of hallucinations or delusions
- To provide structured, goal-directed activity
- To decrease acting-out behavior
- To decrease confusion and disorientation
- To minimize the pt's misperceptions
- To decrease the pt's impulsivity
- To promote the p/f/c's coping with deficits and role changes
- To decrease pt apathy or negativism

Patient Goals

- The pt will report fewer or less severe psychotic symptoms.
- The pt will describe the impact of illness on the self and others.
- The pt will describe situations that increase psychotic symptoms.
- The pt will describe behavioral cues that signal the onset of symptoms.
- The pt talk about negative feelings instead of acting on them.
- The pt will participate in planning the integration of therapeutic regimen into pattern of daily living.
- The pt will demonstrate improved orientation to reality.
- The pt will identify situations that increase anxiety or initiate hallucinations.
- The pt will use self-control strategies to reduce hallucinations.
- The pt will recognize when sensory stimuli are becoming excessive and use time in quiet area.
- The pt will exhibit decreased distrust of others.

Patient and Family/Caregiver Outcomes

The patient will:

- Be free of delusions or demonstrate ability to function without responding to persistent delusional thoughts by _____ (date)
- Verbalize and demonstrate knowledge of hallucinations or illness and safe use of medications by _____ (date)
- Establish contact with reality as demonstrated by _____ within _____ (weeks)
- Demonstrate accurate awareness of surroundings within _____ (weeks)
- Engage in satisfactory interpersonal relationships within limitations as demonstrated by _____ within _____ (weeks)
- Verbally recognize symptoms of psychosis and validate perceptions with f/c when possible as demonstrated by _____ within _____ (weeks)
- Discuss future plans, incorporating the loss or change, as demonstrated by _____ within _____ (weeks)

- Maintain independence within limitations as demonstrated by _____ within _____ (weeks)
- Verbalize abilities and limitations realistically as demonstrated by _____ within _____ (weeks)
- Perform daily routines safely, without taking unnecessary risks as demonstrated by _____ within _____ (weeks)
- Discuss a reality-based interpretation of events that is validated by another person _____ (times) within _____ (weeks)

The family/caregiver will:

- Assist the pt to recognize signs and symptoms that signal psychotic behavior as shown by _____ within _____ (weeks)
- Cue pt to recognize when behaviors are inappropriate or harmful to others (specify)_____ by _____ (date)
- Demonstrate techniques for maintaining a safe environment and reorientation as necessary (specify) _____ by _____ (date)

RESOURCES AND INFORMATION

1. American Psychiatric Association (APA)
   Division of Public Affairs/Code P-H
   1400 K Street, NW
   Washington, DC 20005
   202-336-5500
2. American Psychological Association (APA)
   750 First Street, NE
   Washington, DC 20002
   202-955-7710
   1-800-296-0272
3. National Alliance for the Mentally Ill (NAMI)
   200 N. Glebe Road
   Suite 1015
   Arlington, VA 22203-3754
   703-524-7600
4. National Mental Health Association (NMHA)
   1021 Prince Street
   Alexandria, VA 22314-2971
   703-684-7722
   1-800-969-NMHA
5. National Institute of Mental Health (NIMH)
   Information Resources and Inquiries Branch
   Office of Scientific Information, Room 15C
   5600 Fishers Lane, Room 7C02
   Rockville, MD 20857
   301-443-4513
6. Multiple Sclerosis Association of America
   601-05 White Horse Pike

Oaklyn, NJ 08107
609-858-3211
1-800-822-4MSA (24-hour hotline)
7. National Institute of Neurological Disorders and Stroke (NINDS)
Building 31, Room 8A06
Bethesda, MD 20892
301-496-5751
8. National Institute of Neurological and Communicative Disorders and Stroke (NINCDS)
PO Box 5801
Bethesda, MD 20824
301-496-5751
1-800-352-9424
9. National Rehabilitation Information Center (NARIC)
8455 Colesville Road
Suite 935
Silver Spring, MD 20910
301-588-9284
1-800-34-NARIC

Purpose in Life Problems
(See Meaning in Life Problems)

R

Relationship Problems

PROBLEM DESCRIPTION

People with relationship problems have difficulty establishing and maintaining relationships with others while retaining their separate identity. These problems usually arise from not learning how to trust and form close, intimate relationships (Schwab, Stephenson, & Ice, 1993). Positive, healthy, and satisfying relationships are characterized by sensitivity to each other's needs, open communication of feelings, acceptance of each person in the relationship, validation of the separateness of each one, and empathic understanding (Rogers, 1961; Sullivan, 1953). A relationship problem usually involves conflict between significant persons regarding important issues, such as goals and values, with a resultant lessening of love, mutual support, and enrichment. However, there is insufficient research and consensus on relational problems and disorders to merit a psychiatric diagnosis (Kaslow, 1993).

PROBLEM IDENTIFICATION

Characteristics and Observable Behaviors

- Difficulty providing intimate information during the intake and assessment process
- History of never having had a close relationship with another person or entity
- Limited seeking or initiating of interactions and relationships
- Detachment from others and little interest in others
- Fear of separation from another
- Intense anger toward another
- Domestic abuse and violence
- Affair(s) or other sexual acting out
- Preoccupation with self and minimal conversational skills
- Low motivation and passivity
- Difficulty understanding concepts such as intimacy, love, empathy, responsibility, altruism, gratitude, and remorse
- Changes in self-esteem, appetite, weight, sleep pattern, and sexual interest and activity
- Changes in social and occupational activity and competence
- Relationship conflicts regarding major issues, such as finances and parenting
- Suspicious, manipulative, demanding, or hostile behavior
- Shyness, aloofness, loneliness, and isolation
- Somatic complaints and frequent, various admissions and contacts with and treatments from the health care system

Factors Related to the Problem

- Inadequate communication skills
- Different developmental levels
- Anxiety
- Depression
- Bipolar disorder
- Phobias and panic attacks
- Eating disorders
- Delusions and hallucinations
- Medical disorders and chronic illness
- Loss of body function or loss of body part
- Medications
- PTSD
- Difficulty with impulse control
- Sexual dysfunction
- Personality disorder
- Substance abuse
- Legal problems
- Losses such as divorce and separation
- History of incest, sexual abuse, abandonment, and other abuse
- Inadequate parental role modeling

- Inadequate income, education, health, and other resources necessary for maintaining or substituting roles and relationships (Morgan, 1988)

Assessment Tools and Instruments (see Appendix I)

Administer the:

1. Mini-Mental State Examination
2. Social Dysfunction Rating Scale

Consider administering the:

1. Dyadic Adjustment Scale (Spanier, 1976)
2. Family Adjustment Device (Epstein, Baldwin, & Bishop, 1983)
3. Sarason's Social Support Questionnaire (SSQ-6) (Sarason, Sarason, & Shearin, 1986; Sarason, Sarason, & Shearin, 1987)

PROBLEM LIST

- Communication, Impaired Nonverbal
- Communication, Impaired Verbal
- Helplessness
- Hopelessness
- Parenting Altered, Risk for
- Personal Identity Disturbance
- Powerlessness
- Self Mutilation, Risk for
- Social Interaction, Impaired
- Social Isolation
- Spiritual Distress
- Thought Processes, Altered
- Violence, Risk for, Self-Directed or Directed at Others

PROBLEM MANAGEMENT

Prevention, Maintenance, and Restorative Interventions

- Assess and identify the strengths in the primary relationship.
- Provide concrete feedback regarding the p/f/c's interaction styles.
- Assist the p/f/c to assess their relationship(s) in terms of acceptance, self-disclosure, trust, conflict resolution, affection, affirmation, service, time, listening, initiative, cooperation, recognition, validation, perceptions, shared power, individual and shared needs, shared future, and relatedness.

Medication Management

No specific medications are indicated for this behavior, except for those prescribed for the physical and psychological aspects associated with this problem.

NURSING MANAGEMENT

Nursing Interventions and Rationales

Behavioral

- Observe the p/f/c for behaviors that indicate relationship problems (ie, detachment, indifference, fear of separation, or intense anger). *The provider needs to adequately assess, plan, intervene, and evaluate in-home care services.*
- Role play with the pt various projected relationship scenarios and discussions. *This strengthens pt's relationship skills and enhances effective actions.*

♡ Emotional

- Encourage the pt to verbalize feelings about the relationship problems. *Such verbalization assists the pt to evaluate the current status of the relationship.*
- Acknowledge the p/f/c's emotional pain regarding the relationship problem. *This offers hope and empathy.*
- Assess the pt's feelings toward those near, such as family members, spouse, siblings, children, and pets. *Assessment determines the nature of the pt's emotional involvement with others.*

◬ Cognitive

- Provide or arrange for psychotherapy to assist the pt to obtain insight into the relationship problems(s). *Therapy helps pt to reframe the problem and change behavior.*

☐ Physical

- Assist the pt to evaluate the physical responses to relationship problems. *This reduces anxiety.*

Social

- Instruct the p/f/c about the nature of social relationships. *This sheds light on the relationship problems that might be present.*
- Assess the pt's social involvement with others. *This helps to plan and generate an effective continuing care plan.*
- Identify and refer the p/f/c to appropriate support groups. *This fosters interpersonal relationships, reality testing, and social skill development.*
- Discuss linkages to and ways to contact others as needed. *This conveys knowledge of available resources.*

✳ Spiritual

- Encourage the pt to verbalize beliefs about relationships and the relationship problems. *This assists the pt to view reality and see that change is part of the human condition.*
- Assist the pt to take positive action and assume greater control and responsibility in the relationship. *Such action provides support and decreases ambivalent feelings.*

- Provide or arrange for supportive or relational psychotherapy (Werman, 1984). *This restores or strengthens the pt's defensive, protective, and coping mechanisms* (see Section 1 of this book).

Nursing Goals

- To identify dysfunctional relationship behaviors
- To provide or arrange for supportive, relational therapy

Patient/Client Goals

- The pt will become aware of behavior in relation to others.
- The pt will find appropriate ways to obtain what is needed from and with others.
- The pt will obtain interpersonal satisfaction with others.

Patient and Family/Caregiver Outcomes

The patient will:

- Verbally express concerns regarding relationship problems to the provider by _____ (date)
- Develop a specific plan to deal with, change, or resolve (specify) own part in the relationship problems by _____ (date)
- Establish _____ (specify number) satisfying, healthy interpersonal relationship(s) by _____ (date)
- Identify _____ problematic behavior that interferes with establishing and maintaining a relationship within _____ (weeks)

The family/caregiver will:

- Discuss the history of association with the pt by _____ (date)
- Verbally agree to constructively work on strengthening the relationship with _____ (specify) within _____ (weeks)
- Describe _____ (specify number) of strategies to enhance the relationships among family members by _____ (date)

R

RESOURCES AND INFORMATION

1. See Resources and Information in Social Withdrawal.

REFERENCES

Epstein, H. B., Baldwin, L. M., & Bishop, D. S. (1983). The McMaster Family Assessment Device. *Journal of Marital and Family Therapy, 9,* 171–180.

Kaslow, F. (1993). Relational diagnosis: An idea whose time has come. *Family Process, 32,* 255–259.

Morgan, D. L. (1988). Age differences in social network participation. *Journal of Gerontology, 43,* 5129–5137.

Rogers, C. (1961). *On becoming a person.* Boston: Houghton Miflin.

Sarason, I., Sarason, B., & Shearin, E. (1986). Social support as an individual difference variable: Its stability, origins and relational aspects. *Journal of Personality and Social Psychology, 50,* 845–855.

Sarason, I., Sarason, B., & Shearin, E. (1987). A brief measure of social support: Practical and theoretical implications. *Journal of Personality and Social Psychology, 4,* 497–510.

Schwab, J. J., Stephenson, J. J., & Ice, J. F. (1993). *Evaluating family mental health: History, epidemiology, and treatment issues.* New York: Plenum Press.

Spanier, G. B. (1976). Measuring marital adjustment: New scale for assessing the quality of marriage and similar dyads. *Journal of Marriage and the Family, 38,* 15–28.

Sullivan, H. S. (1953). *The interpersonal theory of psychiatry.* New York: Norton.

Werman, D. S. (1984). *The practice of supportive psychotherapy.* New York: Brunner/Mazel.

Relocation and Retirement Problems

PROBLEM DESCRIPTION

Adjusting to change can be difficult, even when the change is something one is happy about. Relocation and retirement are two such positive changes that may cause problems. Preparing and planning for a change can help with the transition, but the outcome is often in question or it can cause anxiety. Problems adjusting to changes are called adjustment reaction or disorder. An adjustment disorder involves a maladaptive reaction to an identified psychosocial stressor. The problem occurs within 3 months after the onset of the stressor but does not persist for longer than 6 months. The reaction is expected to remit when the stressor is no longer present or when the person reaches a new level of adaptation. There is an ability to cope with daily life effectively. When the change involves stressors that the person is unable to deal with then the adjustment disorder causes an impairment in functioning. Adjustment disorders are described in relation to a primary feature such as anxiety, depression, physical complaints, or withdrawal, although alone they are not severe enough to be diagnosed as anxiety or depression (Busse & Blazer, 1989).

Retirement from work can present significant adjustment challenges financially, socially, and emotionally. The worker who has a balanced work and leisure life is better able to cope with retirement than someone who places little value on leisure time. Research suggests that individuals who have a positive income, good health, and a social support system are better able to adjust to retirement.

As the population over age 65 grows, retirement problems will become more common. According to the U.S. Special Committee on Aging (1987–1988) statistics show that older persons are retiring earlier.

Relocation involves changes similar to retirement. Retirement may involve relocation; some retired persons may have multiple relocations. Relocation is particularly stressful for the older adult. As life-styles change, significant others die, and physical or mental health deteriorates, relocating becomes a problem-solving challenge. Relocation goes more smoothly when the person who is relocating is involved in decision making, has positive feelings about the relocation, and is not being coerced to change.

PROBLEM IDENTIFICATION

Characteristics and Observable Behaviors

- Anger or lack of trust toward family members promoting move
- Anxiety
- Depression: sad, dull affect; sleep disturbance; and change in eating habits
- Change in ability to perform usual roles
- Difficulty with problem-solving
- Emotional reactions disproportionate to life stressors
- Emotional withdrawal and passivity
- Expressed lack of significant purpose in life
- Expressions of loss of control over life situation, perceived lack of control over life situation, and hopelessness
- Expression of unwillingness to relocate
- Feelings of inadequacy, being overwhelmed, and low self-esteem
- Feelings that aloneness is not by choice
- Lack of interest in improving or modifying own care
- Loss of cognitive or self-care capabilities
- Memory deficits or problems
- Unwarranted dependency on others

Factors Related to the Problem

- Any disorder related to inability to live alone
- History of successful coping skills
- Imminent or recent change in life status
- Occurrence of a significant life event within past 3 months
- Recent death of loved one(s) or series of deaths of significant others
- Anxiety
- Depression
- Health problems

Assessment Tools and Instruments (see Appendix I)

Consider administering the:

1. Brief Psychiatric Rating Scale
2. Geriatric Depression Scale
3. Global Assessment of Functioning Scale
4. Mini-Mental Status Examination
5. Social Dysfunction Rating Scale
6. Spiritual Perspectives Clinical Scale
7. Suicide Risk Assessment Tool
8. TRIADS

PROBLEM LIST

- Communication, Impaired Verbal
- Grieving, Anticipatory and Dysfunctional
- Hopelessness
- Mobility, Impaired Physical
- Nutrition, Altered
- Pain, Chronic
- Powerlessness
- Relocation Stress Syndrome
- Self-Care Deficit (specify)
- Sensory/Perceptual Alterations (specify)
- Sexuality Patterns, Altered
- Sleep Pattern Disturbance
- Social Interaction, Impaired
- Social Isolation
- Spiritual Distress
- Thought Process, Altered
- Violence, Risk for, Self-Directed or Directed at Others

PROBLEM MANAGEMENT

Prevention, Maintenance, and Restorative Interventions

R Assess the pt by these indicators to help plan changes and feelings toward relocation or retirement:

- Life history
- Economic status
- Financial status
- Medical Insurance
- Advance directives
- Power of attorney
- Beliefs and values
- Cultural issues
- Recent changes in medical or psychiatric status
- Attitude toward move
- Reason for relocation
- Previous living situations
- Previous coping skills and successes
- Social attachments
- Marital status
- Loss of significant other(s)
- Children, number, location, relationship
- Significant others or relatives, type, location, relationship
- Family traditions and expectations
- Neurologic, sensory, or psychological impairment
- Use of adaptive equipment
- Functional and IADLs
- Functional ability

Medication Management

Antidepressants are rarely used in the treatment of an adjustment disorder. If the pt does not return to previous functioning within a reasonable time, the pt should be evaluated for further complications.

NURSING MANAGEMENT

Nursing Interventions and Rationales
✩ Behavioral

- Give positive feedback about expressing feelings, especially negative ones. *Feedback shows acceptance of feelings related to retirement or relocation and helps the pt see that negative feelings are normal.*
- Teach the pt the problem-solving process, to identify the problem, examine and weigh alternatives, and choose the best approach. *This shows that a logical process for problem-solving works.*
- Instruct the pt in evaluating success or failure of a new approach to _____ and how to select others until pt is satisfied with the results. *This assists the pt in making decisions that do not have to be perfect the first time.*

♡ Emotional

- Encourage the pt to express fears about relocation and possible scenarios that could happen and ways to solve fears. *This decreases fear of the unknown.*

△ Cognitive

- Assist the pt to make a list of the aspects of the relocation that he or she likes and dislikes, then discuss. *A list helps the pt view change objectively with positive and negative aspects.*
- Explore with the pt things to do to make the change more positive. *This focuses on the change that is occurring and the positive alternatives.*
- Avoid giving specific directions to the pt on ways to handle change (let the pt develop own answers). *This makes the pt responsible and allows the pt to develop his or her own suggestions.*

⊐ Physical

- Instruct the pt in establishing a routine activity structure. *This assists in transition to a new life-style.*

◯ Social

- Assist the pt in working with the f/c to get their help in dealing with aspects of life change. *This creates a better chance for success and investment in the change from all involved.*

R

- Assist the p/f/c to identify and anticipate any further changes and ways to deal with further changes before they happen. *Anticipation decreases anxiety and allows planning for future changes.*
- Encourage the p/f/c to visit the new location before the change. *This permits preparation for a move.*

✦ Spiritual

- Assist the pt in writing a list of strengths and limitations and problems in dealing with change. *This assesses previous coping skills and recognizes strengths in problem-solving.*
- Assist the pt to plan what belongings will be taken to the new location and to understand importance of establishing personal space and boundaries. *This elicits a sense of belonging.*

Nursing Goals

- To identify the pt's feelings and thoughts about life change regarding relocation and retirement problems
- To maintain communication between the p/f/c and other treatment team members

Patient Goals

- The pt will exhibit fewer signs of anxiety, anger, depressive mood, or social withdrawal.
- The pt will collaborate with the f/c to make adequate and agreeable plans for relocation.
- The pt will express an understanding of the reasons for relocation.
- The pt will express increased acceptance of a plan for relocation.
- The pt will demonstrate integration of change into daily functioning.

Patient and Family/Caregiver Outcomes

The patient will:

- Discuss relocation and list options regarding living arrangements by _____ (date)
- Discuss the situation with family members and provider without becoming enraged or withdrawn within _____ (weeks)
- Express an understanding of need for relocation as demonstrated by _____ within _____ (weeks)
- Express satisfaction with relocation plans as demonstrated by _____ within _____ (weeks)
- Demonstrate ability to solve problems effectively (specify) _____ within _____ (weeks)
- Demonstrate integration of change into day-to-day functioning (specify) _____ by _____ (date)

- Identify, list, and discuss difficulties of current life change or stress within _____ (weeks)
- Identify aspects of life still under his or her control and accept that some areas are out of his or her control as demonstrated by _____ within _____ (weeks)

The family/caregiver will:

- Participate in discussions about relocation as demonstrated by _____ within _____ (weeks)
- Initiate a process to prepare for relocation as demonstrated by _____ within _____ (weeks)

RESOURCES AND INFORMATION

1. Aging Network Services
   4400 East West Highway
   Suite 907
   Bethesda, MD 20014
   301-986-1608
2. Children of Aging Parents
   Woodbourne Office Campus
   Suite 302-A
   1609 Woodbourne Road
   Levittown, PA 19057
   215-945-6900
3. Family Caregiver (send a large, self-addressed, stamped envelope for information on working with older adults)
   PO Box 15329
   Stamford, CT 06901
4. National Academy of Elder Law Attorneys (send a stamped, self-addressed envelop for "Questions and Answers When Looking for an Elder Law Attorney")
   655 North Alvernon
   Room 108
   Tucson, AZ 85711
5. National Council on Aging (NCOA)
   409 Third Street, SW
   2nd floor
   Washington, DC 20024
   202-479-1200
6. National Institute on Aging (NIA)
   Public Information Office, Building 31
   Room 5C27
   31 Center Drive, MSC 2292
   Bethesda, MD 20892-2292
   301-496-1752
7. American Association for Retired Persons (AARP)
   1909 K Street, NW
   Washington, DC 20049

R

REFERENCES

Busse, E. W., & Blazer, D. G. (1989). *Geriatric psychiatry.* Washington, DC: American Psychiatric Press.

Hogstel, M. O. (1990). *Geropsychiatric nursing.* St. Louis: Mosby-Yearbook.

U.S. Senate Special Committee on Aging. (1987–1988). *Aging America: Trends and projections.* Washington, DC: Department of Health and Human Services.

S

Self-Mutilation

PROBLEM DESCRIPTION

Self-mutilation or self-inflicted injury is the act of deliberate harm to self, severe enough to cause tissue damage, without being a life-threatening event. Forms of self-mutilation include cutting and burning the skin, picking at wounds, chewing fingers, and banging or hitting the head and limbs.

An individual experiencing depression, anxiety, increased tension, anger, loneliness, or rejection and abandonment may perceive these feelings as personal threats that can lead to physical self-mutilation and damage. When the pt is not able to verbally express these feelings, it is known as alexithymia. Self-mutilation provides a grounding in reality; self-injury overcomes feelings of depersonalization. Pts describe self-mutilation as psychological relief that produces calmness and relaxation (Pattison & Kahan, 1983), which enables the individual to reconnect to the body and ego boundary.

Persons with a borderline personality disorder are most prone toward self-injurious behaviors. Inadequate ego development, intense and chaotic relationships, and impulsive behaviors affect the pt with a borderline personality disorder and contribute to feelings that lead to self-mutilation. The person who self-mutilates often has a history of being neglected and sexually and physically abused as a child (Barstow, 1995). Treatment of the pt with a borderline personality disorder is difficult. Traditional therapeutic approaches, which include empathy, warmth, and nurturing, are not effective. A structured, limit-setting, contracted relationship provides clear relationship boundaries and establishes a mutually agreeable process to set and achieve goals. Establishing clear expectations and outcomes assists the pt to develop more adaptive coping skills and decreases the need for self-mutilation (Dyckoff, Goldstein, & Schacht-Levine, 1996).

PROBLEM IDENTIFICATION

Characteristics and Observable Behaviors

- Feelings of worthlessness or hopelessness
- Inability to to solve problems
- Self-destructive behaviors (eg, incisions, scars, lesions, etc)

- Difficulty identifying and expressing emotions
- Frequent use of critical or derogatory remarks against self
- Difficulty accepting positive reinforcement
- Anxiety
- Lack of trust
- Dysfunctional grieving
- Angry or hostile feelings
- Feelings of guilt
- Lack of eye contact
- Inappropriate responses

Factors Related to the Problem

- Withdrawn behavior, social isolation, and poor support system
- Poor self-esteem, sense of identity, and self-image
- Sleep disturbance
- Depression
- Substance use
- Unstable interpersonal relationships
- Dysfunctional family dynamics
- Fatigue
- Post-traumatic stress
- History of physical, sexual, or emotional abuse
- History of using self-mutilation or injury as coping mechanism
- Inability to cope with increased stress
- Psychotic disorder
- Lability of affect
- Real or perceived loss
- Real or perceived crisis in life situations or relationships
- Diagnosis of borderline personality disorder

Assessment Tools and Instruments (see Appendix I)

Consider administering the:

1. Beck Depression Inventory
2. Brief Psychiatric Rating Scale
3. Brief Psychiatric Schizophrenia Rating Scale
4. Geriatric Depression Scale
5. Mini-Mental State Examination
6. Modified Overt Aggression Scale
7. Spiritual Perspective Clinical Scale
8. Suicide Risk Assessment Tool

PROBLEM LIST

- Body Image Disturbance
- Communication, Impaired Verbal

- Community Coping, Ineffective
- Decisional Conflict
- Fatigue
- Grieving, Anticipatory
- Grieving, Dysfunctional
- Hopelessness
- Infection, Risk for
- Nutrition, Altered: Less than Body Requirements
- Nutrition, Altered: More than Body Requirements
- Parenting, Altered
- Parenting, Risk for Altered
- Personal Identity Disturbance
- Post-Trauma Response
- Powerlessness
- Self-Care Deficit, Bathing/Hygiene
- Self-Care Deficit, Feeding
- Self-Mutilation, Risk for
- Sexuality Patterns, Altered
- Skin Integrity, Impaired
- Skin Integrity, Risk for Impaired
- Sleep Pattern Disturbance
- Social Interaction, Impaired
- Social Isolation
- Spiritual Distress
- Thought Processes, Altered
- Trauma, Risk for
- Violence, Risk for, Self-Directed or Directed at Others

PROBLEM MANAGEMENT

Preventive, Maintenance, and Restorative Interventions

- Assess the pt for evidence of previous self-mutilation and assist pt in determining and distinguishing the causes or precipitating factors before the act.
- Assess the pt's mental status and for depression, anxiety, and possible suicidal behaviors.
- Assess the pt's level of understanding about the relationship between self-mutilation and the difficulty expressing feelings.
- Teach the f/c that caring for a pt who exhibits self-mutilating behaviors is difficult and engenders negative feelings and reactions.
- Teach the f/c to cope with the stress of a pt who exhibits self-mutilating behaviors.

Medication Management

No specifically designated medication is prescribed to treat self-mutilation behaviors. Tranquilizing medications such as anxiolytics or antipsychotics may have a calming effect. Favazza (1989) noted that when naloxone HCl (Naloxone), which is an opioid blocker, was administered to pts who are developmentally delayed the incidence of self-mutilation injury was significantly decreased.

NURSING MANAGEMENT

Nursing Interventions and Rationales

☆ Behavioral

- Contract with the pt not to self-mutilate. *This assists the pt in understanding the pt's own responsibility for safety and as a means to follow through with treatment.*
- Instruct f/c that if the pt enters into a dissociative state or is hallucinating that they need to decrease stimuli, remove unsafe materials, remain with the pt, and provide reassurance. *These measures calm and reorient the pt.*
- Develop a behavior modification program with the pt that rewards self-control. *This encourages and reinforces self-control and minimizes or prevents self-mutilation.*

♡ Emotional

- Assist the pt to develop alternatives to reduce feelings related to self-mutilation and to plan for ways to implement strategies. *Such strategies help in having set plans in place during times of emotional crisis.*
- Assist the pt to discuss the secondary gains related to self-mutilation and alternatives for recognition. *Discussion helps the pt understand the dynamics of the negative rewards.*
- Assist the pt to identify feelings related to emotional pain and find ways to positively express emotional pain. *These measures keep the pt from acting impulsively and helps the pt learn to express true feelings.*

△ Cognitive

- Teach the pt cognitive techniques and adaptive coping mechanisms for managing the feelings related to self-mutilation. *These techniques provide basic skills to deal with difficult feelings before or when they occur.*
- Teach p/f/c coping techniques the pt will use to prevent or minimize self-mutilative behavior. *This assists f/c to encourage the pt to practice and use coping mechanisms before or during self-injurious behavior.*
- Teach p/f/c to recognize behaviors that are evident when self-mutilation becomes suicidal and steps to take. *Such intervention in crisis situations helps to prevent self-harm.*

◻ Physical

- Assist the pt to care for injuries without conveying judgment. *This helps pt identify a cause-and-effect relationship of self-injurious actions and consequences.*
- Observe and care for wounds or mutilated sites. *Such care maintains skin integrity and reduces inflammation and infection.*

⬭ Social

- Instruct the pt to identify plans to stop self-mutilative acts and call for help. *This helps the pt recognize that support systems are available and should be used.*
- Encourage the pt to contact support systems to be available during times of stress when self-mutilative behaviors are possible or imminent. *This helps the pt to recognize stressors, when to call for support and help, and prevents or minimizes self-mutilation.*

✴ Spiritual

- Assist the pt to accept and stop blaming events and people in the past as justification for engaging in self-mutilative behavior and assume responsibility for what is happening now. *This promotes responsibility for the self, life, and the future.*
- Teach the p/f/c that the overall goal in preventing self-mutilative behaviors is to assist the pt in maintaining the highest possible degree of autonomy and self-responsibility. *This improves self-esteem, enhances self-worth, and decreases self-injury.*
- Encourage the pt to verbalize recognition that the pt is worthwhile and has significance. *This reduces the need for self-mutilation as the only way to feel and validate one's existence.*

Nursing Goals

- To assist the pt to decrease self-mutilative behaviors
- To assist the pt to decrease obsessive thoughts about harming self
- To teach the pt to express emotional pain appropriately
- To assist the pt to develop insight and increase ability to express emotional pain in a healthy manner

Patient Goals

- The pt will develop coping skills to replace self-mutilative behaviors.
- The pt will develop ways to express anger verbally and reduce the incidence of self-mutilation.

Patient and Family/Caregiver Outcomes

The patient and family/caregiver will:

- Identify and demonstrate positive coping mechanisms to deal with self-mutilative behaviors as demonstrated by _____ within _____ weeks
- Maintain anxiety at a manageable level at which the pt will not feel the need for self-mutilation by _____ (date)
- Plan and rehearse methods for stopping self-mutilation and focus instead on feelings and emotions by _____ (date)

RESOURCES AND INFORMATION

1. See Resources and Information for Abusive Behaviors.
2. Eating Abuse Disorders Hotline: 1-800-888-4673
3. National Suicide Intervention and Prevention Hotline: 1-800-274-2995
4. American Psychological Association (APA; free publications: "Good Mental Health" and "Understanding Stress")
   750 First Street, NE
   Washington, DC 20002
   202-336-5500
   1-800-296-0272
5. Mental Illness Foundation
   7 Penn Plaza
   Suite 222
   New York, NY 10001
   212-629-0755
6. National Alliance For the Mentally Ill (NAMI)
   2101 Wilson Boulevard
   Suite 302
   Arlington, VA 22201
   703-524-7600
   Fax: 703-524-9094
7. National Institute of Mental Health (NIMH)
   Information and Inquiries Branch
   Office of Scientific Information
   5600 Fishers Lane
   Room 7C02
   Rockville, MD 20857
   301-443-4513
8. Survivors of Incest Anonymous, Inc. (SIA)
   PO Box 21817
   Baltimore, MD 21222
   410-433-2365
9. Incest Survivors Helpline: 1-800-551-0008

REFERENCES

Barstow, D. (1995). Self-injury and self-mutilation: Nursing approaches. *Journal of Psychosocial Nursing and Mental Health Services, 33*, 19–22.

Dyckoff, D., Goldstein, L., & Schacht-Levine, L. (1996). The investigation of behavioral contracting in patients with borderline personality disorder. *Journal of the American Psychiatric Nurses Association, 2*(3), 71–76.

Favazza, A. R. (1989). Why patients mutilate themselves. *Hospital and Community Psychiatry, 40*, 137–145.

Pattison, E., & Kahan, J. (1983). The deliberate self-harm syndrome. *American Journal of Psychiatry, 140*, 867–872.

Self-Neglect (See Activities of Daily Living Problems; Aging; Apathy; Body Image Problems and Behaviors; Dementias; Depression and Depressive Behaviors; Psychosis; and Substance Abuse Problems)

Sexual Problems

PROBLEM DESCRIPTION

Sexual problems refer to the presence of physiologic or emotional factors that can alter sexual behavior and may lead to persistent or recurrent distress and a sense of conflict. Sexual problems can be viewed by the pt as unsatisfying, unrewarding, inadequate, or socially inappropriate. The perception or reality of sexual problems can have many causes, depending on age, maturational situation, gender, physical and mental health status, marital status, physical trauma, sexual abuse, and any other number of factors.

Sexual dysfunctions are disorders that compromise sexual activity. Sexual activity can be described through the sexual response cycle. The four phases of the sexual response cycle are:

1. Desire phase
2. Excitement or arousal phase
3. Orgasm phase
4. Resolution phase

Sexual dysfunction and disorders can occur in relation to the sexual response cycle and the activity in each phase.

- Sexual desire disorders stop the sexual response from starting and an individual with problems in this phase has little or no sexual desire or an aversion to sexual contacts.
- Sexual arousal disorders occur at the excitement phase and cause problems such as loss of erection in men and lack of vaginal lubrication in women.
- Orgasm disorders stop the orgasmic process and produce the inability to achieve orgasm, and sometimes in men, the problem of premature ejaculation.
- Sexual pain disorders stop the sexual response cycle at any phase and cause genital pain (dyspareunia) before, during, or after sexual intercourse, or involuntary spasms of the outer third of the vagina (vaginismus).

Sexual disorders define the various types of paraphilias that distinguish the individual nature of sexual interest and intensity of sexual drive. A paraphilia is a sexual disorder in which unusual or bizarre acts or fantasies are required for sexual arousal.

The paraphilias identify various behaviors that are repetitive or preferred sexual acts and fantasies, which are:

1.   Behaviors involving humans and nonhuman objects
2.   Behaviors involving real or simulated suffering
3.   Humiliation with nonconsenting partners

Almost all of those who engage in paraphilias are heterosexual men, many of whom developed their particular paraphilia before the age of 18.

The types of paraphilias include:

- Exhibitionism—exposure of genitals to strangers
- Fetishism—use of nonliving objects such as undergarments
- Frotteurism—touching or rubbing against a nonconsenting person
- Pedophilia—sexual activity with a prepubescent child
- Masochism—the act (real or simulated) of being humiliated, beaten, bound, or made to suffer
- Sadism—inflicting psychological or physical suffering or humiliation on another person
- Transvestite fetishism—cross-dressing (the wearing of women's clothes almost exclusively by heterosexual men)
- Voyeurism—the act of observing unsuspecting people who are naked, disrobing, or engaged in sexual activity

Paraphilias not otherwise specified:

- Telephone scatologia—the desire to place obscene telephone calls
- Necrophilia—sexual attraction to corpses
- Partialism—exclusive sexual focus on parts of the body
- Zoophilia—sexual attraction to animals
- Coprophilia—sexual focus on feces
- Klismaphilia—sexual focus on enemas
- Urophilia—sexual focus on urine

(American Psychiatric Association, 1994)

No matter the cause, a thorough sexual assessment should be obtained to determine physical, emotional, and sexual history; perceived or real problems; and cultural or religious beliefs that may affect the pt's sexual problems.

S

PROBLEM IDENTIFICATION

Characteristics and Observable Behaviors

- Sexual obsessions; chronic masturbation; repeated and obsessive telephone sex; obsessive use of pornography; repeated visits to massage parlors or adult bookstores; persistent violent sexual fantasies; cross-dressing
- Participation in sexual activities that can place the pt or others at serious emotional, medical, or legal risk, such as solicitation of prostitutes; exchange of sexual favors for money; sexual affairs; sexual addiction; anonymous sexual encounters in

public places; exhibitionism; voyeurism; use of drugs during sexual activity; rape and incest; pedophilia; fetishism; stalking; knowing and repeated participation in unsafe sex; and self-erotic asphyxiation

- Inappropriate and provocative sexual comments; inappropriate and excessive physical closeness and touching with peers and others; and inability to adapt sexual behavior to social norms
- General concern about sexual functioning, such as verbalization of problems regarding sexual functioning; questioning of sexual practices; and confusion about the expression of sexual desires
- Sex role conflict or dissatisfaction and negative attitude toward sexuality
- Real or perceived limitations of sexual functioning imposed by disease or treatment of disease
- Altered interpersonal relationships
- Frustration and anger if sexuality is hindered
- Premature or retarded ejaculation and inhibited orgasm
- Reduced sexual pleasure or satisfaction; lack of sexual pleasure or satisfaction; impotence; or painful coitus
- Absence of desire or diminished sexual desire for one's sexual partner
- Disregard for the welfare of the other person, including aggression, violence, coercion, physical force, injury, psychological degradation, or sex with a minor or others unable to give and understand consent
- Anxiety
- Feelings of tension, helplessness, hopelessness, inadequacy, uncertainty, or unmet needs
- Difficulty discussing sexuality
- Disorientation about sense of self
- Altered role performance or poor perception of reality associated with psychological distress

Factors Related to the Problem

- Altered body structure or function from chronic illness; disease processes, especially cancer, diabetes mellitus, epilepsy, multiple sclerosis, and heart disease; injury; chromosomal and genetic factors; congenital anomalies; altered hormonal functioning; and medical treatment-related factors such as surgery, radiation, or medications
- Fatigue
- Physical abuse
- Pain due to organic or psychogenic causes
- Pregnancy and childbirth
- Aging
- Mental illness and psychosis
- Psychosocial issues such as sexual abuse; rape; incest; sexual trauma; negative body image; ambivalence about sexual behavior; overly critical self-appraisal of sexual functioning; performance anxiety; fear of pregnancy; fear of HIV, AIDS, or other STDs; or fear of intimacy
- Lack of privacy

- Lack of knowledge, inadequate sexual techniques, poor communication skills, or ineffective role models
- Lack of sexual partner or significant other, relationship problems with significant other, or pressure from partner
- Unrealistic expectations, values conflict, spiritual factors, religious beliefs, or cultural factors

Assessment Tools and Instruments (see Appendix I)

Consider administering the:

1. Beck Depression Inventory
2. Brief Psychiatric Rating Scale
3. Brief Psychiatric Schizophrenia Rating Scale
4. Geriatric Depression Scale
5. Mini-Mental Status Examination
6. Pain Assessment Tool
7. Sheehan Patient Rated Anxiety Scale
8. Social Dysfunction Rating Scale
9. TRIADS Assessment Tool

PROBLEM LIST

- Body Image Disturbance
- Communication, Impaired Verbal
- Community Coping, Ineffective
- Decisional Conflict
- Diversional Activity Deficit
- Fatigue
- Grieving, Anticipatory
- Grieving, Dysfunctional
- Hopelessness
- Infection, Risk for
- Personal Identity Disturbance
- Post-Trauma Response
- Powerlessness
- Rape-Trauma Syndrome
- Rape-Trauma Syndrome: Compound Reaction
- Rape-Trauma Syndrome: Silent Reaction
- Self-Mutilation, Risk for
- Sexual Dysfunction
- Sexuality Patterns, Altered
- Social Interaction, Impaired
- Social Isolation
- Spiritual Distress
- Thought Processes, Altered

PROBLEM MANAGEMENT

Prevention, Maintenance, and Restorative Interventions

- When counseling the pt with sexual problems, reassure pt that everything said is confidential; pt is believed, not to blame, and can overcome feelings of shame; encourage pt's self-disclosure.
- Educate the pt about the causes of sexual problems and methods to improve or accommodate changes to improve sexual satisfaction and intimate relationships.

- Educate pt that sexual functioning may be adversely affected if one is unable to maintain stable relationships, deal with stress, or has impaired reality.
- Conduct a sexual assessment to determine the sexual problems, physiologic functions, and behavioral, emotional, social and cultural, and spiritual beliefs of sexuality to determine physical problems and the pt's perception of the problem.

Medication Management

Hormones such as testosterone and estrogen may be given alone or in combination to increase sexual drive or lubrication (in women). Research has shown that medroxyprogesterone acetate (Depo-Provera) in sufficient quantity decreases sexual urges and controls sexual behaviors (Berlin, 1985). Side effects or adverse reactions of some medications can cause sexual problems. If this occurs, notify the prescriber. Alcohol and some drugs can cause problems with arousal and performance.

NURSING MANAGEMENT

Nursing Interventions and Rationales

✬ Behavioral

- Set limits on sexual acting-out behaviors. *Limits help the pt to establish control of sexual behavior.*
- Ignore inappropriate sexual comments or innuendoes. *This decreases negative sexual behaviors.*

♡ Emotional

- Encourage the pt to verbalize sexual problems in a nonthreatening manner. *This helps the pt overcome feelings of embarrassment.*
- Provide emotional support for the pt and the pt's significant other. *Such support conveys concern and acceptance.*

◮ Cognitive

- Educate the pt about illness and sexuality and answer specific questions. *This encourages the pt to understand limitations and clarifies misconceptions.*
- Instruct the pt regarding the interaction between depression and sexual desire. *This assists the pt to understand the correlation and decreases feelings of guilt and worthlessness.*
- Educate the pt that some sexually inappropriate or dangerous behaviors are the result of delusional thought systems and that maintaining medication compliance with neuroleptic medications is necessary. *Compliance decreases the inappropriate behaviors and resolves or minimizes the delusions.*

▢ Physical

- Educate the pt and significant other about alternative methods of sexual expression. *This promotes intimacy.*

- Discuss the need for sexual responsibility and safety by using a condom. *Such discussion increases awareness of HIV, AIDS, and other STDs.*

◐ Social

- Encourage the pt to discuss concerns with significant other. *This assists in sharing concerns and improves relationship.*
- Confront the pt about inappropriate sexual behaviors. *This increases awareness about the effect on others and encourages responsibility.*
- Encourage the pt to express self sexually in socially acceptable ways. *This promotes appropriate interactions and behavior.*

✱ Spiritual

- Encourage the pt to identify values and beliefs about sexual problems. *Such identification assists in planning meaningful interventions.*
- Encourage the pt to find an appropriate personal mentor. *This allows pt to discuss sexual choices and outcomes.*
- Support the pt's decisions regarding sexual choices. *Support validates the pt's values and sexuality.*
- Support and assist the pt in seeking a support group. *This encourages a sense of belonging to a group, decreases isolation, and enhances social relationships.*

Nursing Goals

- To build a trusting relationship in which sexual problems will be shared by the pt
- To decrease the pt's anxiety related to sexual functioning and problems
- To provide an assessment and education to the pt related to sexual problems
- To promote the pt's appropriate expression of sexual feelings
- To promote pt learning about changes in sexuality and integrating new strategies for sexual satisfaction and intimacy

Patient Goals

- The pt will regain sexual desire with recovery from depression.
- The pt will reestablish sexual functioning without further sexual or other problems.
- The pt will develop and maintain a positive attitude about sexuality and sexual performance.
- The pt will communicate to significant other about sexual relationship.
- The pt will refrain from sexual behaviors that are emotionally, legally, or medically dangerous.

Patient and Family/Caregiver Outcomes

The patient or family/caregiver will:

- Acknowledge problems in sexual functioning and verbalize methods to adjust or change as demonstrated by _____ within _____ weeks

- Identify stressors that contribute to the sexual problem and methods to correct them as demonstrated by _____ within _____ weeks
- Identify options of sexual expression and communication with the significant other as demonstrated by _____ within _____ weeks
- Report decreased anxiety about sexual functioning as demonstrated by _____ within _____ weeks
- Express feelings about decrease in sexual desire with sexual partner(s) as demonstrated by _____ within _____ weeks
- Explore underlying feelings for sexual acting-out behaviors and demonstrate ways to meet sexual needs in a socially appropriate manner as demonstrated by _____ within _____ weeks

RESOURCES AND INFORMATION

1. Masters and Johnson Institute
   24 South Kings Highway
   St. Louis, MO 63108
   314-361-2377
2. The National Institute for the Prevention and Treatment of Sexual Trauma
   104 East Biddle Street
   Baltimore, MD 21202
   410-955-6292 or 410-539-1661
3. Sexual Disorders Clinic at Johns Hopkins Hospital
   Johns Hopkins Hospital, Meyer 4-181
   600 North Wolfe Street
   Baltimore, MD 21205
   410-955-6292 or 410-539-1661
4. Survivors of Incest Anonymous, Inc. (SIA)
   PO Box 21817
   Baltimore, MD 21222
   410-433-2365
5. Sex Information and Education Council of the United States (SIECUS)
   130 West 42nd Street
   Suite 2500
   New York, NY 10036
   212-819-9770
   Fax: 212-819-9776
6. Incest Survivors Helpline: 1-800-551-0008
7. STDs/VD Helpline: 1-800-227-8922
8. VD Hotline: 1-800-523-1885
9. National Coalition Against Pornography: 513-521-6227
10. American Indian AIDS Institute: 415-626-7639
11. AIDS Hotline: 1-800-545-2437
12. AIDS Information: 1-800-551-2728
13. Centers for Disease Control and Prevention (for books, articles, pamphlets, resources, and information)

S

National Clearing House
PO Box 6003
Rockville, MD 20849-6003
1-800-458-5231

REFERENCES

American Psychiatric Association. (1994). *Diagnostic and statistical manual of mental disorders* (4th ed.). Washington, DC: Author.

Berlin, F. S. (1985). Pedophilia: Medical castration and group counseling sessions help to modify this type of sexual behavior.

Medical Aspects of Human Sexuality, 19(8), 79–88.

Masters, W. H., & Johnson, V. E. (1970). *Human sexual inadequacy.* Boston: Little, Brown.

Sleep Problems

PROBLEM DESCRIPTION

Sleep is a natural periodic state of consciousness during which the powers of the body are restored. When the sleep–wake cycle is interrupted from a physical or emotional influence, sleep is interrupted. The normal sleep cycle lasts about 90 minutes and is repeated four to six times a night. The cycle includes an REM phase and non-REM sleep. Brain waves characterize the different cycles. REM sleep is a rapid side-to-side movement of the eyes with shallow, mixed-frequency brain waves. Non-REM sleep, also called quiet or light sleep, has no rapid eye movements and is represented by slow brain waves. In younger, healthy individuals about 2% to 5% of sleep is spent in transitional sleep, 45% to 55% in light sleep, 13% to 23% in deep sleep, and 20% to 25% in REM sleep (American Nurses Association, 1996).

Sleep restores the mind and body, and without a proper balance, sleep disorders occur. Sleep disorders and sleep disturbances affect as many as one-third of all adults in the United States (American Nurses Association, 1996).

The three common sleep disorders are:

1. Sleep apnea—characterized by chronic heavy snoring concurrent with intervals of not breathing and an absence of air flow for 10 seconds or longer, daytime sleepiness, waking up tired and unrefreshed, and serious morning headaches
2. Narcolepsy—characterized by "sleep attacks" (unexpected falling asleep), cataplexy (sudden loss of muscle tone), sleep paralysis (temporary paralysis of muscles when falling asleep or waking), hypnagogic hallucinations (vivid sensory experiences), or fragmented sleep
3. Insomnia—characterized by inadequate, insufficient, or nonrestorative sleep; can be the result of personal or environmental factors or secondary to medical, psychiatric, or medication effects

Sleep problems can be treated with medications and therapeutic interventions.

PROBLEM IDENTIFICATION

Characteristics and Observable Behaviors

- Early or late awakening
- Difficulty falling asleep, interrupted sleep, or unrefreshing sleep
- Chronic fatigue
- Extreme mood changes
- Obesity, poor nutrition, and lack of exercise
- Changes in behavior or performance, including disorientation, increased irritability, lethargy, listlessness, restlessness, inability to concentrate, and anxiety
- Signs of sleep deprivation: expressionless face, frequent yawning, dark circles under eyes, mild fleeting nystagmus, ptosis of the eyelids, thick speech with mispronunciations and incorrect use of words, and slight hand tremor
- Nightmares and night terrors
- Preoccupation with not obtaining restful sleep

Factors Related to the Problem

- Mental illness
- Increased stress
- Use of prescription or over-the-counter drugs or alcohol to obtain restful sleep
- Excessive use of caffeine products
- Neurologic or physical problems or effects of medications that disrupt the sleep pattern
- Lack of an identifiable psychosocial stressor or physiologic reason for sleep disturbance
- Fear, nervousness, and anxiety
- Feelings of guilt
- Delirium, hallucinations, and delusions
- Inability to exclude unwanted thoughts from the mind
- Boredom
- Discomfort and pain
- Depression
- Failure of coping mechanisms

Assessment Tools and Interventions (see Appendix I)

Consider administering the:

1. Beck Depression Inventory
2. Geriatric Depression Scale
3. Mini-Mental State Examination
4. Pain Assessment Tool

PROBLEM LIST

- Activity Intolerance
- Activity Intolerance, Risk for
- Body Image Disturbance
- Breathing Pattern, Ineffective
- Caregiver Role Strain
- Caregiver Role Strain, Risk for
- Communication, Impaired Verbal
- Fatigue
- Hopelessness
- Memory, Impaired
- Powerlessness

- Self-Care Deficit, Bathing/Hygiene
- Self-Care Deficit, Dressing/Grooming
- Self-Care Deficit, Feeding
- Self-Care Deficit, Toileting
- Sleep Pattern Disturbance
- Social Interaction, Impaired
- Social Isolation
- Spiritual Distress
- Thought Processes, Altered

PROBLEM MANAGEMENT

Prevention, Maintenance, and Restorative Interventions

- Educate the pt regarding tolerance to or withdrawal from drugs that are CNS depressants because they may cause insomnia.
- Instruct the pt that alcohol should not be used as a sleep aid because of the potential for abuse and because it causes sleep disturbances.
- Instruct the pt to avoid caffeine or other stimulants late in the day because they have a tendency to keep people awake.
- Encourage the pt with a sleep disorder to try and stay awake during daylight hours and to sleep only at night to adjust the circadian rhythm.
- Instruct the pt that exercising in the late afternoon or early evening helps induce sleep, but not to exercise or engage in activity too late in the evening, which can stimulate the body and make it difficult for the pt to relax and go to sleep.
- Instruct the pt to use the bedroom only for sleeping, and not watching television or other activities.
- Instruct pts that if they go to sleep and then wake early, or if they have trouble going to sleep, to get up and move to another room, to do something relaxing, and when again tired to go back to bed to condition the whole person to use the bed and bedroom only for sleeping.
- Teach the pt to establish a daily routine of going to bed and awakening at the same time to establish a sleep–wake cycle and to induce a sleepy feeling every night at the same time.
- Instruct the pt in completing a 2-week sleep diary, noting if medications or other agents were taken, recording how many hours were slept, rating the quality of sleep and the level of daytime alertness, noting any naps, and rating mood.

S

Medication Management

Medications used in the treatment of sleep problems include benzodiazepines, sedating antidepressants, barbiturates and barbiturate-like drugs, imidazopyridines, and over-the-counter products. The ideal hypnotic provides rapid GI absorption and optimal brain concentration. Sleeping medications should be used in their lowest possible dose and gradually decreased over a few days when no longer needed.

Medications for sleep can cause dependence and impair cognitive functioning. Alcohol potentiates medications and could possibly cause an overdose. Sleep medications can have a paradoxical reaction in older adults and should be given with caution, after careful assessment.

NURSING MANAGEMENT

Nursing Interventions and Rationales

☆ Behavioral

- Monitor the pt's sleep schedule. *Monitoring determines the sleep–wake cycle and allows planning for interventions.*
- Instruct the pt to structure a daily routine. *A consistent routine promotes regular sleep patterns.*
- Encourage the p/f/c to institute bedtime rituals such as reading a book, taking a hot bath, or listening to soft music. *Rituals stimulate and encourage sleep.*
- Discourage the pt from taking daytime naps, to limit fluids 3 hours before bedtime, and to empty the bladder before bed. *These measures improve the chances for a good night's sleep.*

♡ Emotional

- Encourage the pt to express feelings such as guilt, anxiety, or stress. *This allows planning for interventions and prevents negative emotions from interrupting sleep.*
- Assist the pt to express feelings that may be related to the sleep problem. *Such expression decreases stress and tension that may be interfering with the sleep–wake cycle.*
- Encourage the pt to limit distracting thoughts for a designated time during the day. *This reduces the amount of time spent ruminating before bedtime.*

△ Cognitive

- Discuss with the p/f/c the reasons for the pt's sleep disturbances. *This helps to determine the p/f/c's perceptions of the sleep problem.*
- Teach the p/f/c about sleep and sleep problems. *This enhances awareness of the phenomenon of sleep.*

☐ Physical

- Identify any food allergies the pt has and medications taken that can cause sleeplessness or alertness. *This increases awareness of the sleep problem and permits effective intervention.*

- Teach the p/f/c that medications for sleep disorders can have a paradoxical reaction in older adults and cause them to be awake instead of asleep. *This heightens the awareness and practice of using nonpharmacologic methods of reducing sleep problems.*

⬭ Social

- Instruct the p/f/c to consistently balance solitude and social time. *A regular, life pattern will dovetail with the desired sleep–wake cycle.*
- Encourage the pt to improve relationships with the f/c and friends. *This decreases stress, increases satisfying relationships with others, and eliminates possible stressors that may interrupt the pt's sleep–wake cycle.*
- Instruct the p/f/c to limit social visits in the evening hours. *This decreases stimulation and encourages rest and relaxation, which will enhance sleep.*

✴ Spiritual

- Discuss with the pt the ability to take the time while lying awake, to review life processes, or to plan for a future goal. *This uses the time to focus on something other than not being able to fall asleep.*
- Encourage the pt to express any concerns regarding sleep preparation and rituals. *This helps to determine if the pt has any spiritual barriers to restful sleep.*
- Encourage the pt to select meditative readings for bedtime. *This shifts focus from disturbing or distracting thoughts.*

Nursing Goals

- To promote the pt's development of a bedtime routine
- To facilitate relaxation and alternative methods for stress reduction and sleep induction with the pt
- To increase the quantity, quality, and performance of the pt's sleep

Patient Goals

- The pt will develop an age-appropriate sleep pattern.
- The pt will report restful sleep with few interruptions.
- The pt will decrease the level of anxiety over the loss and quality of sleep.
- The pt will develop comfort measures to promote sleep.

Patient and Family/Caregiver Outcomes

The patient or family/caregiver will:

- Fall asleep within at least 30 minutes of a predetermined bedtime by _____ (date)
- Sleep an adequate number of hours each night (specify) _____ by _____ (date)
- Self-report feeling relaxed, awake, and having no anxiety or stress as evidenced by _____ by _____ (date)

- Identify at least three factors that facilitate sleep (specify) _____ by _____ (date)
- Establish a regular routine for a sleep–wake cycle as evidenced by keeping a sleep chart by _____ (date)

RESOURCES AND INFORMATION

1. National Institutes of Health (NIH)
   Office of Clinical Center Communications (for information and publications on sleep disorders)
   Building 10, Room 1C255
   Bethesda, MD 20892
   301-496-2563
2. Restless Leg Syndrome Foundation
   304 Glenwood Avenue
   Raleigh, NC 27603-1455
3. National Sleep Foundation
   122 South Robertson Boulevard
   Suite 201
   Los Angeles, CA 90048
   310-288-0466
   Fax: 310-288-0570
4. 30 Minute Video and Workbook— "Insomnia" ($19.95)
   Time Life: 1-800-588-9959 (or at a pharmacy)

REFERENCE

American Nurses Association. (1996). Integrating and understanding of sleep knowledge into your practice. *Independent Study Module*. New York: American Journal of Nursing Company.

Smoking (See Substance Abuse Behaviors)

Social Isolation (See Social Withdrawal)

Social Withdrawal

PROBLEM DESCRIPTION

Social withdrawal involves behaviors that are attempts of an individual to withdraw from or avoid interactions and relationships with others. Social withdrawal includes physical avoidance or verbal isolation and results in social isolation. The person who is socially withdrawn might want a relationship but not be able to make the contact; the individual has difficulty interacting spontaneously and appears detached or disinterested. Social withdrawal becomes dysfunctional when interpersonal relationships are impaired or distorted. Behaviors indicative of social withdrawal have many components and may be due to:

- Attempts to control the surroundings or the behavior of another person
- Difficulty developing satisfying relationships and unwanted social isolation, if it is perceived as being imposed by others
- A lack of connection or identification with others
- Physical, psychological, social, or environmental factors
- Alienation or aloneness resulting from inappropriate behavior
- Aloneness as a chosen state to be without others

PROBLEM IDENTIFICATION

Characteristics and Observable Behaviors

- Discomfort in social interactions and feeling threatened in social situations
- Interpersonal difficulties at home and work
- Dissatisfaction with social network
- Frequently feeling misunderstood
- Feelings of loneliness, rejection, abandonment, being unloved and uncared for
- Active avoidance of or isolation from others
- Inability to establish and maintain positive, supportive relationships
- Inability to respond to other's attempts at social interactions
- Ineffective social behaviors
- Excessive social changes
- Lack of close interdependent relationships and superficial relationships
- Reports of problematic patterns of social interaction by f/c
- Bizarre behavior, strange fantasies, and illogical ideas
- Disinterest in previous hobbies or other pleasurable activities
- Feelings of helplessness and hopelessness
- Feelings of frustration and anger
- Failure to use available resources
- Inappropriate or inadequate emotional responses
- Difficulty with verbal communication
- Exaggerated responses to stimuli

S

- Low self-esteem
- Lack of significant meaning and purpose in life
- Lack of supportive family or friends
- Living alone
- Sad, dull affect
- Unavailable (literally and figuratively) and uncommunicative
- Preoccupation with own thoughts
- Performance of repetitive, meaningless actions
- Reluctance to engage in social activities

Factors Related to the Problem

- Use of alcohol, tranquilizers, or other mood-altering drugs
- Alteration in mental status and altered thought processes
- Unacceptable social behavior
- Impaired reality testing
- Lack of contact with reality
- Disordered, illogical thinking
- Lack of supportive significant others
- Low self-esteem
- Sensory deficits
- Speech impediments and other physical anomalies
- Severe pain
- Limited physical mobility
- Developmental handicaps
- Psychiatric disorders
- Poor impulse control
- Severe aggression
- Treatment-related factors such as surgery, radiation, or medications
- Extreme emotions such as panic
- Inadequate social and communication skills
- Lack of opportunity to interact with others
- Maturational crisis
- Cultural barriers and language barriers
- Self-concept disturbance
- Environmental and geographic barriers such as having been in a long-term care facility in another area
- Debilitating physical illness such as terminal cancer
- Recent divorce, death in family, or loss of job

Assessment Tools and Instruments (see Appendix I)

Consider administering the:

1. Beck Depression Inventory
2. Brief Psychiatric Rating Scale

3. Brief Psychiatric Schizophrenia Rating Scale
4. Geriatric Depression Scale
5. Mini-Mental State Examination
6. Social Dysfunction Rating Scale

PROBLEM LIST

- Activity Intolerance
- Activity Intolerance, Risk for
- Body Image Disturbance
- Caregiver Role Strain
- Caregiver Role Strain, Risk for
- Communication, Impaired Verbal
- Community Coping, Ineffective
- Decisional Conflict
- Diversional Activity Deficit
- Fatigue
- Grieving, Anticipatory
- Grieving, Dysfunctional
- Growth and Development, Altered
- Hopelessness
- Memory, Impaired
- Noncompliance
- Pain
- Pain, Chronic
- Personal Identity Disturbance
- Powerlessness
- Self-Care Deficit, Bathing/Hygiene
- Self-Care Deficit, Dressing/Grooming
- Sleep Pattern Disturbance
- Social Interaction, Impaired
- Social Isolation
- Spiritual Distress
- Thought Processes, Altered

PROBLEM MANAGEMENT

Prevention, Maintenance, and Restorative Interventions

- To increase the pt's awareness of dynamics involved in socially withdrawn behaviors, instruct the pt that low self-esteem, anxiety, and feelings of shame and guilt can cause an individual to avoid contact with others and initiate self-isolation as a self-protective mechanism against being hurt or rejected.

- Instruct the pt that repeated failures and rejection increase behaviors related to social withdrawal and that learning defense, protective, and coping mechanisms will decrease negative social interactions and social withdrawal.

Medication Management

No specific medication is indicated for this behavior problem.

NURSING MANAGEMENT

Nursing Interventions and Rationales

⭐ Behavioral

- Assess the pt's level and tolerance of stimulation. *This helps in designing interventions that will increase the pt's tolerance to stimulation in a nonthreatening manner.*
- Assess the nature of the pt's behavior and social interactions. *Assessment assists in designing interventions that allow the pt to gradually increase the amount of time spent with others to decrease social withdrawal.*
- Instruct the pt in assertiveness skills. *This improves the pt's self-esteem, increases coping skills, and increases social interaction.*

♡ Emotional

- Praise the pt for expressing feelings related to engaging in social interactions. *This assesses the pt's feeling state, increases self-esteem, and improves social skills.*
- Discuss interpersonal relationships and explore the pt's fears of intimate relationships. *Such discussion increases awareness of lack of social interactions and establishes goals for improvement of interactions.*
- Educate the pt that new behaviors will increase anxiety. *This allows pt to prepare and plan for new social experiences and uncomfortable feelings.*
- Discuss with the pt the characteristics of a healthy relationship. *This helps the pt form realistic expectations of self and others.*

△ Cognitive

- Assist the pt to identify when perceptions are unrealistic. *This helps the pt to recognize misperceptions.*
- Educate the pt regarding the defense, protective, and coping mechanisms. *This assists the pt in choosing strategies to anticipate and deal with social interactions.*

▯ Physical

- Instruct the pt in the skills necessary to maintain physical integrity and treatment protocols. *These skills provide concrete plans and actions to prevent further social withdrawal.*
- Treat the pt's somatic complaints matter of factly. *This promotes physical well-being without focusing on secondary gains.*

⬭ **Social**

- Teach social skills and encourage the pt to practice interactions with f/c, and then choose another person outside the home to interact with. *Gradually introduce other people into the home milieu and minimize the perception of a threat.*
- Assist the pt to create a list of persons he or she feels comfortable interacting with and a schedule for implementing spending time together. *Such activity increases awareness of a support system and prevents social withdrawal behaviors in the future.*
- Instruct the pt to differentiate between social and intimate relationships. *This differentiation teaches healthy social and emotional boundaries.*
- Encourage the f/c and friends to strengthen their relationship with the pt. *This helps the pt maintain and enhance the social support systems.*
- Assist the pt to identify factors that contribute to social withdrawal. *Such identification helps match needs to available resources.*

✴ **Spiritual**

- Encourage the pt to review positive relationships with others. *Such review helps the pt to recognize progress and reduces feelings of rejection.*
- Assist the pt to recognize own sense of value in life. *Restoring faith and optimism in the self encourages feelings of worth and importance.*
- Educate the p/f/c regarding the benefits of social interaction. *This increases the understanding and practice of engaging in regular social interaction.*
- Assist the pt in identifying activities that can be initiated independently. *Independence encourages feelings of control and contact with others.*

Nursing Goals

- To assist the pt to establish a relationship with another
- To assist the pt to decrease behaviors related to social withdrawal
- To promote a socially supportive and secure environment for the pt
- To assist the pt to maintain interactions and social contact with the f/c and the environment

Patient Goals

- The pt will increase social interactions.
- The pt will identify problems in social interactions.
- The pt will report increased comfort with acting assertively in social settings.
- The pt will describe decreased feelings of anxiety and fear of rejection related to social interactions.
- The pt will demonstrate increased skills in personal interactions.
- The pt will identify goals and plans for increasing social interactions.
- The pt will verbalize increased trust in others.
- The pt will demonstrate willingness to maintain community contacts.
- The pt will report an increase in social contacts.

Patient and Family/Caregiver Outcomes

The patient or family/caregiver will:

- Prepare plans and set goals to achieve an increase in social interactions by _____ (date)
- Practice and use assertiveness and problem-solving skills to decrease behaviors related to social withdrawal as demonstrated by _____ within _____ weeks
- Describe aspects of healthy social interactions as demonstrated by _____ within _____ weeks
- Demonstrate comfortable interactions with the f/c and others as evidenced by _____ within _____ weeks
- Report improvement in social relationships and decreased feelings of social isolation and self-esteem as evidenced by _____ within _____ weeks

RESOURCES AND INFORMATION

1. National Alliance for the Mentally Ill (NAMI; for information about social support and opportunities for social interaction)
   2101 Wilson Boulevard
   Suite 302
   Arlington, VA 22201
   703-524-7600
   Fax: 703-524-9094

2. National Mental Health Association (NMHA; for information about social support and opportunities for social interaction)
   1021 Prince Street
   Alexandria, VA 22314-2971
   703-684-7722
   1-800-969-NMHA
   Fax: 703-684-5968

3. National Institute of Mental Health (NIMH)
   Information Resources and Inquiries Branch
   Office of Scientific Information, Room 15C
   5600 Fishers Lane
   Room 7C02
   Rockville, MD 20857
   301-443-4513

S

Somatization Problems

PROBLEM DESCRIPTION

Somatization problems, the conversion of mental states to physical or bodily symptoms, are a result of the mind–body connection in relation to stress. Physical symptoms are primarily what led the individual to seek health care. The more common symptoms that individuals seek help for are chronic pain, hypertension, irritable bowel syndrome, migraine headaches, and temporomandibular disorder or temporomandibular joint syndrome. A thorough physical assessment is necessary when any pt complains of physical symptoms. When no physiologic explanation can be found, it is necessary to assess for the presence of a somatoform disorder, which is a mental disorder manifested by symptoms seen in physical diseases. This group of disorders is so widespread that it may involve 30% to 40% of medical pts seen in general and family practice settings (Fava, 1992).

Somatoform disorders, not voluntarily produced by the pt, include:

- Body dysmorphic disorder—preoccupation with imagined defects in appearance or excessive concern with a slight physical anomaly
- Conversion disorder—one or more symptoms or deficits affecting voluntary motor or sensory function that suggests a neurobiologic or other general medical condition that can be precipitated by conflict or stress, is not intentionally produced, and has no known medical cause
- Hypochondriasis—fear of having a serious disease based on a misinterpretation of bodily symptoms despite medical evaluation and reassurance
- Somatization disorder—history of physical complaints beginning before age 30 and having each of these four symptoms: four different sites of pain, two GI symptoms, one sexual symptom, and one pseudoneurologic symptom suggesting a neurologic condition
- Pain disorder—pain in one or more anatomic sites that is of sufficient severity to warrant clinical attention and is not associated with a general medical condition

(American Psychiatric Association, 1994)

PROBLEM IDENTIFICATION
Characteristics and Observable Behaviors
- Chronic fatigue and worry
- Poor coping and problem-solving skills
- Inability to meet basic needs and lack of independence
- Need for immediate gratification
- Need for immediate relief of pain
- Frequent complaints of physical symptoms not confirmed by medical assessment
- Denial or anger regarding a diagnosis of a psychiatric illness
- Difficulty asking for and accepting help

- Denial of change in health status
- Compulsive behavior or obsessive thoughts
- Avoidance of activity
- Helplessness and despair
- Persistent fatigue that interferes with daily activities
- Inability to function in job and other roles
- Myalgia
- Impaired cognition
- Anxiousness
- Sleep disorder
- Change in communication patterns
- Excessive consumption of alcohol
- Insomnia
- Irritability and impulsiveness
- Irritable bowel syndrome
- Lack of insight and judgment
- Low self-esteem and perceived self-victimization
- Muscular tension
- Overeating or lack of appetite
- Inadequate resources and support systems
- Psychosocial stressors
- Verbal manipulation
- Physical dysfunction
- Constantly vigilant for new illness manifestations
- Exacerbation of physical symptoms with stressful situations
- Unable to fulfill family and other role responsibilities
- Unexpected intensification of symptoms when asked to participate in undesirable activities
- Bores others with a litany of complaints
- Displaces depressive affect to somatic symptoms
- Obsessed with fears of illness

Factors Related to the Problem

- Impaired cognition
- Inadequate resources and support systems
- Psychosocial stressors
- Lack of insight and judgment
- Poor coping and problem-solving skills
- Severe level of anxiety
- Repressed anxiety
- Low self-esteem
- Difficulty asking for and accepting help
- Unmet dependency needs
- History of self or a loved one having experienced a serious illness or disease
- Being at an earlier level of development
- Delayed ego development

- Inadequate coping skills
- Psychological stress

Assessment Tools and Instruments (see Appendix I)

Consider administering the:

1. Beck Depression Inventory
2. Geriatric Depression Scale
3. Global Assessment of Functioning Scale
4. Mini-Mental State Examination
5. Pain Assessment Tool
6. Sheehan Patient-Related Anxiety Scale
7. Suicide Risk Assessment Tool

PROBLEM LIST

- Activity Intolerance
- Activity Intolerance, Risk for
- Body Image Disturbance
- Caregiver Role Strain
- Caregiver Role Strain, Risk for
- Communication, Impaired Verbal
- Community Coping, Ineffective
- Community, Ineffective Management of Therapeutic Regimen
- Constipation, Perceived
- Decisional Conflict
- Diarrhea
- Fatigue
- Growth and Development, Altered
- Hopelessness
- Memory, Impaired
- Mobility, Impaired Physical
- Noncompliance
- Pain
- Pain, Chronic
- Parenting, Altered
- Parenting, Risk for Altered
- Powerlessness
- Sensory/Perceptual Alterations (specify)
- Sexual Dysfunction
- Sexuality Patterns, Altered
- Sleep Pattern Disturbance
- Social Interaction, Impaired
- Social Isolation
- Spiritual Distress
- Swallowing, Impaired
- Thought Processes, Altered

PROBLEM MANAGEMENT

Prevention, Maintenance, and Restorative Interventions

- Instruct the p/f/c that hypochondria is a physical manifestation of the need to be nurtured and a secondary gain is usually derived from the attention.

- Instruct the pt that individual beliefs and thoughts can create physical illness and that symptoms can be altered with grasping the process and recognition of feelings.
- Educate the pt that a fear of failure might exhibit itself in physical symptoms, with the sick role providing justification for the failure to live up to potential.
- Understand that a pt with a somatic disorder is difficult to treat, will engender negative emotions, and often reject the provider to protect the pt from unwanted feelings by distancing from a therapeutic relationship.

Medication Management

There is no specific medication identified for the treatment of somatic disorders.

NURSING MANAGEMENT

Nursing Interventions and Rationales

☆ Behavioral

- Minimize the amount of time and attention given to physical complaints. *This decreases the number of problems verbalized.*
- Avoid interpreting or confronting somatic symptom behavior. *Symptoms serve a purpose and as the pt learns new behaviors it will not be necessary to maintain the symptoms as a defense.*

♡ Emotional

- Encourage the pt to recognize and discuss fears rather than to somatize fear. *This focuses on feelings of fear and not the physical problem.*
- Discuss with the pt satisfaction with life and relationships. *This assists the pt's self-assessment and awareness of the nature of the physical symptoms.*
- Respond when the pt expresses feelings and personal issues. *A response provides positive reinforcement for expression of feelings and not somatization.*

△ Cognitive

- Avoid implying that physical symptoms are imaginary. *This prevents an increase in anxiety as a result of the pt not feeling that he or she is believed.*
- Provide attention when the pt is not complaining, and teach the f/c to do so. *This reinforces noncomplaining behaviors.*
- Encourage the pt to make his or her own decisions. *This reduces somatization and unhealthy dependency, and increases self-care.*
- Teach thought stopping techniques. *These techniques decrease obsessive thoughts about somatic complaints.*

⊐ Physical

- Discuss the potential harmful effects of polypharmacy. *Such discussion increases knowledge and awareness of medication interactions and keeps the pt from seeking medications from many different prescribers.*

- Encourage the pt to participate in diversional activities and exercise as much as is possible. *The expectation of involvement in physical activity allows the pt to focus on activities rather than on the self and somatic sensations.*
- Provide a thorough physical assessment. *This is needed to rule out any health or medical problems or complications.*

◯ Social

- Teach the p/f/c that somatic illness indicates the pt has human needs that have to be met and done so in a direct manner. *This provides for satisfaction in behavior and creates an awareness that somatization is a reflection of an unmet human need.*
- Encourage the pt to participate in social activities as much as is possible. *Involvement in role responsibilities enables the pt to focus on others' needs rather than on the self and somatic sensations.*

✦ Spiritual

- Explore with the pt feelings about the perceived lack of control in life. *This recognizes pt's feelings and allows the pt to gain control.*
- Instruct pts in their ability to make choices about how they express themselves. *Pts are responsible for their own behavior and their own conscious choices.*
- Focus on past successes and stay oriented to the present. *Such focus maintains a here-and-now perspective and teaches that the past cannot be changed but the present can.*
- Instruct the pt not to blame the past for present somatic sensations and behavior. *The pt should take responsibility for his or her own feelings and actions.*
- Discuss the pt's values and belief systems, and their meaning and purpose in life. *Discussion determines the level of commitment and recognition of the need to change.*

Nursing Goals

- To accurately assess and treat the pt's somatic problems
- To promote the pt's expression of feelings related to somatization
- To decrease secondary gains obtained from the somatoform disorder
- To decrease the pt's unwarranted reliance on medications and treatments
- To assist the pt to identify and express feelings of stress and somatization

Patient Goals

- The pt will decrease the number and frequency of somatic problems.
- The pt will improve social relationships with others to focus on others and not on somatic sensations.
- The pt will develop healthy habits and feelings rather than being involved in self-pity and somatization.

Patient and Family/Caregiver Outcomes

The client or family/caregiver will:

- Decrease the number of somatic complaints as demonstrated by _____ within _____ weeks

- Express self verbally and identify stress and somatization as demonstrated by _____ within _____ weeks
- Demonstrate coping skills to deal with stress or other feelings related to somatization as evidenced by _____ within _____ weeks

RESOURCES AND INFORMATION

1. Bodymind Systems (for audiotapes and booklets on relaxation, imagery, music therapy, and touch)
   910 Dakota Drive
   Temple, TX 76504
2. American Psychiatric Association (APA; for information on somatoform disorders)
   Division of Public Affairs/Code P-H
   1400 K Street, NW
   Washington, DC 20005
   202-682-6220
3. American Psychological Association (APA; for a brochure, "The Mind–Body Connection")
   750 First Street, NE
   Washington, DC 20002
   202-336-5500
   1-800-296-0272
4. National Institutes of Health (NIH; for a publication, "Behavior Patterns and Health," NIH Publication No. 83-2625)
   Office of Clinical Center Communications
   Building 10, Room 1C255
   Bethesda, MD 20892
   301-496-2563

REFERENCES

American Psychiatric Association. (1994). *Diagnostic and statistical manual of mental disorders* (4th ed.). Washington, DC: Author.

Fava, G. (1992). The concept of psychosomatic disorder. *Psychotherapy Psychosomatic, 58,* 1–12.

Spiritual Distress (See Meaning and Purpose in Life Problems)

Stress (See Post-Traumatic Stress Disorder)

Substance Abuse Behaviors

PROBLEM DESCRIPTION

Substance abuse and addictive disorders are major health and social problems in today's society. Substance use disorders and substance-induced disorders are the two categories of substance-related disorders. Substance use disorders include substance dependence and substance abuse. Substance-induced disorders include substance intoxication and substance withdrawal. Substances include alcohol, amphetamines, caffeine, cannabis, cocaine, hallucinogens, inhalants, nicotine, opioids, PCP, sedatives, hypnotics, and anxiolytics.

Substance use disorders have predictable physical symptoms and behavior patterns that are associated with the voluntary ingestion of a psychoactive substance. Use of substances is compulsive and compelling and has negative consequences. Changes in behavior occur as a result of the drug's effect on normal brain transmissions. Addiction is a state of chronic intoxication produced by repeated consumption of a substance. Most substances cause a physical dependence; other addictions can cause emotional dependence with similar behaviors and consequences. Physical dependence is a physical need for the psychoactive substance that when not available causes withdrawal symptoms, such as, but not limited to, nausea, vomiting, delusions and hallucinations, and fever. Intoxication occurs when clinically significant s/s are associated with recent ingestion of the substance. Detoxification is a process by which the substance is withdrawn over a period of time to allow the body to reestablish a drug-free state. Toxicity refers to taking too much of the substance and can lead to overdose in those who have not built up a tolerance to heavy doses. Tolerance is the body's ability to adjust to higher levels of substances and creates a potential for dependence.

When a person with a substance abuse disorder receives an intervention for the problem, either voluntarily or not, detoxification will be necessary. Once the body is rid of the physical substance and is stable, the issue of psychological dependence must be addressed. Psychological dependence is obsessive thinking about the substance that can cause the individual to seek the substance despite the negative consequences. Cravings for the substance can be great as remembrances of the positive effects produced compel the individual to initiate use of the substance again.

Persons who have attended a treatment process and have maintained a physical and psychological abstinence of the substance are said to be in recovery. Relapse is always a possibility for any person in recovery, and preventive techniques are used to assist during difficult and stressful times that might precipitate a relapse. Relapse prevention is important during the first few months after intensive treatment and during the stressful times that could potentiate a relapse. Education, intervention, group therapy, behavioral therapy, enhancing social skills, having a plan for continuing care and relapse, aftercare, and developing a solid community support system are necessary to assist persons with substance abuse problems to maintain their recovery.

PROBLEM IDENTIFICATION

Characteristics and Observable Behaviors

- Isolative behaviors and frequent vague and withdrawn moods
- Low self-esteem and disregard for personal appearance
- Lack of impulse control and getting into fights
- Difficulty with authority and stealing
- Frequent use of drugs or alcohol
- Denial of the illness and feelings
- Minimization of chemical or substance use
- Blaming others for one's problems
- Lack of insight
- Failure to accept responsibility for behavior and inability to follow through with commitments
- Views self as different from others
- Lack of social skills
- Superficial relationships and an inability to form and maintain personal relationships
- Ineffective coping skills
- Increasing anxiety
- Avoidance of problems and conflicts
- Difficulty making decisions
- Dissatisfied with life, hopeless, and despairing
- Inability to trust others and secretiveness
- Excessive need or desire to control others, situations, and emotions
- Intolerant of changes

Factors Related to the Problem

- Intellectualization and rationalization of problems
- Marital and family problems
- Inadequate support system, dysfunctional relationships, and increased isolation
- Financial, work, school, or legal problems
- Physical symptoms or problems
- Exacerbation of preexisting chronic illnesses
- Stress-related physical problems
- Lowered pain threshold
- Accident proneness
- History of self-medication
- Sleep problems

- Personality disorder
- Major psychiatric illness
- Psychosis, delusions, or hallucinations
- Suicidal ideas or actions
- Addictive behaviors
- Impaired nutrition or eating disorder
- Chemical dependence

Assessment Tools and Instruments (see Appendix I)

Consider administering the:

1. Beck Depression Inventory
2. Clinical Inventory Withdrawal Assessment
3. Geriatric Depression Scale
4. Global Assessment of Functioning Scale
5. Mini-Mental State Examination
6. Modified Overt Aggression Scale
7. Pain Assessment Tool
8. Sheehan Patient Rated Anxiety Scale
9. Social Dysfunction Rating Scale
10. Spiritual Perspective Clinical Scale
11. Suicide Risk Assessment Tool

PROBLEM LIST

- Alcoholism, Altered Family Process
- Body Image Disturbance
- Caregiver Role Strain
- Caregiver Role Strain, Risk for
- Communication, Impaired Verbal
- Community Coping, Ineffective
- Confusion, Acute
- Confusion, Chronic
- Decisional Conflict
- Diarrhea
- Diversional Activity Deficit
- Fatigue
- Fluid Volume Deficit
- Fluid Volume Deficit, Risk for
- Fluid Volume Excess
- Grieving, Anticipatory
- Grieving, Dysfunctional
- Hopelessness
- Incontinence, Bowel
- Memory, Impaired
- Mobility, Impaired Physical
- Noncompliance
- Nutrition, Altered: Less than Body Requirements
- Pain
- Pain, Chronic
- Parental Role Conflict
- Parenting, Altered
- Peripheral Neurovascular Dysfunction, Risk for
- Personal Identity Disturbance
- Poisoning, Risk for
- Post-Trauma Syndrome
- Powerlessness
- Relocation Stress Syndrome
- Self-Care Deficit, Bathing/Hygiene
- Self-Care Deficit, Dressing/Grooming
- Self-Care Deficit, Feeding
- Self-Care Deficit, Toileting

- Self Mutilation, Risk for
- Sensory/Perceptual Alterations (specify)
- Sexual Dysfunction
- Sexuality Patterns, Altered
- Skin Integrity, Risk for Impaired
- Sleep Pattern Disturbance
- Social Interaction, Impaired
- Social Isolation
- Spiritual Distress
- Swallowing, Impaired
- Thermoregulation, Ineffective
- Therapeutic Regimen, Ineffective Management of (Individuals)
- Thought Processes, Altered
- Tissue Integrity, Impaired
- Trauma, Risk for
- Urinary Elimination, Altered
- Violence, Risk for, Self-Directed or Directed at Others

PROBLEM MANAGEMENT

Prevention, Maintenance, and Restorative Interventions

- Assess the pt entering treatment for the stage of readiness and motivation for change (Sullivan, 1995):
  1. Precontemplation—pt's complete denial of an addiction problem
  2. Contemplation—pt admits wanting to change without following through
  3. Preparation—pt makes feeble attempts to change
  4. Action—pt makes overt behavioral changes
  5. Maintenance—pt continues behavioral changes
- Determine the nature the pt's stage of readiness and match the intervention with this stage for effective treatment.
- Contract between the provider and the pt to determine the expected behaviors to plan for problems that will be encountered.
- Educate the p/f/c about alcoholism and chemical dependency, a critical component of treatment for substance abuse behavior, to demystify and inform the p/f/c about the disease process, instill hope for recovery, and involve the pt's whole f/c system in treatment.
- Plan and arrange for pt enrollment in a 12-step program such as AA and NA to provide a supportive milieu network through attendance and education.
- Plan and arrange for f/c enrollment in 12-step program such as Al-Anon, Alateen, or Families Anonymous to provide a supportive milieu network through attendance and education.
- Encourage family therapy for the p/f/c so they can understand the role and impact of substance abuse behaviors on the support system.
- Plan and arrange for vocational counseling services with the pt to assess and provide vocational opportunities, skills training, or job development because often the pt has no marketable skills and may have a history of difficulty with employers.
- Educate the pt in leisure skills and diversional activities as alternatives to substance abuse behaviors.
- Teach or refer for relapse prevention strategies, such as cognitive and behavioral approaches, to assist the pt in identifying high-risk situations and behaviors, develop alternatives, and identify, recognize, and intervene in relapse before actually using a substance.

- Assist the pt to seek spiritual counseling as a method for developing personal strengths that can include a new connection or reconnection with a religious belief system.
- Teach the p/f/c that recovery from substance abuse includes abstinence and lifestyle changes, and requires support and participation from the p/f/c.
- Educate the pt about the physiologic factors, psychological state, and warning signs of relapse that are critical for the continued success of recovery.

Medication Management

Pharmacotherapy for substance abuse treatment is used for detoxification, reducing drug cravings, substitution of a substance, aversive therapy, symptomatic treatment of withdrawal, and treating comorbid psychiatric and medical disorders.

Detoxification is the process of withdrawal from a substance with a physical dependence. Detoxification treatment and approach depends on type of substance abused, social supports, detoxification history, medical and psychiatric problems, and relapse history. Medications for detoxification are given to lower the seizure threshold and to decrease s/s of withdrawal. Benzodiazepines frequently used for alcohol detoxification include chlordiazepoxide (Librium), diazepam (Valium), clonazepam (Klonopin), lorazepam (Ativan), and oxazepam (Serax). Vitamin B_1 (thiamine) is given to prevent the occurrence of Wernicke-Korsakoff syndrome (a thiamine deficiency caused by inadequate diet).

Medications may be used to reduce the reinforcing effects of a substance. Naltrexone (Trexan) is an opiate antagonist that blocks the euphoric effects of opiates such as heroin and cocaine. Bromocriptine (Parlodel) is used for cocaine withdrawal and clonidine (Catapres) for heroin, cocaine, and nicotine addictions. Carbamazepine (Tegretol), fluoxetine (Prozac), mazindol (Mazanor), and bromocriptine (Parlodel) are being tested to reduce the craving for cocaine.

Methadone is used as a substitution drug to provide maintenance therapy for heroin. Disulfiram (Antabuse) is an antidipsotropic agent that causes an unpleasant reaction when combined with alcohol (Sullivan, 1995).

NURSING MANAGEMENT

Nursing Interventions and Rationales

✫ Behavioral

- Instruct the p/f/c on firm and consistent limit setting for substance abuse behaviors. *Limits make expectations clear, nonpunitive, and in the best interests of the pt.*
- Focus on the "here-and-now" situation to assist the pt in directing behavior and life. *Such focus initiates change and requires pt to take responsibility.*
- Discuss the circumstances of relapse with the p/f/c. *Such discussion may identify the events that led to substance use and to avoid similar circumstances in the future.*
- Assess pt's unstructured time and plan for events that are purposeful. *Planning assists the pt in finding activities to replace substance abusive behaviors.*

Emotional

- Instruct the pt in journaling techniques. *Writing provides an outlet and focus for thoughts, feelings, and activities that may provide useful information in future planning.*
- Allow the pt to ventilate feelings about the behavioral contract and limits, but do not become engaged in power struggles or attempt to rationalize the treatment plan. *This verifies and validates feelings and reinforces limits as necessary.*

Cognitive

- Confront the pt's denial of any substance abuse problem with a matter-of-fact approach, focusing on the present, stating the problem in objective terms, probing for details, and returning to the issue at hand. *Confrontation assists the pt in recognizing substance abuse behaviors and the impact substance abuse has on significant others.*
- Assist the pt to focus discussions on the issue of the substance abuse problem. *Such focus avoids the pt's denial of the involvement and the blaming of others.*
- Provide factual information on substance abuse to the p/f/c in a matter-of-fact manner, without argument. *Facts dispel myths and focus on the substance abuse behaviors.*
- Explore alternative methods of dealing with stress and difficult situations with the p/f/c. *This helps p/f/c to learn coping skills without the use of substances.*

Physical

- Assess the pt's substance abuse history, sleep patterns, nutrition, physical complications, and effects of substance abuse behaviors on others. *Assessment establishes a baseline for evaluation and treatment planning.*
- Monitor vital signs on a scheduled basis during in-home detoxification, observe for physical symptoms and changes, ensure that food and fluids are available, instruct the p/f/c in medications to be administered and their effects, and inform the p/f/c when to call the prescriber or physician for an emergency. *This provides for a safe and effective withdrawal process.*
- Educate the p/f/c about HIV, AIDS, and STDs and the prevention of disease transmission. *Those who abuse substances are at increased risk for HIV and STDs infection through sharing needles or by sexual activity during periods of impaired judgment.*
- Inform the p/f/c of drug interactions between medications and other substances. *Factual information may avoid potential medication interaction problems.*
- Assess the pt for s/s that indicate other psychiatric disturbances. *Assessment may reveal as yet undiagnosed or undertreated problems that need treatment.*

Social

- Encourage the pt to focus on behaviors that have caused family problems. *This helps the pt see the relationship between substance abuse problem and behavior.*
- Involve the pt in a group of peers to provide feedback, confront, and share feelings. *Peers provide an honest and supportive system.*
- Refer the p/f/c to support organizations such as AA, Al-Anon, Alateen, Adult Children of Alcoholics, or NA. *These groups provide continued support services in the community.*

- Instruct the pt in social skills such as attentive listening, eye contact, or assertiveness. *This increases knowledge of social interaction skills, models appropriate behaviors, and enhances socialization attempts during recovery.*

✦ Spiritual

- Refer the pt to a spiritual advisor. *This individual may assist the pt in dealing with feelings of guilt or despair, maintaining sobriety, and finding spiritual and social support.*
- Assist the pt to realistically view self in the present to allow the past to become history. *This allows the pt to sort through past feelings and experiences and to "let go," and move on.*

Nursing Goals

- To provide information and education about substance abuse to the p/f/c
- To promote realistic pt self-evaluation about substance abuse behaviors and self-responsibility
- To promote the pt's development of alternative coping strategies
- To direct the therapeutic focus to the here-and-now problems and issues related to substance abuse behaviors
- To provide information and education about medication, alcohol, drugs, and associated risks to the p/f/c
- To promote safe in-home detoxification procedures and accurate reporting of symptoms and compliance with therapeutic regimen
- To facilitate substituting of substance abuse behaviors with the development of social and diversional skills

Patient Goals

- The pt will abstain and change life-style (recover) from substance abuse behaviors.
- The pt will initiate plans for relapse and further prevention.
- The pt will participate in an organized community support program.
- The pt will verbalize knowledge of prevention of HIV, AIDS, and STDs transmission.
- The pt will accept responsibility for own behaviors related to substance abuse.
- The pt will demonstrate effective communication and socialization skills with others without ingesting substance(s).
- The pt will verbalize knowledge of information related to substance use and related family problems.
- The pt will demonstrate alternative methods of problem-solving that do not involve substances.
- The pt will demonstrate control of aggressive behaviors and effective use of coping skills.
- The pt will follow through with commitments and chosen obligations.

Patient and Family/Caregiver Outcomes

The patient or family/caregiver will:

- Detoxify safely in the home as demonstrated by _____ within _____ days

- Demonstrate decreased aggressive or threatening behaviors related to substance abuse behaviors as demonstrated by _____ within _____ weeks
- Identify negative effects of their substance abuse behavior on others as demonstrated by _____ within _____ weeks
- Abstain from substance use as demonstrated by _____ within _____ weeks
- Verbalize responsibility for own behavior as demonstrated by _____ within _____ weeks
- Participate in realistic self-evaluation regarding substance abuse behaviors as evidenced by _____ within _____ weeks
- Verbalize a process for problem-solving without use of chemicals as demonstrated by _____ within _____ weeks
- Identify difficulties (specify) _____ associated with substance abuse by _____ (date)
- Develop plans to manage unstructured time as demonstrated by _____ within _____ weeks
- Demonstrate the ability to manage conflict situations without use of substances as demonstrated by _____ within _____ weeks
- Identify a community support system, location, times of meetings, and attend _____ (state number) within _____ weeks

RESOURCES AND INFORMATION

1. Adult Children of Alcoholics (ACOA) Interim
World Service Organization
2522 West Sepulveda Boulevard
Suite 200
PO Box 3216
Torrance, CA 90510
310-534-1815
2. Al-Anon Family Groups Headquarters, Inc.
PO Box 862
Midtown Station
New York, NY 10018-0862
212-302-7240
Fax: 212-869-3757
24-Hour Toll-Free: 1-800-356-9996
3. Alateen
PO Box 862
Midtown Station
New York, NY 10018-0862
212-302-7240
Fax: 212-869-3757
24-Hour Toll-Free: 1-800-356-9996
4. Alcohol, Drug Abuse, and Mental Health Administration
Parklawn Building
5600 Fishers Lane

S

Rockville, MD 20857
301-443-4795

5. Alcohol Rehab for the Elderly
PO Box 267
Hopedale, IL 61747
Hotline: 1-800-354-7089

6. Alcoholics Anonymous (AA)
475 Riverside Drive
11th Floor
New York, NY 10115
212-870-3400
Fax: 212-870-3003

7. Families Anonymous (FA)
PO Box 3475
Culver City, CA 90231
1-800-736-9805

8. National Clearinghouse for Alcohol and Drug Information (NCADI)
PO Box 2345
Rockville, MD 20852
301-468-2600

9. National Council on Alcoholism and Drug Dependence (NCADD)
Attn: Information Director
12 West 21st Street
New York, NY 10010
212-206-6770
Fax: 212-645-1690
1-800-NCA-CALL

10. SOS/Secular Organization for Sobriety/Save Our Selves
PO Box 5
Buffalo, NY 14215-0005
24-Hour Phone: 310-821-8430

11. National Institute on Alcohol Abuse and Alcoholism (NIAAA): http://www.niaaa.nih.gov

12. National Nurses Society on Addictions (NNSA): 919-783-5871
4101 Lake Boone Trail, Suite 201
Raleigh, NC 27607

13. American Psychological Association (APA; request free publications: "Understanding and Dealing with Alcoholism" and "What You Should Know About Drug Abuse")
750 First Street, NE
Washington, DC 20002
202-336-5500
1-800-296-0272

14. Alcohol/Cocaine, Crack and Drug Abuse-Addiction Hotline Referrals: 1-800-252-6465; 1-800-962-8963; 1-800-888-9383

15. Cocaine Abuse Lines (24-Hour): 1-800-234-0420; 1-800-262-2463

16. Alcohol Abuse Lines (24-Hour): 1-800-ALCOHOL

17. National Institute of Drug Abuse Helpline: 1-800-662-4357

S

18. Women for Sobriety: 1-800-333-1606
19. 30-minute video and workbook: "Alcoholism" ($19.95)
    Time Life: 1-800-588-9959 (or at a pharmacy)
20. Injury Prevention for the Elderly
    Preventing Problem Use of Alcohol (0-8342-0825-3, #20825)
    Aspen Publishers, Inc.
    200 Orchard Ridge Drive
    Gaithersburg, MD 20878
    1-800-638-8437
    Fax: 301-417-7650
    http://www.aspen.pub.com
21. Schmall, V. L., Gobeli, C. L. , & Stiehl R. E. (1989). *Alcohol problems in later life.*
    Pacific Northwest Extension Publication—#PNW 246 (Single copy —$0.75, plus
    S&H of $0.25 up to $2.50)
    Agricultural Communications
    Publications Orders
    Oregon State University
    Corvallis, OR 97331-2119
    503-737-2513

REFERENCE

Sullivan, E. J. (1995). *Nursing care of clients with substance abuse.* St. Louis: Mosby-Yearbook.

Suicidal and Homicidal Behaviors

PROBLEM DESCRIPTION

Suicidal and homicidal behaviors are disturbances in the balance of life and disruptive interactions in the physical, psychological, social, and spiritual variables of relationships with the self or others. When an individual feels that life is unbalanced and has no meaning, a conflict arises as to the continuation of life for the self or others. Abusive, aggressive, or assaultive behaviors are indicators of actions toward others with or without homicidal ideation. Homicidal feelings are hostile and violent acts in which death could be the objective. Most individuals are able to control their feelings and actions with only thoughts of harm. When feelings are overwhelming, situations are intolerable, or psychosis is involved, the person is sometimes unable to distinguish right from wrong or use internal or external controls to stop the action. Homicidal behaviors have obvious legal implications. A person with or without a psychiatric diagnosis can be prosecuted for homicidal actions.

A person commits suicide in the United States every 15 minutes. Suicide is now one of the leading causes of death and surpasses murder. More than 30,000 people commit suicide a year by official statistics, although the actual number may be more than three to five times higher. Among college-age students, suicide is the second leading cause of death, after accidents. In older adults the suicide rate for those over 65 years old, rose 9% between 1980 and 1992, after a 40-year decline. Suicide in the elderly is not impulsive but carefully planned for months (Carson, 1996).

The majority of persons who commit suicide gives clues that they are contemplating suicide. Any and all talk of suicide is of concern. The pt who is suicidal often verbalizes intent or ideation regarding self-harm. Suicidal behaviors occur on a continuum from low to high lethality: indirect self-destructive behaviors, direct self-destructive behaviors, suicide attempts or gestures, suicidal ideation, or completed suicide.

Populations at High Risk

Persons with psychotic depression have a higher risk for completing violent suicides. Pts identified with major depression are at high risk for suicide, especially those who have feelings of anxiety, worthlessness, delusions, sleep problems, or a history of previous suicide attempts. Pts with a diagnosis of bipolar disorder are at greatest risk for suicide during their depressive phase. Schizophrenic pts have a 10% to 13% rate of completed suicide. People with schizophrenia are at high risk because of the enduring and persistent nature of the illness and their tendency to feel hopeless and not to disclose information about suicidal thoughts. Alcohol and substance abuse are contributing factors to 25% to 50% of all completed suicides (Forster, 1994).

The cause of suicide is not attributable to any one factor. Physical evidence shows that serotonin levels are low in persons who have attempted suicide (Roy, 1989). Psychological theories propose that suicide is aggression and anger directed toward others that is turned inward on the self (Menninger, 1938). Filstead (1980) explains that indirect self-destructive behaviors are related to despair and that when individuals try to cope with serious personal problems they feel suicide is the only possible resolution. Social and cultural influences affect suicidality and relate to a sense of not belonging, alienation, aloneness, lack of freedom, or an altruistic and honorable death. Spiritual factors can also influence suicide and the strength of the personal belief system in that there is a sense or purpose in life.

Assessment of suicidal or homicidal ideation requires an in-depth review of possible factors and lethality of plans. A thorough assessment is completed and documented. The one exception to the Mental Health Systems Act (1980) for confidentiality is the *Tarasoff* decision (*Tarasoff v. the Regents of the University of California*, 1976). This decision clearly established that a therapist has the duty to use reasonable care to protect a known, intended victim of a pt's threat to harm—known as "the duty to warn." The *Tarasoff* decision applies to the pt who is threatening homicidal actions toward another. The provider has a duty to protect the pt and maintain safety by ensuring that the pt is assessed for the appropriate level and location of care.

PROBLEM IDENTIFICATION

Characteristics and Observable Behaviors

- Dysfunctional grieving
- Perceived or observable loss

- Social isolation and loneliness
- Feelings of dependency on others
- Feelings of worthlessness, hopelessness, despair, or rejection
- Verbalization of low self-esteem, guilt, and shame
- Lack of future orientation
- Inability to solve problems
- Difficulty concentrating
- Inability to deal with feelings of anger or hostility
- Inability to control behaviors and lack of impulse control
- Difficulty identifying and expressing emotions and lack of insight
- Self-destructive behaviors or tendencies
- Feelings of anxiety, fear, panic, or ambivalence
- Lack of trust
- Denial and projection of feelings
- Actual or potential physical acting out of violence
- Aggressive behaviors
- Destruction of property
- Homicidal or suicidal ideation
- Agitation or restlessness
- Delusions, hallucinations, or other psychotic behaviors
- Disorientation, disorganization, and confusion
- Awareness of effect of threats or attempts on others

Factors Related to the Problem

- History of suicides in the family
- Personality disorders, especially a diagnosis of borderline personality disorder or antisocial personality disorder
- Substance abuse
- Manic behaviors
- Post-traumatic behavior
- Depression
- Withdrawn behaviors
- Manipulative behaviors
- Fatigue and sleep disturbance
- Social isolation
- Living in subculture where social cohesion is lacking with few community ties
- Family, financial, legal, and physical problems or stressors
- Lack of support systems

Assessment Tools and Instruments (see Appendix I)

Consider administering the:

1. Beck Depression Inventory
2. Brief Psychiatric Rating Scale
3. Brief Psychiatric Schizophrenia Rating Scale
4. Geriatric Depression Scale
5. Global Assessment of Functioning

6. Mini-Mental State Examination
7. Modified Overt Aggression Scale
8. Sheehan Patient Rated Anxiety Scale
9. Social Dysfunction Rating Scale
10. Spiritual Perspective Clinical Scale
11. Suicide Risk Assessment Tool
12. TRIADS

PROBLEM LIST

- Alcoholism, Altered Family Process
- Body Image Disturbance
- Caregiver Role Strain
- Caregiver Role Strain, Risk for
- Communication, Impaired Verbal
- Community Coping, Ineffective
- Confusion, Acute
- Confusion, Chronic
- Decisional Conflict
- Diversional Activity Deficit
- Fatigue
- Grieving, Anticipatory
- Grieving, Dysfunctional
- Hopelessness
- Mobility, Impaired Physical
- Noncompliance
- Nutrition, Altered: Less than Body Requirements
- Pain
- Pain, Chronic
- Personal Identity Disturbance
- Poisoning, Risk for
- Post-Trauma Response
- Powerlessness
- Rape-Trauma Syndrome
- Rape-Trauma Syndrome: Compound Reaction
- Rape-Trauma Syndrome: Silent Reaction
- Relocation Stress Syndrome
- Self Mutilation, Risk for
- Sensory/Perceptual Alterations (specify)
- Sleep Pattern Disturbance
- Social Interaction, Impaired
- Social Isolation
- Spiritual Distress
- Suffocation, Risk for
- Thought Processes, Altered
- Trauma, Risk for
- Violence, Risk for, Self-Directed or Directed at Others

PROBLEM MANAGEMENT

Prevention, Maintenance, and Restorative Interventions

- Assess and monitor the pt for homicidal or suicidal thoughts or behaviors on every home visit.
- Assess pt for imminent harm or danger to self or others.
- Educate p/f/c about changes in behaviors related to suicidal or homicidal actions and inform the physician, other providers, and police if necessary to provide immediate intervention.

- Educate the p/f/c that a death wish is exhibited through anger and aggression toward the self or others and that when it is repressed and turned inward, self-destructive behaviors result.
- Assess the pt for feelings related to loss, depression, rejection, abandonment, frustration, dependency, guilt, or hopelessness to provide early intervention in suicide threats, gestures, or ideation.
- Instruct the f/c to observe the pt for devaluation of self, negative interpretation of life and experiences, and a pessimistic view of the future.
- Inform the f/c that suicide preceded by homicide is an act of revenge and to discuss feelings related to anger with the pt.
- Instruct p/f/c that an indicator of the intent to commit suicide is often shown beforehand by giving away personal possessions, threats, discussions of suicide methods, depression, direct and indirect verbal cues, or suicide notes.

Medication Management

No specific medications are indicated for persons with suicidal or homicidal behaviors.

NURSING MANAGEMENT

Nursing Interventions and Rationales

✦ **Behavioral**

- Establish a written contract with the pt stating that the pt will not harm self intentionally or unintentionally. *This may prevent impulsive actions.*
- Assess the p/f/c for suicidal or homicidal ideation at every visit. *This determines the seriousness and lethality of intent.*
- Remove harmful objects from the home situation. *This provides safety and reduces risk of harmful behavior to the pt or others.*
- Educate the p/f/c that physical and diversional activities are methods to redirect and refocus attention when suicidal or homicidal thoughts threaten behaviors. *Such activities provide alternative methods of reducing anger and anxiety as well as preventing suicide.*
- Prepare a plan of emergency action with the p/f/c for when suicidal or homicidal intent is first expressed. *A specific plan provides a means of crisis intervention in case of imminent danger.*

♡ **Emotional**

- Observe and assess the pt for changes in the level of depression and feelings that might indicate increased suicidal potential. *Assessment allows intervention before potential self-harm.*
- Encourage expression of feelings. *Openness relieves feelings of anger and guilt related to suicidal and homicidal behaviors.*

Cognitive

- Assist the pt in refocusing thoughts when anxiety level is high. *Refocusing prevents scattered, disorganized thinking.*
- Encourage independent decision making. *This prevents the pt's dependence on others.*
- Encourage the pt to seek out f/c or significant others to clarify thoughts and feelings, assist in decision making, and help in achieving goals. *These individuals provide a support structure that is aware of potentially harmful situations and assists the pt in becoming aware of behaviors.*
- Discuss with the pt the effect of threats or attempts of suicidal or homicidal thoughts on others and the results of secondary gains or manipulative efforts. *This increases awareness of behavior and the rewards gained for manipulative behaviors and prevents suicide.*

Physical

- Assess medications, interactions, and function and instruct p/f/c about potential harm if medications are not monitored, stored, or administered properly. *This promotes safe medication administration through awareness and education.*

Social

- Assist the pt in planning a strategy for mobilizing a support system to be available when the pt feels in danger of hurting self or others. *Planning identifies supportive persons and prevents suicide or homicide.*
- Assist the pt in developing a plan to adapt to changes from loss and reinforce actions that indicate a will to live. *This provides a realistic plan that increases the pt's involvement in own care and reduces the chance of suicide.*

Spiritual

- Encourage forgiveness of the self and others. *This relieves feelings of anger and guilt.*
- Discuss with the pt the meaning and purpose in life and identify what the pt plans to do. *Discussion determines positive aspects of life and plans to achieve goals.*
- Assist the pt in creating a life with meaning. *This allows the pt to assume responsibility for valuing life and decreasing feelings of hopelessness.*
- Discuss religious values and beliefs. *Strengthening beliefs about life may decrease the chance of suicidal or homicidal behaviors.*
- Discuss realities of death and reasons for living. *This promotes life and prevents an unrealistic view of death.*

Nursing Goals

- To decrease the pt's suicidal or homicidal behaviors
- To maintain close supervision or monitoring behaviors of the pt with the f/c
- To decrease p/f/c feelings of depression, anxiety, fear, and anger related to suicidal or homicidal behaviors

S

- To help the pt develop insight and acknowledge responsibility for own behavior
- To decrease social withdrawal and increase communication and social interaction with others
- To help the pt identify and decrease self-destructive behaviors
- To facilitate appropriate expression of angry, hostile feelings

Patient Goals

- The pt will not harm the self or others.
- The pt will demonstrate alternative ways of dealing with stress and anger.
- The pt will express angry feelings in a safe manner.
- The pt will establish meaningful relationships with others.
- The pt will state the value of own life and life in general.

Patient and Family/Caregiver Outcomes

The patient or family/caregiver will:

- Identify and verbalize the early s/s of self-destructive behaviors
- Identify and verbalize plans for emergency crisis intervention regarding suicidal and homicidal behaviors
- Identify and develop positive coping skills to replace self-destructive behavior or such behavior toward others
- Verbalize ways in which the future will be better or different
- Verbalize expectations and plans for future behavioral changes
- Express an awareness of the consequences of suicidal or homicidal behaviors
- Learn social skills that allow for involvement and focus on others rather than on self

RESOURCES AND INFORMATION

1. Local resources in the telephone white pages under "Suicide Prevention" and "Crisis Prevention"
2. Suicide Intervention and Prevention: 1-800-274-2995
3. American Association of Suicidology (for a publication, "Understanding and Helping the Suicidal Person")
   2459 South Ash
   Denver, CO 80222
   303-692-0985
   or
   4201 Connecticut Avenue, NW
   Suite 310
   Washington, DC 20008
   202-237-2280
4. American Suicide Foundation
   1045 Park Avenue
   New York, NY 10028
   1-800-273-4042

5. Hemlock Society
   PO Box 11830
   Eugene, OR 97440
   503-342-5748
   1-800-247-7421
6. Injury Prevention for the Elderly
   Preventing Suicide and Depression: (0-8342-0831-8, #20831)
   Aspen Publishers, Inc.
   200 Orchard Ridge Drive
   Gaithersburg, MD 20878
   1-800-638-8437
   Fax: 301-417-7650
   http://www.aspen.pub.com
7. American Psychological Association (APA; request free publication: "Depression: What You Need To Know")
   750 First Street, NE
   Washington, DC 20002
   202-336-5500
   1-800-296-0272

REFERENCES

Carson, V. B. & Arnold, E. N., eds (1996). *Mental health nursing: The nurse-patient journey*. Philadelphia: Saunders.

Filstead, W. J. (1980). Despair and its relationship to indirect self-destructive behavior. In N. L. Faberow (Ed.), *The many faces of suicide: Indirect self-destructive behavior*. New York: McGraw-Hill.

Forster, P. (1994). Accurate assessment of short-term suicide risk in a crisis. *Psychiatric Annals, 24*, 571–578.

Mental Health Systems Act. (1980). 96th Congress, Publication L. 96-398, Section 9501.

Menninger, A. (1938). *Man against himself*. Orlando, FL: Harcourt Brace.

Roy, A. (1989). Suicide. In H. I. Kaplan & B. J. Sadock (Eds.), *Comprehensive textbook of psychiatry* (5th ed.). Baltimore: Williams & Wilkins.

Tarasoff v. Regents of the University of California. 17 Cal., 3d. 425, 551. P. 2d 334, 1976.

Toileting Problems (See Activities of Daily Living Problems)

T

V

Violence, Directed at Self, Other(s), or Property (See Abusive Behaviors, Aggressive Behaviors, Self-Mutilation, and Suicidal and Homicidal Behaviors)

W

Wandering

PROBLEM DESCRIPTION

Wandering behavior is a response to a variety of pt needs and conditions. Synonyms for wandering include roving, straying, and strolling without a regular or fixed course (*American Heritage Dictionary*, 1980). A definition of wandering behavior in home care is any change in physical location that results in a pt's inability to return to the immediate area (or home), with or without prosthetic devices, independently of the usual and customary reasons for leaving the home (Hussian, 1981; Hussian & Davis, 1985). The phenomenon of wandering behavior is not well understood (Beck and Heacock, 1988; Fopma-Loy, 1988). The timing or duration of wandering behavior may be related to external events, such as the setting sun, changes in the seasons, or mealtime. If pts who engage in wandering behavior are unsupervised or unobserved, they may leave the home and become lost or hurt. However, wandering behavior has some positive effects. Wandering behavior stimulates circulation and oxygenation, promotes exercise and activity, decreases skin breakdown and contractures, decreases stress, promotes a feeling of freedom, and provides dignity to the pt (Heim, 1986).

PROBLEM IDENTIFICATION

Characteristics and Observable Behaviors

The pt who is wandering is in motion. Snyder, Rupprecht, Pyrck, Brekhus, and Moss (1978) identify three types or patterns of wandering behavior and Hussian and Davis

(1985) identify four categories of pts who engage in wandering behavior, which when combined produce five types of wandering behavior:

1. Overtly goal directed—searching: pt is constantly searching for an object or a person (such as a deceased parent) that is not attainable; frequently calls out for the object or person.
2. Overtly goal directed—industrious: pt engages in a constant drive to engage in activities; often the goal is to get away or escape from the home; frequently gestures; and may believe that he or she is somewhere else.
3. Apparently nongoal directed: pt is drawn aimlessly to random stimuli; walks a particular course or circuit without purpose or thought; may constantly, aimlessly ambulate; and may exhibit other forms of self-stimulation such as rocking, clapping, singing, or patting walls.
4. Only with others: pt has no intention of leaving the home, but will model behavior and meander if someone else goes through the door.
5. From akathisia: pt continuously ambulates or paces; usually the result of long-term, high-dose use of psychotropic medications.

Factors Related to the Problem

- Inability to appropriately communicate
- Lack of social involvement and activity
- Cognitive deficits, especially confusion, and memory, orientation, and judgment deficits
- Irreversible dementia
- Mental retardation
- Pain and discomfort
- CV disease, especially dizziness and orthostatic hypotension
- Hunger or thirst
- Allergies
- Perceptions of heat and cold in the home environment with a need for warmth or cooling
- Somatic complaints
- Responses to touching
- Need to urinate or defecate
- Over- or understimulating environment
- Illusions, delusions, and hallucinations
- Mental illnesses, particularly restlessness associated with depression and anxiety
- Boredom
- Feelings of being lost
- Injuries, falls, or trauma
- Medications, especially psychotropic ones
- Prior history of a stressful life with walking and wandering as a way to cope with stress
- Previous work roles that involved physical activity

W

- Previous social and leisure activities that involved the expenditure of physical energy and travel
- Precursor to catastrophic reaction

Assessment Tools and Instruments (see Appendix I)

Consider administering the:

1. At Risk for Falls Assessment
2. Geriatric Depression Scale
3. Mini-Mental State Examination

PROBLEM LIST

- Caregiver Role Strain
- Caregiver Role Strain, Risk for
- Communication, Impaired Verbal
- Confusion, Acute
- Confusion, Chronic
- Diversional Activity Deficit
- Environmental Interpretation Syndrome, Impaired
- Grieving, Anticipatory
- Grieving, Dysfunctional
- Memory, Impaired
- Pain
- Pain, Chronic
- Personal Identity Disturbance
- Post-Trauma Response

- Powerlessness
- Protection, Altered
- Relocation Stress Syndrome
- Sensory/Perceptual Alterations (specify)
- Sleep Pattern Disturbance
- Social Interaction, Impaired
- Social Isolation
- Spiritual Disorders
- Thermoregulation, Ineffective
- Thought Processes, Altered
- Trauma, Risk for
- Violence, Risk for, Self-Directed or Directed at Others

PROBLEM MANAGEMENT

Prevention, Maintenance, and Restorative Interventions

- Assess to determine if the pt engages in wandering behavior, and if so, obtain further information (eg, what the f/c do to manage this behavior, pt's hobbies, etc) for the treatment plan.
- Determine what the pt is demonstrating, communicating, or responding to by engaging in wandering behavior.
- Observe when pt is engaging in wandering behavior to determine the type or pattern of wandering behavior and the need the behavior may be meeting (Rader, Doan, & Schwab, 1985).
- Eliminate or modify any conditions or factors that contribute to, intensify, or are associated with the wandering behavior to minimize wandering behavior and prevent harm or injury to the p/f/c.

W

- Provide a safe selection of items that can be manipulated easily (but not put into the mouth) and are satisfying to the pt for self-stimulation to meet the pt's need and prevent harm.
- Instruct the f/c to anticipate the pt's wandering behavior or ambulation patterns and provide gratification before onset of wandering behavior.

Medication Management

No specific medications are indicated for this behavior. However, low-dose antipsychotic medications may be helpful to the pt who is engaging in wandering behavior if it is due to disorganized thinking or agitation. Antianxiety medication can be effective if the wandering behavior is caused by anxiety.

NURSING MANAGEMENT

Nursing Interventions and Rationales

☆ Behavioral

- Instruct the f/c to place multiple visual cues (such as signs in the shape of a stop sign, that say "no exit," and mirrors on doors), actual barriers (such as double locks or chairs in front of doors), and safe articles of interest at exits. *These measures prevent the pt from leaving the home and provide stimulation.*
- Provide points of interest (eg, a window with a view or available finger foods) and a stimulating environment. *This prevents or minimizes wandering behavior.*
- Assess f/c actions to manage pt's wandering behavior. *This assessment determines if such actions improve or worsen the wandering behavior.*
- Instruct the f/c to observe and record pt's wandering behavior. *This assesses what type or category of wandering the pt engages in, and where, when, how, and with whom the pt ambulates, to determine if it is a problem and design effective interventions.*
- Assist the f/c to establish a routine and schedule and minimize their own stress. *These interventions provide a home atmosphere that is conducive to the elimination or reduction of wandering behavior.*
- Provide a safe area with adequate lighting for the pt to wander within the home. *This meets the pt's need to engage in wandering behavior.*

🜪 Emotional

- Determine if a relationship exists between the pt's wandering behavior and feelings of frustration, fear, and boredom (Burnside, 1980; Hiatt, 1980), or of feeling lost (Mace & Rabins, 1981). *This provides a basis for understanding the pt's behavior, attempts to communicate feelings, and designs effective emotional interventions.*
- Instruct the f/c that wandering behavior might be a precursor to a catastrophic reaction. *This prevents or minimizes the duration, frequency, and intensity of a catastrophic reaction.*

W

▲ Cognitive

- Determine if a relationship exists between the pt's wandering behavior and self-stimulation. *This provides a basis for understanding the pt's behavior and designing effective cognitive interventions.*
- Instruct the pt, and instruct the f/c to instruct the pt, only to ambulate in designated areas of the home and not to leave the home. *This prevents the pt from leaving the home and possibly becoming lost or injured.*
- Teach the f/c about wandering behavior and not to impede the pt's movements while pt is sitting or sleeping. *This enhances an understanding of the behavior and assists the pt in maintaining function and independence.*
- Develop with the f/c a plan to follow, and to have recent photographs of the pt available, in the event that the pt leaves the home. *Such an approach will more efficiently locate the wandering pt.*

☐ Physical

- Refrain from the use of restraints and sedation of the pt. *This minimizes wandering behavior, falls, excess dependence, the hazards of immobility, sensory deprivation, and loss of control* (Hussian, 1981).
- Seek to eliminate or reduce the amount of psychotropic medication the pt is taking. *This minimizes the wandering and pacing caused by akathisia.*
- Teach the f/c about the benefits of wandering and incorporate regular physical exercise, stretching, range-of-motion exercises, rhythmic movements, and periods of time for the pt to ambulate into the daily routine. *These measures decrease the need and desire of the pt to wander, especially wandering caused by anxiety and agitation* (Wolanin & Phillips, 1981).

◖ Social

- Determine if a relationship exists between the pt's wandering behavior and previous work roles or leisure activities. *This provides a basis for understanding the pt's behavior and designing effective social interventions.*
- Assess if the pt is using wandering behavior when lonely because the pt may be less sociable and verbal (Hiatt, 1980; Rader et al., 1985). *Assessment provides a basis for understanding the pt's behavior and designing effective social interventions.*

✴ Spiritual

- Determine if a relationship exists between the pt's wandering behavior and possible search for security, a sense of purpose, comfort, safety, connectedness, personal identity, belonging, or a desire to explore or rediscover experiences. *This provides a basis for understanding the pt's behavior and designing effective spiritual interventions.*
- Instruct the f/c that facilitating the pt's safe wandering behavior is important. *This gives a feeling of freedom and imparts autonomy and dignity to the pt.*
- Provide measures that preserve the identity of the pt. *These reduce the pt's feelings of separation and minimizes the need or desire to wander.*

Nursing Goals

- To prevent pt accidents and fatal falls
- To prevent exposure of the pt to adverse weather conditions
- To assess the f/c for risk of physical and mental decompensation

Patient Goals

- The pt will ambulate safely.
- The pt will have needs and desires met by wandering.
- The pt will experience a balance of rest and motion.

Patient and Family/Caregiver Outcomes

The patient and family/caregiver will:

- Ambulate _____ times a day for _____ (specify the amount of time) by _____ (date)
- Engage in physical or other _____ (specify) activities that are satisfying to the pt as demonstrated by _____ within _____ weeks
- Attend a support group to learn interventions that will positively affect the pt's wandering behavior by _____ (date)
- Ensure that the pt remains safely in the home due to _____ (specify measures), and is able to ambulate, as demonstrated by _____ by _____ (date)

RESOURCES AND INFORMATION

1. Alzheimer's Association (for information on managing wandering behavior) in the white pages for local chapters and 1-800-272-3900
   919 N. Michigan Avenue
   Suite 1000
   Chicago, IL 60611-1676
2. Head Injury Foundation: 1-800-444-6443
3. Mental Retardation Association: 1-800-424-3688
4. Protection and Advocacy for People with Disabilities: 1-800-432-4682

REFERENCES

American Heritage Dictionary (Eds.) (1980). *Roget's II The New Thesaurus*. Boston: Houghton Mifflin.

Beck, C., & Heacock, P. (1988). Nursing intervention for patients with Alzheimer's disease. *Nursing Clinics of North America, 23*(1), 95–124.

Burnside, I. (1985). Symptomatic behaviors in the elderly. In J. E. Birren & R. B. Sloan (Eds.), *Handbook of mental health and aging*. Englewood Cliffs, NJ: Prentice Hall.

Fopma-Loy, J. (1988). Wandering: Causes, consequences, and care. *Journal of Psychosocial Nursing and Mental Health Services, 26*(5), 8–18.

Heim, K. M. (1985). Wandering behavior. *Journal of Gerontological Nursing, 12*(11), 4–7.

Hiatt, L. G. (1980). The happy wanderer. *Nursing Homes, 29*(1), 27–31.

Hussian, R. (1981). *Geriatric psychology: A behavioral perspective*. New York: Van Nostrand Reinhold.

W

Hussian, R. A., & Davis, R. L. (1985). *Responsive care behavioral interventions with elderly persons.* Champaign, IL: Research Press.

Mace, N. L., & Rabins, P. V. *The 36-hour day.* Baltimore: Johns Hopkins University Press.

Rader, J., Doan, J., & Schwab, Sr. M. (1985). How to decrease wandering: A form of agenda behavior. *Geriatric Nursing, 6,* 196–199.

Snyder, L. H., Rupprecht, P., Pyrck, J., Brekhus, S., & Moss, T. (1978). Wandering. *The Gerontologist, 18,* 272–280.

Wolanin, M. O., & Phillips, L. R. (1981). *Confusion: Prevention and care.* St. Louis: Mosby.

W

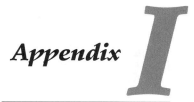

Assessment Tools and Instruments

ABNORMAL INVOLUNTARY MOVEMENT SCALE (AIMS)

Complete this form at start of care, once a month, when medications or dosages are changed, and at discharge for all patients on antipsychotic medications.

Movement Ratings: Circle the highest level of severity observed.

Level of Severity:

0 = None
1 = Minimal, may be extreme normal
2 = Mild
3 = Moderate
4 = Severe

Facial and Oral Movements
1. Muscles of facial expression   0 1 2 3 4
   Movements of forehead, eyebrows, periorbital area,
   cheeks (include frowning, blinking, smiling, grimacing)
2. Lips and perioral areas   0 1 2 3 4
3. Jaw   0 1 2 3 4
   Biting, clenching, chewing, mouth opening, lateral
   movement
4. Tongue   0 1 2 3 4
   Rate only increase in movement both in and out of
   mouth, *NOT* inability to sustain movement

Extremity Movements
5. Upper (arms, wrists, hands, fingers)   0 1 2 3 4
   Include choreoid movements such as rapid, objectively purposeless, irregular, or spontaneous, and
   athetoid movements such as slow, irregular, complex,
   or serpentine
6. Lower (legs, knees, ankles, toes)   0 1 2 3 4
   Lateral knee movement, foot tapping, heel dropping,
    foot squirming, inversion and eversion of foot

Trunk Movements
7. Neck, shoulders, hips   0 1 2 3 4
   Rocking, twisting, squirming, pelvic gyrations

Global Judgments
8. Severity of abnormal movements   0 1 2 3 4
9. Incapacitation due to abnormal movements   0 1 2 3 4
10. Patient's awareness of abnormal movements   0 1 2 3 4

Dental Status   **Total Score**
11. Current problems with teeth or dentures   No   Yes
12. Does patient usually wear dentures?   No   Yes

Examination Procedure

Either before or after completing the examination procedure, observe the patient unobtrusively, at rest.

The chair to be used in this examination should be a hard, firm one without arms.

1. Ask patient to remove shoes and socks.
2. Ask patient whether there is anything in his or her mouth (ie, gum, candy, etc) and if there is, to remove it.
3. Ask patient about the current condition of his or her teeth. Ask patient if he or she wears dentures. Do teeth or dentures bother patient now?
4. Ask patient whether he or she notices any movements in mouth, face, hands, or feet. If yes, ask to describe and to what extent the movements currently bother patient or interfere with activities.
5. Have patient sit in chair with hands on knees, legs slightly apart, and feet flat on floor. (Look at entire body for movements while in this position.)
6. Ask patient to sit with hands hanging unsupported—if male, between legs, if female and wearing a dress, hanging over knees. (Observe hands and other body areas.)
7. Ask patient to open mouth. (Observe tongue at rest in mouth.) Do this twice.
8. Ask patient to protrude tongue. (Observe abnormalities of tongue movement.) Do this twice.
9. Ask patient to tap thumb, with each finger, as rapidly as possible for 10 to 15 seconds, separately with right hand, then with left hand. (Observe facial and leg movements.)
10. Flex and extend patient's left and right arms (one at a time). (Note any rigidity.)
11. Ask patient to stand up. (Observe in profile. Observe all body areas again, hips included.)
12. Ask patient to extend both arms outstretched in front with palms down. (Observe trunk, legs, and mouth.)
13. Have patient walk a few paces, turn, and walk back to chair. (Observe hands and gait.) Do this twice.

Psychopharmacology Research Branch, National Institute of Mental Health (1976). Abnormal involuntary movement scale (AIMS). In W. Guy (Ed.). *ECDEU assessment manual for psychopharmacology* (Revised, pp. 534–537). (DHEW Publication No. ADM 76-338). Rockville, MD: Author. (The publication is in the public domain.)

BARTHEL INDEX—FUNCTIONAL EVALUATION OF ACTIVITIES OF DAILY LIVING

Action	With Help	Independent
1. Feeding (if food needs to be cut up—help)	5	10
2. Moving from wheelchair to bed and return (includes sitting up in bed)	5–10	15
3. Personal toilet (wash fash, comb hair, shave, clean teeth)	0	5
4. Getting on and off toilet (handling, clothes, wipe, flush)	5	10
5. Bathing self	0	5
6. Walking on level surface (or if unable to walk, propel wheelchair)	0	5*
7. Ascend and descend stairs	5	10
8. Dressing (includes tying shoes, fastening fasteners)	5	10
9. Controlling bowels	5	10
10. Controlling bladder	5	10

Patients scoring 100 BDI are continent, feed themselves, get up out of bed and chairs, bathe themselves, walk at least a block, and can ascend and descend stairs. This does not mean that they are able to live alone. They may not be able to cook, keep house, and meet the public, but are able to get along without attendant care.

Definition and Discussion of Scoring

1. Feeding
    10 = Independent. The patient can feed self a meal from a tray or table when someone puts the food within reach. Patient must put on assistive device if this is needed, cut up the food, use salt and pepper, spread butter, etc; must accomplish this in a reasonable time.
    5 = Some help is necessary (with cutting up food, etc, as listed above).
2. Moving from Wheelchair to Bed and Return
    15 = Independent in all phases of this activity. Patient can safely approach the bed in wheelchair, lock brakes, lift footrests, move safely from bed, lie down, come to a sitting position on the side of the bed, change the position of the wheelchair, if necessary, to transfer back into it safely and return to the wheelchair.
    10 = Either some minimal help is needed in some step of this activity or the patient needs to be reminded or supervised for safety of one or more parts of this activity.
    5 = Patient can come to a sitting position without the help of a second person but needs to be lifted out of bed, or, if transfers, with a great deal of help.

3. Doing Personal Toilet

   5 = Patient can wash hands and face, comb hair, clean teeth, and shave. Patient may use any kind of razor but must put in blade or plug in razor without help as well as get it from the drawer or cabinet. Female patients must put on own makeup, if used, but need not braid or style hair.

4. Getting on and off toilet

   10 = Patient is able to get on and off toilet, fasten and unfasten clothes, prevent soiling of clothes, and use toilet paper without help. Patient may use a wall bar or other stable object for support if needed. If it is necessary to use a bed pan instead of toilet, patient must be able to place it on a chair, empty it, and clean it.

   5 = Patient needs help because of imbalance or in handling clothes or in using toilet paper.

5. Bathing Self

   5 = Patient may use a bathtub, a shower, or take a complete sponge bath. Patient must be able to do all the steps involved in whichever method is used without another person being present.

6. Walking on a Level Surface

   15 = Patient can walk at least 50 yards without help or supervision. Patient may wear braces or prosthesis and use crutches, canes, or a walkerette but not a rolling walker. Patient must be able to lock and unlock braces if used, assume the standing position and sit down, get the necessary mechanical aids into position for use, and dispose of them when they sit. (Putting on and taking off braces is scored under Dressing.)

6a. Propelling a Wheelchair

   5 = If a patient cannot ambulate but can propel a wheelchair independently, must be able to go around corners, turn around, maneuver the chair to a table, bed, toilet, etc. Patient must be able to push a chair at least 50 yards. Do not score this item if the patient gets a score for walking.

7. Ascending and Descending Stairs

   10 = Patient is able to go up and down a flight of stairs safely without help or supervision. Patient may and should use handrails, canes, or crutches when needed. Patient must be able to carry canes or crutches while ascending or descending stairs.

   5 = Patients needs help with or supervision of any one of the above items.

8. Dressing and Undressing

   10 = Patient is able to put on and remove and fasten all clothing, and tie shoelaces (unless it is necessary to the adaptations for this). This activity includes putting on and removing and fastening corset or braces when these are prescribed. Such special clothing as suspenders, loafer shoes, dresses that open down the front may be used when necessary.

   5 = Patients need help in putting on and removing or fastening any clothing. They must do at least half the work. They must accomplish this in a reasonable time.

Women need not be scored on use of a brassiere or girdle unless these are prescribed garments.

9. Continence of Bowels
      10 = Patient is able to control bowels and have no accidents. Patient can use a suppository or take an enema when necessary (as for spinal cord injury patients who have had bowel training).
       5 = Patient needs help in using a suppository or taking an enema or has occasional accidents.
10. Controlling Bladder
      10 = Patient is able to control bladder day and night. Spinal cord injury patients who wear an external device and leg bag must put them on independently, clean and empty bag, and stay dry day and night.
       5 = Patient has occasional accident, or cannot wait for the bed pan, or get to the toilet in time, or needs help with an external device.

The total score is not as significant or meaningful as the breakdown into individual items because these indicate where the deficiencies are.

Mahoney, F. I., & Barthel, D. W. (1965). Functional evaluation: The Barthel Index. *Maryland State Medical Journal, 14,* 62.

BECK DEPRESSION INVENTORY

The Beck Depression Inventory is a self-rating scale that measures depression. The patient can complete the questionnaire in about 10 minutes. The total score provides an estimate of the degree of severity of the depressed mood. Add the raw scores. The mean scores can be interpreted as follows:

Total Score	Levels of Depression
1–10	Normal ups and downs
11–16	Mild mood disturbance
17–20	Borderline clinical depression
21–30	Moderate depression
30–40	Severe depression
Over 40	Extreme depression

(A persistent score of 17 or above indicates professional treatment might be necessary.)

1.
   0 I do not feel sad.
   1 I feel sad.
   2 I am sad all the time and I can't snap out of it.
   3 I am so sad or unhappy that I can't stand it.
2.
   0 I am not particularly discouraged about the future.
   1 I feel discouraged about the future.
   2 I feel I have nothing to look forward to.
   3 I feel that the future is hopeless and that things cannot improve.
3.
   0 I do not feel like a failure.
   1 I feel I have failed more than the average person.
   2 As I look back on my life, all I can see is a lot of failures.
   3 I feel I am a complete failure as a person.
4.
   0 I get as much satisfaction out of things as I used to.
   1 I don't enjoy things the way I used to.
   2 I don't get real satisfaction out of anything anymore.
   3 I am dissatisfied or bored with everything.
5.
   0 I don't feel particularly guilty.
   1 I feel guilty a good part of the time.
   2 I feel quite guilty most of the time.
   3 I feel guilty all of the time.
6.
   0 I don't feel I am being punished.
   1 I feel I may be punished.
   2 I expect to be punished.
   3 I feel I am being punished.
7.
   0 I don't feel disappointed in myself.
   1 I am disappointed in myself.
   2 I am disgusted with myself.
   3 I hate myself.
8.
   0 I don't feel I am worse than anybody else.
   1 I am critical of myself for my weaknesses or mistakes.
   2 I blame myself all the time for my faults.
   3 I blame myself for everything bad that happens.

9. 0   I don't have any thoughts of killing myself.
    1   I have thoughts of killing myself, but I would not carry them out.
    2   I would like to kill myself.
    3   I would kill myself if I had the chance.
10. 0   I don't cry any more than usual.
    1   I cry more now than I used to.
    2   I cry all the time now.
    3   I used to be able to cry, but now I can't even though I want to.
11. 0   I am no more irritated by things than I ever am.
    1   I am slightly more irritated now than usual.
    2   I am quite annoyed or irritated a good deal of the time.
    3   I feel irritated all the time now.
12. 0   I have not lost interest in other people.
    1   I am less interested in other people than I used to be.
    2   I have lost most of my interest in other people.
    3   I have lost all of my interest in other people.
13. 0   I make decisions about as well as I ever could.
    1   I put off making decisions more than I used do.
    2   I have greater difficulty in making decisions than before.
    3   I can't make decisions at all anymore.
14. 0   I don't feel that I look any worse than I used to.
    1   I am worried that I am looking old or unattractive.
    2   I feel that there are permanent changes in my appearance that make me look unattractive.
    3   I believe that I look ugly.
15. 0   I can work about as well as before.
    1   It takes an extra effort to get started as doing something.
    2   I have to push myself very hard to do anything.
    3   I can't do any work at all.
16. 0   I can sleep as well as usual.
    1   I don't sleep as well as I used to.
    2   I wake up 1–2 hours earlier than I used to and cannot get back to sleep.
    3   I wake up several hours earlier than I used to and cannot get back to sleep.
17. 0   I don't get more tired than usual.
    1   I get tired more easily than I used to.
    2   I get tired from doing almost anything.
    3   I am too tired to do anything.
18. 0   My appetite is no worse than usual.
    1   My appetite is not as good as it used to be.
    2   My appetite is much worse now.
    3   I have no appetite at all anymore.
19. 0   I haven't lost much weight, if any, lately.
    1   I have lost more than 5 pounds.
    2   I have lost more than 10 pounds.
    3   I have lost more than 15 pounds.
20. 0   I am no more worried about my health than usual.
    1   I am worried about physical problems such as aches and pains, or upset stomach, or constipation.

2   I am very worried about physical problems and it's hard to think of much else.

3   I am so worried about my physical problems that I cannot think about anything else.

21.   0   I have not noticed any recent change in my interest in sex.

1   I am less interested in sex than I used to be.

2   I am much less interested in sex now.

3   I have lost interest in sex completely.

Beck, A. T., Ward, C. H., Mendelson, M., Mock, J. & Erbaugh, J. (1961). Inventory for measuring depression. *Archives of General Psychiatry, 4,* 561–571. (This was written by an employee of the federal government and is in the public domain.)

BRIEF PSYCHIATRIC RATING SCALE

Instruction: This form consists of 18 symptom constructs, each to be rated on a 7-point scale of severity, ranging from "not present" to "extremely severe." If a specific symptom is not rated, mark "0" = Not assessed. Score each item as follows:

0 = Not assessed
1 = Not present
2 = Very mild
3 = Mild
4 = Moderate
5 = Moderately severe
6 = Severe
7 = Extremely severe

Check the appropriate number ranking.

1	2	3	4	5	6	7	Description
							Somatic Concern—Degree of concern over present bodily health. Rate the degree to which physical health is perceived as a problem by the patient, whether complaints have a realistic basis or not.
							Anxiety—Worry, fear, or overconcern for present or future. Rate solely on the basis of verbal report of patient's own subjective experiences. Do not infer anxiety from physical signs or from neurotic drefense mechanisms.
							Emotional Withdrawal—Deficiency in relating to the interviewer and to the interviewer situation. Rate only the degree to which the patient gives the impression of failing to be in emotional contact with other people in the interview situation.
							Conceptual Disorganization—Degree to which the thought processes are confused, disconnected, or disorganized. Rate on the basis of integration of the verbal products of the patient; do not rate on the basis of patient's subjective impression of own level of functioning.
							Guilt Feelings—Overconcern or remorse for past behavior. Rate on the basis of the patient's subjective experiences of guilt as evidenced by verbal report with appropriate affect; do not infer guilt feelings from depression, anxiety, or neurotic defenses.
							Tension—Physical and motor manifestations of tension, "nervousness," and heightened activation level. Tension should be rated solely on the basis of physical signs and motor behavior and not on the basis of subjective experiences of tension reported by the patient.

1	2	3	4	5	6	7	Description
							Mannerisms and Posturing—Unusual and unnatural motor behavior, the type of motor behavior that causes certain mental patients to stand out in a crowd of normal people. Rate only abnormality of movements; do not rate simple heightened motor activity here.
							Grandiosity—Exaggerated self-opinion, conviction of unusual ability or powers. Rate only on the basis of patient's statements about self or self in relation to others, not on the basis of demeanor in the interview situation.
							Depressive Mood—Despondency in mood, sadness. Rate only degree of despondency; do not rate on the basis of inferences concerning depression based on general retardation and somatic complaints.
							Hostility—Animosity, contempt, belligerence, disdain for other people outside the interview situation. Rate solely on the basis of the verbal report of feelings and actions of the patient toward others; do not infer hostility from neurotic defenses, anxiety, or somatic complaints. (Rate attitude toward interviewer under "uncooperativeness.")
							Suspiciousness—Belief (delusional or otherwise) that others have now, or have had in the past, malicious or discriminatory intent toward the patient. On the basis of verbal report, rate only those suspicions that are currently held whether they concern past or present circumstances.
							Hallucinatory Behavior—Perceptions without normal external stimulus correspondence. Rate only those experiences that are reported to have occurred within the last week and are described as distinctly different from the thought and imagery processes of normal people.

1	2	3	4	5	6	7	Description
							Motor Retardation—Reduction in energy level evidenced in slowed movements. Rate on the basis of observed behavior of the patient only; do not rate on basis of patient's subjective impression of own energy level.
							Uncooperativeness—Evidence of resistance, unfriendliness, resentment, and lack of readiness to cooperate with the interviewer. Rate only on the basis of the patient's attitude and responses to the interviewer and the interview situation; do not rate on basis of reported resentment or uncooperativeness outside the interview situation.
							Unusual Thought Content—Unusual, odd, strange, or bizarre thought content. Rate here the degree of unusualness, not the degree of disorganization of thought processes.
							Blunted Affect—Reduced emotional tone, apparent lack of normal feeling or involvement.
							Excitement—Heightened emotional tone, agitation, increased reactivity.
							Disorientation—Confusion or lack of proper association for person, place, or time.

Score: _____

Score interpretations:

  0 = Absence symptomatology
18 = Very mild psychiatric impairment
36 = Mild psychiatric impairment
54 = Moderate psychiatric impairment
72 = Moderately severe psychiatric impairment
90 = Severe psychiatric impairment
108 = Extremely severe psychiatric impairment

Overall, J. E., & Gorham, D. R. (1962; modified, 1966). The Brief Psychiatric Rating Scale. *Psychological Reports, 10,* 799–812.

Overall, J. E. (Chair), & Gorham, D. R. (1988). The Brief Psychiatric Rating Scale (BPRS): Recent developments in ascertainment and scaling. *Psychopharmacology Bulletin, 24* (1), 97–100. Reprinted with permission.

BRIEF PSYCHIATRIC SCHIZOPHRENIC RATING SCALE (BPSRS)

The Brief Psychiatric Schizophrenic Rating Scale measures the level of severity observed for 21 indicators of schizophrenic behavior. The scale may be administered on admission, periodically throughout treatment, and at discharge, to assess the level of progress or decline in individual indicators. Treatment interventions are directed toward improving the problems identified by the indicators.

Instructions: Circle the highest severity observed.

Level of severity:

1 = Not present
2 = Very mild
3 = Mild
4 = Moderate
5 = Moderately severe
6 = Severe
7 = Extremely severe

1	2	3	4	5	6	7	Description
							Somatic Concern—Degree of concern over present bodily health. Rate the degree to which physical health is perceived as a problem by the patient (whether complaints have a realistic basis or not).
							Anxiety—Worry, fear, or overconcern for present or future. Rate solely on the basis of verbal report of patient's own subjective experiences. Do not infer anxiety from physical signs or from neurotic defense mechanisms.
							Depression—Despondency in mood, sadness. Rate only degree of despondency. Do not rate on the basis of interferences concerning depression based on general retardation and somatic complaints.
							Guilt Feelings—Overconcern or remorse for past behavior. Rate on the basis of the patient's subjective experiences of guilt as evidenced by verbal report with appropriate affect. Do not infer guilt feelings from depression, anxiety, or neurotic defenses.
							Hostility—Animosity, contempt, belligerence, disdain for people outside the interview situation. Rate solely on the basis of the verbal report of feelings and actions of the patient toward others. Do not infer hostility from neurotic defenses, anxiety, or somatic complaints. (Rate attitude toward interviewer under "uncooperativeness.")
							Suspiciousness—Belief (delusional or otherwise) that others have now, or have had in the past, malicious or discriminatory intent toward the patient. On the basis of verbal report, rate only those suspicions that are currently held whether they concern past or present circumstances.

1	2	3	4	5	6	7	Description
							Unusual Thought Content—Unusual, odd, strange, or bizarre thought content. Rate here the degree of unusualness, not the degree of disorganization of thought processes.
							Grandiosity—Exaggerated self-opinion, conviction of unusual ability or powers. Rate only on the basis of patient's statements about self or self in relation to others, not on the basis of demeanor in the interview situation.
							Hallucinatory Behavior—Perceptions without normal external stimulus correspondence. Rate only those experiences that are reported to have occurred within the last week and are described as distinctly different from the thought and imagery processes of normal people.
							Disorientation—Confusion or lack of proper association for person, place, or time.
							Conceptual Disorganization—Degree to which the thought processes are confused, disconnected, or disorganized. Rate only on the basis of integration of the verbal products of the patient. Do not rate on the basis of patient's subjective impression of own level of functioning.
							Excitement—Heightened emotional tone, agitation, increased reactivity.
							Motor Retardation—Reduction in energy level evidenced in slow movements. Rate on the basis of observed behavior of the patient only. Do not rate on the basis of patient's subjective impression of own energy.

1	2	3	4	5	6	7	Description
							Blunted Affect—Impairment in emotional expressiveness of face, voice, and gestures. Marked indifference or flatness even when discussing distressing topics.
							Tension—Physical and motor manifestations of tension "nervousness" and heightened activation level. Tension should be rated solely on the basis of physical signs and motor behavior, and not on the basis of subjective experiences of tension reported by the patient.
							Mannerisms and Posturing—Unusual and unnatural motor behavior, the type of motor behavior that causes certain mental patients to stand out in a crowd of normal people. Rate only abnormality of movements. Do not rate simple heightened motor activity here.
							Uncooperativeness—Evidence of resistance, unfriendliness, resentment, and lack of readiness to cooperate with the interviewer. Rate only on the basis of the patient's attitude and responses to the interviewer and the interview situation. Do not rate on the basis of reported resentment or uncooperativeness outside the interview situation.
							Emotional Withdrawal—Deficiency in relating to the interviewer and to the interview situation. Rate only the degree to which the patient gives the impression of failing to be in emotional contact with other people in the interview situation.
							Suicidiality—Expressed desire, intent, or actual actions to harm or kill self.
							Self-Neglect—Hygiene, appearance, or eating behavior below usual expectations, below socially acceptable standards, or life-threatening.

1	2	3	4	5	6	7	Description
							Bizarre Behavior—Reports of behaviors that are odd, unusual, or psychotically criminal. Not limited to interview period.

Total Score: _____

Department of Health and Welfare. Brief Psychiatric Schizophrenic Rating Scale. (This was written by an employee of the federal government and is in the public domain.)

CLINICAL INVENTORY WITHDRAWAL ASSESSMENT FOR ALCOHOL

The Clinical Inventory Withdrawal Assessment for Alcohol quantifies the severity of alcohol withdrawal and designates potential levels of care.

Instructions: Assess daily during detoxification, note date and time assessment completed, record pulse/heart rate for 1 full minute, and record blood pressure.

Total score 65

Score of:		
<20	=	No medications necessary for withdrawal
20–30	=	Potential for medications during detoxification
30–40	=	Medications necessary for detoxification/withdrawal
>40	=	Potential for hospitalization for detoxification/withdrawal

Nausea and Vomiting—Ask "Do you feel sick to your stomach? Have you vomited?"
Observation:
0 ☐ No nausea and no vomiting
1 ☐ Mild nausea with no vomiting
2 ☐
3 ☐
4 ☐ Intermittent nausea with dry heaves
5 ☐
6 ☐
7 ☐ Constant nausea, freuqent dry heaves and vomiting

Tremor—Arms extended and fingers spread apart. Observation:
0 ☐ No tremor
1 ☐ Not visible, but can be felt fingertip to fingertip
2 ☐
3 ☐
4 ☐ Moderate, with patient's arms extended
5 ☐
6 ☐
7 ☐ Severe, even with arms not extended

Paroxysmal Sweats—Observation:
0 ☐ No sweat visible
1 ☐ Barely perceptible sweating, palms moist
2 ☐
3 ☐
4 ☐ Beads of sweat obvious on forehead
5 ☐
6 ☐
7 ☐ Drenching sweats

Anxiety—Ask "Do you feel nervous?" Observation:
0 ☐ No anxiety, at ease
1 ☐ Mildly anxious
2 ☐
3 ☐
4 ☐ Moderately anxious, or guarded, no anxiety is inferred
5 ☐
6 ☐

Agitation—Observation:
0 ☐ Normal activity
1 ☐ Somewhat more than normal activity
2 ☐
3 ☐
4 ☐ Moderately fidgety and restless
5 ☐
6 ☐
7 ☐ Paces back and forth during most of the interview or constantly thrashes about

Tactile Disturbances—Ask "Do you have any itching, pins and needles sensations, any burning, any numbness or do you feel bugs crawling on or under your skin?" Observation:

0 ☐ None
1 ☐ Very mild itching, pins and needles, burning or numbness
2 ☐ Mild itching, pins and needles, burning or numbness
3 ☐ Moderate itching, pins and needles, burning or numbness
4 ☐ Moderately severe hallucinations
5 ☐ Severe hallucinations
6 ☐ Extremely severe hallucinations
7 ☐ Continuous hallucinations

Auditory Disturbances—Ask "Are you more aware of sounds around you? Are they harsh? Do they frighten you? Are you hearing anything that is disturbing to you? Are you hearing things you know are not there?" Observation:

0 ☐ Not present
1 ☐ Very mild harshness or ability to frighten
2 ☐ Mild harshness or ability to frighten
3 ☐ Moderate harshness or ability to frighten
4 ☐ Moderately severe hallucinations
5 ☐ Severe hallucinations
6 ☐ Extremely severe hallucinations
7 ☐ Continuous hallucinations

Visual Disturbances—Ask "Does the light appear to be too bright? Is its color different? Does it hurt your eyes? Are you seeing anything that is disturbing to you? Are you seeing things you know are not there?" Observation:

0 ☐ Not present
1 ☐ Very mild sensitivity
2 ☐ Mild sensitivity
3 ☐ Moderate sensitivity
4 ☐ Moderately severe hallucinations
5 ☐ Severe hallucinations
6 ☐ Extremely severe hallucinations

Headache, Fullness in Head—Ask "Does your head feel different? Does it feel like there is a band around your head?" Do not rate for dizziness or lightheadedness. Otherwise, rate severity.

0 ☐ Not present
1 ☐ Very mild
2 ☐ Mild
3 ☐ Moderate
4 ☐ Moderately severe
5 ☐ Severe
6 ☐ Very severe
7 ☐ Extremely severe

Orientation and Clouding of Sensorium—Ask "What day is this?" "What are you?" "What am I?"

0 ☐ Oriented and can do serial additions
1 ☐ Cannot do serial additions or is uncertain about date
2 ☐ Disoriented for date by no more than 2 calendar days
3 ☐ Disoriented for date by more than 2 calendar days
4 ☐ Disoriented for place and/or person

Total Score _____

Maximum Possible Score _____

FALLS RISK ASSESSMENT

The At Risk of Falls and the Falls Risk Factors Assessment measure the potential for possible falls and injury.

At Risk of Falls (ARF)

Age
55–65 years	1 point	_____
65–75 years	2 points	_____
76 years or older	3 points	_____

Number of Days of Home Care
0–14 days	1 point	_____
15–30 days	2 points	_____
Over 31 days	3 points	_____

Mental Status/Activity Status
Assistance required for ambulation	1 point	_____
Confusion at all times	2 points	_____
Intermittent confusion	3 points	_____

Medications
With diuretic effects	1 point	_____
That increase GI motility	2 points	_____
That suppress thought process, level of consciousness, or create hypertensive effects	3 points	_____

General Data
History of seizures	1 point	_____
Falls prior to admission	2 points	_____
Falls during this or previous admission	3 points	_____

Detoxification

Potential for seizures due to alcohol or drug withdrawal	1 point	_____
Use of mood-altering drugs prior to admission	2 points	_____
Potential for withdrawal symptoms	3 points	_____

Total of Points

If total points are 10 or above, institute At Risk of Falls precautions.

Falls Risk Factors Assessment

Yes   **No**   **Description**

Information from History, Assessment, and Other Objective Sources

1. Does the patient have a history of falls, with or without result of injury? If yes, approximately how many? _____
2. Does the patient have a history of CV disorders that would alter blood pressure and cause dizziness, syncope, or paresis?
3. Does the patient have a history of neurologic dysfunction that could affect sensation, blood pressure, or muscular control or cause confusion?
4. Does the patient have a history of musculoskeletal disorders or use orthopedic devices?
5. Does the patient have a history of visual impairment?
6. Does the patient have a history of hearing loss?
7. Does the patient have a history of urinary urgency or incontinence?

Observational Data

1. Does the patient show postural instability with a tendency toward loss of balance (ie, inability to maintain an upright position)?
2. Does the patient exhibit gait changes with a tendency to trip or an inability to recover from a stumble or an unexpected step?
3. Does the patient exhibit impaired muscular control or strength?
4. Does the patient complain of or show behavior indicating pain or stiffness on movement?
5. Does the patient show hyperactivity? (If yes, please explain in the Comments section below.)
6. Does the patient misjudge depth or distance? (If yes, please explain in the Comments section below.)

7. Does the patient, due to confusion, show decreased ability to comprehend and follow instructions or guidance?

8. Does the patient, due to confusion, place the self in danger (eg, climbing on furniture, falling asleep while standing)?

9. Does the patient engage in activities that are self-harming (eg, pulling hair or scratching skin)?

10. Does the patient refuse to stay in bed during sleeping hours?

11. Does the patient show a decreased level of cooperation, increased agitation, or denial of need for assistance?

12. Does the patient ambulate on the toes or balls of feet?

Number of yeses   _____

Number of nos   _____

ARF score at this time: _____

Comments:

Adapted from Hendrich, A. Nyhuis, A., Kippenbrock, T., & Soja, M. E. (1995). Hospital falls: Development of a predictive model for clinical practice. *Applied Nursing Researh, 8 (3)*, 129–139.

GERIATRIC DEPRESSION SCALE

The Geriatric Depression Scale can be used as a self-rating or observer-rated measurement.

During the past 2 weeks:		
1. Have you been sad or tearful?	☐ Yes	☐ No
2. Have there been changes or problems with appetite or sleep?	☐ Yes	☐ No
3. Have you lost pleasure in previously pleasurable activities?	☐ Yes	☐ No
4. Have you thought about death?	☐ Yes	☐ No
5. Have you thought about suicide?	☐ Yes	☐ No
6. Do you have a plan?	☐ Yes	☐ No

**If the patient answers yes to two or more of the above,
the following scale is to be completed.**

1. Are you basically satisfied with your life?	☐ Yes	☐ No
2. Have you dropped many of your activities and interests?	☐ Yes	☐ No
3. Do you feel that your life is empty?	☐ Yes	☐ No
4. Do you often get bored?	☐ Yes	☐ No
5. Are you hopeful about the future?	☐ Yes	☐ No
6. Are you bothered by thoughts you can't get out of your head?	☐ Yes	☐ No
7. Are you in good spirits most of the time?	☐ Yes	☐ No
8. Are you afraid that something bad is going to happen to you?	☐ Yes	☐ No
9. Do you feel happy most of the time?	☐ Yes	☐ No
10. Do you feel helpless?	☐ Yes	☐ No
11. Do you often get restless and fidgety?	☐ Yes	☐ No
12. Do you prefer to stay at home, rather than going out and doing new things?	☐ Yes	☐ No
13. Do you frequently worry about the future?	☐ Yes	☐ No
14. Do you feel you have more problems with memory than most?	☐ Yes	☐ No
15. Do you think it is wonderful to be alive now?	☐ Yes	☐ No
16. Do you feel downhearted and blue?	☐ Yes	☐ No
17. Do you feel pretty worthless the way you are now?	☐ Yes	☐ No
18. Do you worry a lot about the past?	☐ Yes	☐ No
19. Do you find life very exciting?	☐ Yes	☐ No
20. Is it hard for you to get started on new projects?	☐ Yes	☐ No
21. Do you feel full of energy?	☐ Yes	☐ No
22. Do you feel that your situation is hopeless?	☐ Yes	☐ No
23. Do you think that most people are better off than you?	☐ Yes	☐ No
24. Do you frequently get upset over little things?	☐ Yes	☐ No
25. Do you frequently feel like crying?	☐ Yes	☐ No
26. Do you have trouble concentrating?	☐ Yes	☐ No
27. Do you enjoy getting up in the morning?	☐ Yes	☐ No
28. Do you prefer to avoid social gatherings?	☐ Yes	☐ No
29. Is it easy for you to make decisions?	☐ Yes	☐ No
30. Is your mind as clear as it used to be?	☐ Yes	☐ No

Total Scoring: Count 1 point for each depressive answer.

Total:_____

0–10 = normal, 11–20 = mild depression, 21–30 = moderate to severe depression

Yesavage, J. A., Brink, T. L., Rose, T. L., Lum, O., Huang, V., & Adey, M. (1983). Development and validation of a Geriatric Depression Screening Scale: A preliminary report. *Journal of Psychiatric Research, 17,* 37–49. Elsevier Science Ltd., Oxford, England. Reprinted with permission.

GLOBAL ASSESSMENT OF FUNCTIONING SCALE

The Global Assessment of Functioning Scale measures an individual's ability to function in a psychological, social, and occupational continuum of mental health-illness, and does not include impairment in functioning due to physical or environmental limitations.

Instructions: Rate lowest level of functioning in the past week, giving consideration to psychological, social and occupational (or scholastic) factors. Ranges may be used (eg, 22–26, 45–49) as appropriate. Rating based on information from any source.

91–100   Relatively **symptom free** and functioning well in all areas. Interested and involved in wide range of activities, generally being satisfied and experiencing no more than ordinary, everyday problems and concerns.

81–90   **Transient symptoms** that would be expected to occur given certain psychosocial stressors (eg, difficulty concentrating after family argument), but any problems in functioning are only temporary.

71–80   **Minimal symptoms** may be present, but no more than slight impairment in everyday functioning. Occasional worries and problems that sometimes get out of hand.

61–70   **Mild symptoms** (eg, intermittent, but mild depression and insomnia) *or* minor difficulty in daily functioning, but overall managing fairly well and maintaining some meaningful interpersonal relationships.

51–60   **Moderate symptoms** (eg, flat affect, depressed mood, pathologic self-doubt or euphoric mood and pressure of speech) or generally functioning with some difficulty in social, school, or occupational settings. (eg, numerous conflicts with family or coworkers).

41–50   **Serious symptoms** (eg, suicidal ideation, obsessive/compulsive rituals, panic attacks, frequent shoplifting) *or* serious impairment in day-to-day functioning in social, home, or work settings (eg, few friends, unable to maintain employment); child exhibits chronic academic and behavior problems that necessitate family or school intervention (eg, often angry and resentful, refuses to comply with requests of those in authority).

31–40   **Discretionary supervision recommended because of critical impairment** in several areas such as cognition, mood, judgment, or relationships (eg, clinically depressed, avoids friends, neglects family, unable to work, continuous alcohol or drug abuse); child displays consistent pattern of conduct that violates the rights of others or societal norms (eg, stealing, fire setting, physical cruelty to people and animals).

21–30   **Moderate degree of supervision** indicated due to behavior being considerably influenced by delusions or hallucinations; major impairment in communication, judgment, or reality testing (eg, incoherent at times, acts grossly inappropriately, suicidal threats) *or* unable to function in almost all areas of life (eg, stays in bed all day).

11–20   **Frequent amount of supervision** necessary due to some degree of danger of hurting self or others (eg, suicide attempts without clear expectation of death, periodic violence, manic excitement) *or* ability to communicate is severely impaired (eg, primarily incoherent or mute).

0–10   **Intensive supervision** required due to clear and imminent danger of hurting oneself or others (eg, recurrent violence or lethal suicide attempt).

Endicott, J., Spitzer, R. L., Fleiss, J. L., & Cohen, J. (1976). The Global Assessment Scale: A procedure for measuring overall severity of psychiatric disturbance. *Archives of General Psychiatry, 33,* 766–771. "Copyrighted 1976, American Medical Association." Reprinted with permission.

MINI-MENTAL STATE EXAMINATION

The Mini-Mental State Examination is a measurement indicator of mental status and orientation.

Instructions: Ask the client the questions and score one point for each correct answer.

Maximum Score	Score	
		Orientation
5	( )	What is the (year) (season) (date) (month)? (Ask about omitted parts).
5	( )	Where are we: (state) (country) (town) (street) (building)?
		Registration
3	( )	Name these three objects (hat, car, tree): a second to say each. Then ask the patient for all three after you have said them. Give 1 point for each correct answer. Then repeat them until he learns all three. Count trials and record.
		Trials _____
		Attention and Calculation
5	( )	Serial 7's backward from 100 (stop after five answers: 93, 86, 79, 72, 65). 1 point for each correct. Alternatively spell "world" backwards. Score is number of letters in correct order (DLROW = 5).
		Recall
3	( )	Ask for three objects repeated above. Give 1 point for each correct.
		Language
9	( )	Show a pencil and a watch. Ask patient to name them (2 points). Repeat the following "No ifs, ands, or buts" (1 point). Follow a three-stage command:
		a. "Take a paper in your right hand, fold it in half, and put it on the floor." (3 points total, 1 for each part correctly executed).
		b. Reading: Give patient the following page. Tell the patient to read and obey the following: CLOSE YOUR EYES (1 point).
		c. Writing: Give the patient a blank piece of paper and ask him to WRITE A SENTENCE (1 point).

d. Copying: On a clean piece of paper, draw intersecting pentagons, each side about 1 inch, and ask him to COPY THE DESIGN (1 point)

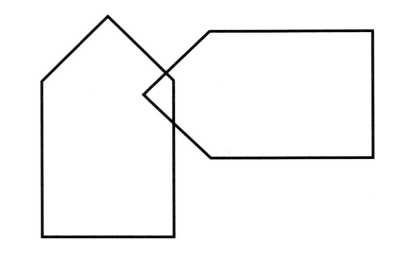

_____ Total Score   Maximim score = 30
Score of 24 or less considered positive for cognitive disorders.

Assess level of consciousness along a continuum.

Alert _____ Drowsy _____ Stupor _____ Coma _____

Folstein, M. F., Folstein, S. E., & McHugh, P. R. (1975). Mini-mental state: A practical method for grading the cognitive state of patients for the clinician. *Journal of Psychiatric Research, 12,* 189. Elsevier Science Ltd., Oxford, England. Reprinted with permission.

MODIFIED OVERT AGGRESSION SCALE (MAOS)

The MAOS is an indicator of the severity of aggressive behaviors.

Instructions: Circle the highest severity observed. The total score is determined by multiplying the four individual scales by their specific weights and then adding the four weighted scores.

Verbal Aggression

Verbal hostility, such as statements or invectives that seek to inflict psychological harm on another through devaluation or degradation, and threats of physical attack

0. No verbal aggression
1. Shouts angrily, curses mildly, or makes personal insults
2. Curses viciously, is severely insulting, has temper outbursts
3. Impulsively threatens violence toward others or self
4. Threatens violence toward others or self repeatedly or deliberately (such as to gain money or sex)

Autoaggression

Physical injury toward oneself, such as self-mutilation or suicide attempt

0. No autoaggression
1. Picks or scratches skin, pulls out hair, hits self (without injury)
2. Bangs heads, hits fists into walls, throws self on floor
3. Inflicts minor cuts, bruises, burns, or welts oneself
4. Inflicts major injury to oneself or makes a suicide attempt

Aggression Against Property

Wanton and reckless destruction of home or others' possessions

0. No aggression against property
1. Slams door angrily, rips clothing, urinates on floor
2. Throws objects down, kicks furniture, defaces walls
3. Breaks objects, smashes windows
4. Sets fires, throws objects dangerously

Physical Aggression

Violent action intended to inflict pain, bodily harm, or death on another

0. No physical aggression
1. Makes menacing gestures, swings at people, grabs at clothing
2. Strikes, kicks, pushes, scratches, pulls hair of others (without injury)
3. Attacks others, causing mild injury (bruises, sprains, or welts)
4. Attacks others, causing serious injury (fracture, loss of teeth, deep cuts, or loss of consciousness)

Rating Summary

Scale	Scaled Score	Weighted Score
Verbal aggression	X 1 =	
Aggression against property	X 1 =	
Autoaggression	X 1 =	
Physical aggression	X 1 =	

Kay, S. (1988). Profiles of aggression among psychiatric patients. *The Journal of Nervous & Mental Disease, 176* (9), 539–546. Reprinted with permission.

NIMH DEMENTIA MOOD ASSESSMENT SCALE (DMAS)

Instructions: Based on a clinical interview and objective information from family or professional staff, select the description that comes closest to portraying the patient. Comparison should be made to the expected level of functioning for his or her age group. Each item is to be rated on a continuum of "0" (within normal limits) to "6" (most severe). The descriptors are intended as general indicators of severity. The presence of any particular descriptive term is not required to place an individual in a certain range, nor is its absence a reason to lower a rating. When the subject falls between descriptors, the half-steps (ie, 1, 3, and 5) should be used.

1. Self-Directed Motor Activity
    0 = Remains active in day-to-day pursuits (irrespective of skills or ability).
    1 =
    2 = Participates in planned activities but may need some guidance structuring free time.
    3 =
    4 = Needs much direction with unstructured time but still participates in planned free time.
    5 =
    6 = Little or no spontaneous activity initiated. Does not willingly participate in activities even with much direction.

2. Sleep (Rate A and B)
    A. Insomnia
    0 = No insomnia/restlessness
    1 =
    2 = Restlessness at night or occasional insomnia (>1 hour). May complain of poor sleep.
    3 =
    4 = Intermittent early awakening or frequent difficulty falling asleep (>1 hour). May get out of bed briefly for purposes other than voiding.
    5 =
    6 = Almost nightly sleep difficulties, insomnia, frequent awakening, or agitation, which is profoundly disturbing the patient's sleep–wake cycle.

    B. Daytime Drowsiness
    0 = No apparent drowsiness
    1 =
    2 = May appear drowsy during the day with occasional napping.
    3 =
    4 = May frequently nod off during the day.
    5 =
    6 = Continuously attempts to sleep during the day.

3. Appetite (Rate either A or B)
    A. Decreased Appetite
    0 = No decreased appetite

1 =
2 = Shows less interest in meals.
3 =
4 = Reports loss of appetite or shows greater than 1 pound/week weight loss.
5 =
6 = Requires urging or assistance in eating or shows greater than 2 pounds/week weight loss.

B. Increased Appetite
0 = No increased appetite
1 =
2 = Shows increased interest in meals and meal planning.
3 =
4 = Snacking frequently in addition to regular meal schedule or weight gain of greater than 1 pound/week.
5 =
6 = Excessive eating throughout the day or weight gain of greater than 2 pounds/week.

4. Psychosomatic Complaints
0 = Not present or appropriate for physical condition.
1 =
2 = Overconcern with health issues (ie, real or imaginary medical problems).
3 =
4 = Frequent physical complaints or repeated requests for medical attention out of proportion to existing conditions.
5 =
6 = Preoccupied with physical complaints. May focus on specific complaints to the exclusion of other problems.

5. Energy
0 = Normal energy level
1 =
2 = Slight decrease in general energy level
3 =
4 = Appears tired often. Occasionally misses planned activities because of "fatigue."
5 =
6 = Attempts to sit alone in a chair or lie in bed much of the day. Appears exhausted despite low activity level.

6. Irritability
0 = No more irritable than normal
1 =
2 = Overly sensitive, showing low tolerance to normal frustration; sarcastic.
3 =
4 = Impatient, demanding, frequent angry reactions.
5 =
6 = Global irritability that cannot be relieved by diversion or explanation.

7. Physical Agitation

   0 = No physical restlessness or agitation noted.

   1 =

   2 = Fidgetiness (ie, plays with hands or taps feet) or bodily tension

   3 =

   4 = Has trouble sitting still. May move from place to place without obvious purpose.

   5 =

   6 = Hand wringing or frequent pacing. Unable to sit in one place for structured activity.

8. Anxiety

   0 = No apparent anxiety

   1 =

   2 = Apprehension or mild worry noted but able to respond to reassurance

   3 =

   4 = Frequent worries about minor matters or overconcern about specific issues. Tension usually obvious in facial countenance or manner. May require frequent reassurances.

   5 =

   6 = Constantly worried and tense. Requires almost constant attention and reassurance to maintain control of anxiety.

9. Depressed Appearance

   0 = Does not appear depressed and denies when questioned directly.

   1 =

   2 = Occasionally seems sad or downcast. May admit to "spirits" being low from time to time.

   3 =

   4 = Frequently appears depressed, irrespective of ability to express or explain underlying thoughts.

   5 =

   6 = Shows mostly depressed appearance, even to casual observer. May be associated with frequent crying.

10. Awareness of Emotional State

   0 = Fully acknowledges emotional condition. Expressed emotions are congruent with current situation.

   1 =

   2 = Occasionally denies feelings appropriate to situation.

   3 =

   4 = Frequently denies emotional reactions. May display some appropriate feelings with focused discussion of individual issues.

   5 =

   6 = Persistently denies emotional state, even with direct confrontation.

11. Emotional Responsiveness

   0 = Smiles and cries in appropriate situations. Establishes eye contact regularly. Speaks and jokes spontaneously in groups.

1 =

2 = Occasionally avoids eye contact but able to respond appropriately when addressed by others. Sometimes may appear distant when sitting in social situations, as if not paying attention.

3 =

4 = Often sitting with blank stare while with others. Responses usually show limited variation of facial expression.

5 =

6 = Does not seek social interaction. Shows little emotion, even when in the presence of loved ones. Seems unable to react to emotional situations, either positively or negatively (ie, calm or bland).

12. Sense of Enjoyment

   0 = Appears to enjoy activities, friends, and family normally.

   1 =

   2 = Reduced animation. May display less pleasure.

   3 =

   4 = Infrequent display of pleasure. May show less enjoyment of family or friends.

   5 =

   6 = Rarely expresses pleasure or enjoyment, even when taking part in formerly consuming interests.

13. Self-Esteem

   0 = No obvious loss of self-esteem or sense of inferiority

   1 =

   2 = Mild decrease in self-esteem noted occasionally. May be unable to identify strengths and accomplishments.

   3 =

   4 = Spontaneously self-deprecating. May display feeling of worthlessness out of proportion to objective observations.

   5 =

   6 = Persistent feelings of worthlessness that cannot be dispelled with reassurance

14. Guilt Feelings

   0 = Absent

   1 =

   2 = Self-reproach. Admits on questioning to feeling like a burden to family or friends.

   3 =

   4 = Spontaneously talks of being a burden to the family or caretakers. May be overly concerned with ideas of guilt or past errors but can be reassured by others.

   5 =

   6 = Preoccupied with guilty thoughts or feelings of shame.

15. Hopelessness/Helplessness

   0 = No evidence of hopelessness or helplessness

   1 =

   2 = Questions ability to cope with life and future. May ask for assistance with simple tasks or decisions that are within own capacity.

3 =

4 = Pessimistic about the future but can be reassured. Frequently seeks assistance regardless of need.

5 =

6 = Feels hopeless about the future. Expresses belief of having little or no control over life.

16. Suicidal Ideation

0 = Absent. Denies any thoughts of suicide.

1 =

2 = Feels life is not worth living or states that others would be better off without him or her. Not consciously pursuing any plans for self harm.

3 =

4 = Thoughts of possible death to self; may wish to die during sleep or pray for "God to take me now."

5 =

6 = Any attempt, gesture, or specific plan of suicide.

17. Speech

0 = Normal rate and rhythm with usual tonal variability. Speech is audible, clear, and fluent.

1 =

2 = Noticeable pauses during conversation. Voices may be low, soft, or monotonous.

3 =

4 = Reduced spontaneous speech. Responses to direct questions are less fluent or mumbled. Initiates little conversation; difficult to hear.

5 =

6 = Rarely speaks spontaneously. Speech is difficult to understand.

18. Diurnal Mood Variation

A. Note whether mood appears worse in morning or evening. If no diurnal variation, mark "none."

0 = None

1 = Worse in morning

2 = Worse in evening

B. When present, mark the severity of the variation. Mark "none" if no variation is present.

0 = None

1 =

2 = Mild

3 =

4 = Moderate

5 =

6 = Severe

19. Diurnal Cognitive Variation

A. Note whether general cognitive abilities appear worse in morning or evening. If no diurnal variation, mark "none."

0 = None
1 = Worse in morning
2 = Worse in evening

B. When present, mark the severity of the variation. Mark "none" if no variation present.
0 = None
1 =
2 = Mild
3 =
4 = Moderate
5 =
6 = Severe

20. Paranoid Symptoms
0 = None
1 =
2 = Occasionally suspicious of harm or watching others closely. Guarded with personal questions.
3 =
4 = Shows intermittent ideas of reference or frequent suspiciousness.
5 =
6 = Paranoid delusions or overt thoughts of persecution

21. Other Psychotic Symptoms
0 = None
1 =
2 = Occasionally misinterprets sensory input or experiences illusions.
3 =
4 = Frequently misinterprets sensory input.
5 =
6 = Overt hallucinations or nonparanoid delusions

22. Expressive Communication Skills
0 = Able to make self understood, even to strangers.
1 =
2 = Sometimes has difficulty communicating with others, but is able to make self understood with additional effort (eg, visual cues).
3 =
4 = Frequently has trouble expressing ideas to others.
5 =
6 = Marked difficulty communicating ideas to others, even family members and significant others.

23. Receptive Cognitive Capacity
0 = Appears to grasp ideas normally.
1 =
2 = Experiences occasional difficulty understanding complex statements expressed by others.

3 =

4 = Frequently misunderstands or fails to comprehend issues when addressed directly, despite repeated attempts.

5 =

6 = Needs multiple modalities of communication (eg, verbal, visual, or physical prompts) to comprehend basic task.

24. Cognitive Insight

0 = Normal cognitively or shows insight into deficits

1 =

2 = Admits to some, but not all of his or her cognitive difficulties.

3 =

4 = Intermittently denies cognitive deficits even when pointed out by others.

5 =

6 = Denies cognitive difficulties even when they are obvious to casual observers.

Functional impairment _____   Depression _____

Cognitive impairment _____   Sadness _____

Psychosis _____   Anxiety _____

Mania _____   Anger _____

Produced by the Unit on Geriatric Psychopharmacology, Laboratory of Clinical Science, National Institute of Mental Health, Bethesda, MD, 1984 (last update: July 1988).

Sunderland, T., Hill, J. L., Lawlor, B. A., & Molchan, S. E. (1988). NIMH Dementia Mood Assessment Scale (DMAS). *Psychopharmacology Bulletin, 24*(4), 747–754. (This was written by an employee of the federal government and is in the public domain.)

OBSESSIVE-COMPULSIVE DISORDER SCREENING CHECKLIST

The Obsessive-Compulsive Disorder Screening Checklist is an indicator of the potential for obsessive-compulsive disorder (OCD).

OCD Screener

Obsessive-Compulsive Disorder Screening Questions

Yes No

☐ ☐ Do you have thoughts that bother you or make you anxious and that you can't get rid of regardless of how hard you try?

☐ ☐ Do you have a tendency to keep things extremely clean or to wash your hands very frequently, more than other people you know?

☐ ☐ Do you check things over and over to excess?

☐ ☐ Do you have to straighten, order, or tidy things so much that it interferes with other things you want to do?

☐ ☐ Do you worry excessively about acting or speaking more aggressively than you should?

☐ ☐ Do you have great difficulty discarding things even when they have no practical value?

Obsessive-Compulsive Screening Checklist

People with OCD usually have difficulty with some of the following activities. Answer each question by circling the appropriate number next to it.

0   No problem with activity—takes me same time as average person. I do not need to repeat or avoid it.

1   Activity takes me twice as long as most people, or I have to repeat it twice, or I tend to avoid it.

2   Activity takes me three times as long as most people, or I have to repeat it three or more times, or I usually avoid it.

Score			Activity
0	1	2	Taking a bath or shower
0	1	2	Washing hands and face
0	1	2	Care of hair (eg, washing, combing, brushing)
0	1	2	Brushing teeth
0	1	2	Dressing and undressing
0	1	2	Using toilet to urinate
0	1	2	Using toilet to defecate
0	1	2	Touching people or being touched
0	1	2	Handling waste or waste bins
0	1	2	Washing clothes
0	1	2	Washing dishes
0	1	2	Handling or cooking food
0	1	2	Cleaning the house

0	1	2	Keeping things tidy
0	1	2	Bed making
0	1	2	Cleaning shoes
0	1	2	Touching door handles
0	1	2	Touching own genitals, petting or sexual intercourse
0	1	2	Throwing things away
0	1	2	Visiting a hospital
0	1	2	Turning lights and taps on or off
0	1	2	Locking or closing doors or windows
0	1	2	Using electrical appliances (eg, heaters)
0	1	2	Doing arithmetic or accounts
0	1	2	Getting to work
0	1	2	Doing own work
0	1	2	Writing
0	1	2	Form filing
0	1	2	Mailing letters
0	1	2	Reading
			Total

Total score > 10 increases the possibility of OCD, and further evaluation is recommended.

Total score > 20 is highly suggestive of OCD.

Modified from Greist, J. H., Jefferson, J.W., & Marks, I. M. (1986). *Anxiety and its treatment: Help is available.* Washington, DC: American Psychiatric Press.

PAIN ASSESSMENT TOOL

The Pain Assessment Tool is a clinical practice measurement of a patient's perception of pain and factors that contribute or reduce the level of pain.

1. Location: Patient or nurse mark drawing:

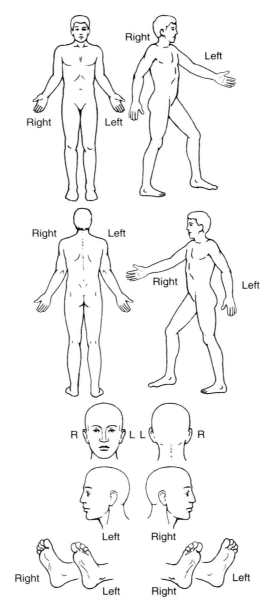

II. Intensity: Patient rates the pain. Scale used _____

   Present: _____

   Worse pain gets: _____

   Best pain gets: _____

   Acceptable level of pain: _____

III. Quality: (Use patient's own words, eg, prick, ache, burn, throb, pull, sharp) _____

IV. Onset, duration variations, rhythms: _____

_____

V. Manner of expressing pain: _____

_____

VI. What relieves the pain? _____

VII. What causes or increases the pain? _____

VIII. Effects of pain: (Note decreased function, decreased quality of life)

   Accompanying symptoms (eg, nausea) _____

   Sleep _____

   Appetite _____

   Physical activity _____

   Relationship with others (eg, irritability) _____

   Emotions (eg, anger, suicidal, crying) _____

   Concentration _____

   Other _____

IX. Other comments: _____

_____

X. Plan: _____

_____

Daily Diary

NAME: _____   DATE: _____

Time	Pain Rating Scale	Medication Type and Amount Taken	Other Pain Relief Measures Tried, or Anything That Influences Your Pain	Major Activity Being Done, Lying, Sitting, Standing/ Walking
12 midnight				
1 AM				
2				
3				
4				
5				
6				
7				
8				
9				
10				
11				
12 noon				
1				
2				
3				
4				
5				
6				
7				
8				
9				
10				
11				

Comments: _____

_____

McCaffery, M., & Beebe, A. (1989). *Pain clinical manual for nursing practice.* St. Louis: Mosby.

SHEEHAN PATIENT RATED ANXIETY SCALE

The Sheehan Patient Rated Anxiety Scale is a 46-question, self-rated measurement of a patient's level of anxiety.

Scoring and Interpretation: Assign a value of 0 to the first answer column ("Not at all"), 1 to the second column, 2 to the third, and so on. Scores above 30 are usually considered abnormal and scores above 80 are severe. The mean score in panic disorder and agoraphobia is 57 ± 20. The goal of treatment is to bring the score below 10.

Instructions: Below is a list of problems and complaints that people sometimes have. Part 1 asks about how you have felt during *the past week;* Part 2 asks about how you feel *right now.* Mark only one box for each problem, and do not skip any items.

Part 1—During the past week, how much did you suffer from . . .

	Not at all	A little	Moderately	Markedly	Extremely
1. Difficulty in getting your breath, smothering, or overbreathing					
2. Choking sensation or lump in throat					
3. Skipping, racing, or pounding of your heart					
4. Chest pain, pressure, or discomfort					
5. Bouts of excessive sweating					
6. Faintness, lightheadedness, or dizzy spells					
7. Sensation of rubbery or "jelly" legs					
8. Feeling off balance or unsteady like you might fall					
9. Nausea or stomach problems					
10. Feeling that things around you are strange, unreal, foggy, or detached from you					
11. Feeling outside or detached from part or all of your body or a floating feeling					

	Not at all	A little	Moderately	Markedly	Extremely
12. Tingling or numbness in parts of your body					
13. Hot flashes or cold chills					
14. Shaking or trembling					
15. Having a fear that you are dying or that something terrible is about to happen					
16. Feeling you are losing control or going insane					
17. Situational Anxiety Attack Sudden anxiety attacks with four or more symptoms listed previously that occur when you are in or about to go into a situation that is likely, from your experience, to bring on an attack.					
18. Unexpected Anxiety Attack Sudden unexpected anxiety attacks with four or more symptoms (listed previously) that occur with little or no provocation (ie, when you are *not* in a situation that is likely, from your experience, to bring on an attack).					
19. Unexpected Limited Symptom Attack Sudden unexpected spells with only one or two symptoms (listed previously) that occur with little or no provocation (ie, when you are *not* in a situation that is likely, from your experience, to bring on an attack).					

	Not at all	A little	Moderately	Markedly	Extremely
20. Anticipatory Anxiety Episode Anxiety episodes that build up as you anticipate doing something that is likely, from your experience, to bring on anxiety that is more intense than most people experience in such situations.					
21. Avoiding situations because they frighten you					
22. Being dependent on others					
23. Tension and inability to relax					
24. Anxiety, nervousness, restlessness					
25. Spells of increased sensitivity to sound, light, or touch					
26. Attacks of diarrhea					
27. Worrying about your health too much					
28. Feeling tired, weak, and exhausted easily					
29. Headaches or pains in neck or head					
30. Difficulty in falling asleep					
31. Waking in the middle of the night or restless sleep					
32. Unexpected waves of depression occurring with little or no provocation					
33. Emotions and moods going up and down a lot in response to changes around you					

	Not at all	A little	Moderately	Markedly	Extremely
34. Recurrent and persistent ideas, thoughts, impulses, or images that are intrusive, unwanted, senseless, or repugnant					
35. Having to repeat the same action in a ritual (eg, checking, washing, counting repeatedly) when it is not really necessary					

Part 2—Right now, at this moment . . .

	Not at all	A little	Moderately	Markedly	Extremely
1. Mouth drier than usual					
2. Worried, preoccupied					
3. Nervous, jittery, anxious, restless					
4. Afraid, fearful					
5. Tense, "uptight"					
6. Shaky inside or out					
7. Fluttery stomach					
8. Warm all over					
9. Sweaty palms					
10. Rapid or heavy heart beat					
11. Tremor of hands or legs					

Printed with permission courtesy of David V. Sheehan, MD, University of South Florida, Institute for Research in Psychiatry, Tampa, Florida.

SOCIAL DYSFUNCTION RATING SCALE (SDRS)

The SDRS was developed to assess the dysfunctional aspects of adjustment in areas of self, interpersonal, and performance systems.

The SDRS can evaluate patient change based on the total score, or it may be assessed on the five factor scores.

Factor 1: Apathetic detachment—Lack of goals, relationships, participation, interest
Factor 2: Dissatisfaction—Lack of leisure activities, need for friends
Factor 3: Hostility—Suspiciousness, hostility, anxiety
Factor 4: Health/finance concern—Self-health concern, financial insecurity
Factor 5: Manipulative dependency—Manipulation, overdependency

Instructions: Score each of the items as follows:
1. Not present   2. Very mild   3. Mild   4. Moderate   5. Severe   6. Very severe

	Score	Self-System
1.		Low self-concept (feelings of inadequacy, not measuring up to self ideal)
2.		Goallessness (lack of inner motivation and sense of future orientation)
3.		Lack of a satisfying philosophy or meaning of life (a conceptual framework for integrating past and present experiences)
4.		Self-health concern (preoccupation with physical health, somatic concerns)
		Interpersonal System
5.		Emotional withdrawal (degree of deficiency relating to others)
6.		Hostility (degree of aggression toward others)
7.		Manipulation (exploiting of environment, controlling at others' expense)
8.		Overdependency (degree of parasitic attachment to others)
9.		Anxiety (degree of feeling of uneasiness, impending doom)
10.		Suspiciousness (degree of distrust or paranoid ideation)
		Performance System
11.		Lack of satisfying relationships with significant persons (spouse, children, kin, significant persons serving in family role)
12.		Lack of friends, social contacts
13.		Expressed need for more friends, social contacts
14.		Lack of work (remunerative or nonremunerative, productive work activities that normally give a sense of usefulness, status, confidence)
15.		Lack of satisfaction from work
16.		Lack of leisure time activities
17.		Expressed need for more leisure, self-enhancing, satisfying activities
18.		Lack of participation in community activities
19.		Lack of interest in community affairs/activities that influence others
20.		Financial insecurity
21.		Adaptive rigidity (lack of complex coping patterns to stress)

Linn, M. W., Sculthorpe, W. B., Evge, M., Slater, P.H., & Goodman, S. P. (1969). A Social Dysfunction Rating Scale. *Journal of Psychiatric Research, 6,* 299–306.

Address inquiries regarding this scale to: Margaret W. Linn, PhD, Director, Social Science Research (151), Veterans Administration Medical Center, 1201 NW 16th Street, Miami, FL 33125. Reprinted with permission.

SPIRITUAL PERSPECTIVE CLINICAL SCALE (SPCS)

The SPCS is a self-rated instrument that measures a person's spiritual perspective as it relates to a transcendent or nonphysical realm, or to something greater than the self without disregarding the value of the individual.

Instruct the patient to answer the following questions by marking an "X" in the space above the group of words that best describes his or her feeling.

1. In talking with others, how often do you typically mention spiritual matters?

Not at all	Less than once a year	About once a year	About once a month	About once a week	About once a day
1	2	3	4	5	6

2. How often do you engage in private prayer?

Not at all	Less than once a year	About once a year	About once a month	About once a week	About once a day
1	2	3	4	5	6

3. To what extent do you agree or disagree that having a spiritual perspective is an important part of your life?

Strongly disagree	Disagree	Disagree more than agree	Agree more than disagree	Agree	Strongly agree
1	2	3	4	5	6

4. To what extent do you agree or disagree that you seek guidance in making decisions at this time of your life?

Strongly disagree	Disagree	Disagree more than agree	Agree more than disagree	Agree	Strongly agree
1	2	3	4	5	6

5. To what extent do you agree or disagree that you feel a sense of connectedness to God or a higher power in your life?

Strongly disagree	Disagree	Disagree more than agree	Agree more than disagree	Agree	Strongly agree
1	2	3	4	5	6

6. To what extent do you agree or disagree that your spiritual perspective helps to answer questions about the meaning of life?

Strongly disagree	Disagree	Disagree more than agree	Agree more than disagree	Agree	Strongly agree
1	2	3	4	5	6

Please feel free to express any views you may have about your spiritual perspective that have not been addressed by these six questions.

_____

_____

Scoring instructions: The SPCS is scored by calculating the arithmetic mean across all items, for a total score that ranges from 1.0 to 6.0. Responses to each item are selected using a 6-point Likert-type scale that is anchored with descriptive words for each of the six items. The instrument can be administered as a questionnaire or, better, in an interview format. The score may be compared with other scales previously reported in the literature based on the Spiritual Perspective Scale data, even though this clinically adapted instrument is being used here.

Reed, P. G. (1991). Spirituality and mental health of older adults: Extant knowledge for nursing. *Family and Community Health, 14*(2), 14. Reprinted with permission.

SUICIDE RISK ASSESSMENT TOOL

The following tool was developed by the Los Angeles Suicide Prevention Center to help identify persons at risk for suicide. Scores are given in each of several categories, then totaled and averaged based on the number of categories rated. An average score of 1 or 2 indicates that the patient is at low risk for suicide, a score of 3 to 6, at medium risk, and a score of 8 or 9, at high risk.

Low   Medium   High
1   2   3   4   5   6   7   8   9

Suicide Potential

_____ Age and sex   _____ Resources   _____ Total

_____ Symptoms   _____ Prior suicidal behavior   _____ Number of
                                                                                            categories related

_____ Stress   _____ Medical status   _____ Average

_____ Acute vs. chronic   _____ Communication aspects

_____ Suicidal plan   _____ Reaction of significant
                                                  other

Category		Rate	Rate for Category
Age and Sex (1–9)			
Male:	50 plus (7–9)		
	35–49 (4–6)		
	15–34 (1–3)		
Female:	50 plus (5–7)		
	35–49 (3–5)		
	15–34 (1–3)		
Symptoms (1–9)			
Severe depression, sleep disorder, anorexia, weight loss, withdrawal, despondent, loss of interest, apathy (7–9)			
Feelings of hopelessness, helplessness, exhaustion (7–9)			
Delusions, hallucination, loss of contact, disorientation (6–8)			
Compulsive gambler (6–8)			
Disorganization, confusion, chaos (5–7)			
Alcoholism, drug addiction, homosexuality (4–7)			
Agitation, tension, anxiety (4–6)			
Guilt, shame, embarrassment (4–6)			
Feelings of rage, anger, hostility, revenge (4–6)			
Poor impulse control, poor judgment (4–6)			
Frustrated dependency (4–6)			
Other (describe)			
Stress (1–9)			
Loss of loved person by death, divorce, separation (5–9)			
Loss of job, money, prestige, status (4–8)			
Sickness, serious illness, surgery, accident, loss of limb (3–7)			
Threat of prosecution, criminal involvement, exposure (4–6)			
Change(s) in life, environment, setting (4–6)			
Success, promotion, increased responsibilities (2–5)			
No significant stress (1–3)			
Other (describe)			

Category	Rate	Rate for Category
Acute versus Chronic (1–9)		
Sharp, noticeable, and sudden onset of specific symptoms (1–9)		
Recurrent outbreak of similar symptoms (4–9)		
Recent increase in long-standing traits (4–7)		
No specific recent change (1–4)		
Other (describe)		
Suicidal Plan (1–9)		
Lethality of proposed method—gun, jump, hanging, drowning, knife, poison, pills, aspirin (1–9)		
Availability of means in proposed method (1–9)		
Specific detail and clarity in organization of plan (1–9)		
Specificity in time planned (1–9)		
Bizarre plans (4–6)		
Rating of previous suicide attempts (1–9)		
No plans (1–3)		
Other (describe)		
Resources (1–9)		
No sources of support (family, friends, agencies, employment) (7–9)		
Family and friends available, unwilling to help (4–7)		
Available professional help, agency, or therapist (2–4)		
Family or friends willing to help (1–3)		
Stable life history (1–3)		
Physician or clergy available (1–3)		
Employed (1–3)		
Finances no problem (1–3)		
Other (describe)		
Prior Suicidal Behavior (1–7)		
One or more prior attempts of high lethality (6–7)		
One or more prior attempts of low lethality (4–5)		
History of repeated threats and depression (3–5)		

Category	Rate	Rate for Category
No prior suicidal or depressed history (1–3)		
Other (describe)		
Medical Status (1–7)		
Chronic debilitating illness (5–7)		
Pattern of failure in previous therapy (4–6)		
Many repeated unsuccessful experiences with doctors (4–6)		
Psychosomatic illness (such as asthma, ulcer) (2–4)		
Chronic minor illness complaints, hypochondria (1–3)		
No medical problems (1–2)		
Other (describe)		
Communication Aspects (1–7)		
Communication broken with rejection of efforts to reestablish by both patient and others (5–7)		
Communications have internalized goal (such as to cause guilt in others or to force behavior) (2–4)		
Communications directed toward world and people in general (3–5)		
Communications directed toward one or more specific persons (1–3)		
Other (describe)		
Reaction of Significant Other (1–7)		
Defensive, paranoid, rejected, punishing attitude (5–7)		
Denial of own or patient's need for help (5–7)		
No feelings of concern about the patient, does not understand the patient (4–6)		
Indecisiveness, feelings of helplessness (3–5)		
Alternation between feelings of anger and rejection and feelings of responsibility and desire to help (2–4)		
Sympathy and concern plus admission of need for help (1–3)		
Other (describe)		

From Los Angeles Suicide Prevention Center. (1980). *Assessment of suicidal potentiality.* Los Angeles: Author.

TRIADS

The TRIADS Assessment Tool was developed by A. Burgess (1990) at the University of Pennsylvania School of Nursing and refined by S. Brown (1991) to evaluate sexual abuse. It is also applicable to other types of abuse. It determines the severity of abuse and, therefore, can help to direct treatment strategies (Finkelhor, 1986).

TRIADS Assessment Tool

I. **T**ype of Abuse
   1. Physical abuse
   2. Sexual abuse
   3. Emotional abuse
   4. Spiritual abuse
II. **R**ole Relationship of Patient to Abuser
   1. Intrafamilial
   2. Extrafamilial
   3. Authority of abuse
III. **I**ntensity of Abuse
   1. Number of acts
   2. Number of abuses
   3. Types of abuse(s)
IV. **A**ffective State
   1. Expressed style (anxious, angry, sad)
   2. Controlled style (blank, calm, denial)
   3. Mixed style
V. **D**uration
   1. Length of time
VI. **S**tyle of Abuse
   1. Blitz style of abuse
   2. Repetitive/patterned abuse
   3. Ritualistic/ceremonial abuse
   4. Mutual abuse

Burgess, A. W., Hartman, C. R., & Kelley, S. J. (1990). Assessing child abuse: The TRIADS Checklist. *Journal of Psychosocial Nursing, 28*(4), 7.

Finkelhor, D. (1986). *A sourcebook on child sexual abuse.* Newbury Park, CA: Sage.

Brown, S. (1991). *Counseling victims of violence.* Alexandria, VA: American Counseling Association. Modified and used with permission.

Appendix *II*

Bibliography and Background Readings

Aguilera, D. C. (1990). *Crisis intervention: Theory and methodology* (6th ed.). St. Louis: Mosby-Yearbook.

American Psychiatric Association. (1994). *Diagnostic and statistical manual of mental disorders* (4th ed.). Washington, DC: Author.

Backman, M. E. (1989). *The psychology of the physically ill patient: A clinician's guide.* New York: Plenum Press.

Barry, P. D. (1996). *Psychosocial nursing: Care of physically ill patients and their families* (3rd ed.). Philadelphia: Lippincott-Raven.

Beattie, M. (1987). *Codependent no more.* Center City, MN: Hazelden.

Bulechek, G. M., & McCloskey, J. C. (Eds.) (1992). *Nursing interventions: Essential nursing treatments* (2nd ed.). Philadelphia: Saunders.

Burgess, W. (1983). *Community health nursing.* East Norwalk, CT: Appleton-Century-Crofts.

Busch, P. E. (1996). Panic disorder: The overlooked problem. *Home Healthcare Nurse, 14*(2), 111–116.

Busse, E. W., & Blazer, D. G. (1989). *Geriatric psychiatry.* Washington, DC: American Psychiatric Press.

Butler, R. N., Lewis, M., & Sunderland, T. (1991). *Aging and mental health: positive psychosocial and biomedical approaches* (4th ed.). New York: Merrill.

Carpenito, L. J. (1992). *Nursing diagnosis application to clinical practice* (4th ed.). Philadelphia: Lippincott.

Carson, V. B., & Arnold, E. N. (1996). *Mental health nursing: The nurse-patient journey.* Philadelphia: Saunders.

Chandler, S. C. (1993). Crisis theory and intervention. In B. S. Johnson (Ed.), *Psychiatric-mental health nursing: adaptation and growth* (3rd ed., pp. 661–674). Philadelphia: Lippincott.

Chenitz, W. C., Stone, J. T., & Salisbury, S. A. (1991). *Clinical gerontological nursing: a guide to advanced practice.* Philadelphia: Saunders.

Doenges, M. E., Townsend, M. C., & Moorhouse, M. F. (1989). *Psychiatric care plans guidelines for client care.* Philadelphia: Davis.

Dossey, B. M., Keegan, L., Guzzetta, C. E., & Kolkmeier, L. G. (1995). *Holistic nursing: a handbook for practice* (2nd ed.). Gaithersburg, MD: Aspen.

Dyer, J. G., Sparks, S. M., & Taylor, C. M. (1994). *Psychiatric nursing diagnoses: A comprehensive manual of mental health care.* Springhouse, PA: Springhouse.

Esser, A. H., & Lacey, S. D. (1989). *Mental illness: A homecare guide.* New York: Wiley.

Friel, J. C., & Friel, L. D. (1988). *Adult children: The secrets of dysfunctional families.* Deerfield Beach, FL: Health Communications.

Goldberg, T. E. (1995, October). Cognitive deficits in schizophrenia. *Current Approaches to Psychoses Diagnosis and Management, 4,* pp. 12–13.

Gorman, L. M., Sultan, D., & Luna-Raines, M. (1989). *Psychosocial nursing handbook for the nonpsychiatric nurse.* Baltimore: Williams & Wilkins.

Guze, S. B., & Robins, E. (1970). Suicide and primary affective disorders. *British Journal of Psychiatry, 117,* 437–438.

Harris, A. C. (1981). *Mental health practice for community nurses.* New York: Springer.

Hogstel, M. O. (Ed.). (1990). *Geropsychiatric nursing.* St. Louis: Mosby.

Huttunen, M. O. (1995, April). The expanding role of serotonin-dopamine antagonists in psychoses treatment. *Current Approaches to Psychoses Diagnosis and Management, 4,* pp. 2–3.

Johnson, B. S. (Ed.). (1993). *Psychiatric-mental health nursing adaptation and growth* (3rd ed.). Philadelphia: Lippincott.

Kaplan, H. I., & Sadock, B. J. (1988). *Clinical psychiatry from synopsis of psychiatry.* Baltimore: Williams & Wilkins.

Katon, W., Berg, A. O., & Robins, A. J. (1986). Depression—Medical utilization and somatization. *Western Journal of Medicine, 144,* 564–568.

Keys, M. (1985). *Four communication styles.* Conference presentation, Houston, TX. Miller Keys Associates.

Klebanoff, N. A. (1996). Psychosocial home care nursing. In B. S. Johnson (Ed.), *Psychiatric-mental health nursing: adaptation and growth* (4th ed.). Philadelphia: Lippincott.

Lederer, J. R., Marculescu, G. L., Mocnik, B., & Seaby, N. (1990). *Care planning pocket guide: A nursing diagnosis approach* (3rd ed.). Redwood City, CA: Addison-Wesley Nursing.

Lewis, S., Grainger, R. D. K., McDowell, W. A., Gregory, R. J., & Messner, R. L. (1989). *Manual of psychosocial nursing interventions promoting mental health in medical-surgical settings.* Philadelphia: Saunders.

Loftis, P. A. & Glover, T. L. (Eds.). (1993). *Decision making in gerontological nursing.* St. Louis: Mosby-Yearbook.

Maas, M., Buckwalter, K. C., & Hardy, M. (1991). *Nursing diagnoses and interventions for the elderly.* Redwood City, CA: Addison-Wesley Nursing.

McBride, A. B., & Austin, J. K. (1996). *Psychiatric-mental health nursing: Integrating the behavioral and biological sciences.* Philadelphia: Saunders.

McCloskey, J. C., & Bulechek, G. M. (1992). *Nursing interventions classification (NIC) Iowa intervention project.* St. Louis: Mosby-Yearbook.

McFarland, G. K., Wasli, E., & Gerety, E. K. (1992). *Nursing diagnosis and process in psychiatric mental health nursing* (2nd ed.). Philadelphia: Lippincott.

National Institute of Mental Health/National Institutes of Health. (1985). Consensus Development Conference Statement. Mood disorders: Pharmacologic prevention of recurrences. *American Journal of Psychiatry, 142,* 469–476.

Newman, D. K., & Smith, D. A. J. (1991). *Geriatric care plans.* Springhouse, PA: Springhouse.

North American Nursing Diagnosis Association (NANDA). (1994). *NANDA nursing diagnoses: Definitions and classification 1995–1996.* Philadelphia: Author.

Rawlins, R. P., & Heacock, P. E. (1993). *Clinical manual of psychiatric nursing* (2nd ed.). St. Louis: Mosby-Yearbook.

Reighley, J. W. (Ed.). (1988). *Nursing care planning guides for mental health.* Baltimore: Williams & Wilkins.

Rieger, D. A., Boyd, J. H., & Burke, J. D. (1988). One-month prevalence of mental disorders in the United States. *Archives of General Psychiatry, 45,* 977–986.

Roy, A. (1995, October). Risk factors for suicide in patients with schizophrenia. *Current Approaches to Psychoses Diagnosis and Management, 4,* pp. 10–11.

Schultz, J. M., & Videbeck, S. D. (1994). *Manual of psychiatric nursing care plans* (4th ed.). Philadelphia: Lippincott.

Shader, R. I. (Ed.). (1994). *Manual of psychiatric therapeutics* (2nd ed.). Boston: Little, Brown.

Siegel, D. (1992, June). The role of behavioral styles in communication. *DFW Nursing,* 18–20.

Skidmore-Roth, L. (1996). *Mosby's 1996 nursing drug reference.* St. Louis: Mosby-Yearbook.

Stanhope, M., & Knollmueller, R. N. (1996). *Handbook of community and home health nursing tools for assessment, intervention, and education* (2nd ed.). St. Louis: Mosby-Yearbook.

Stuart, G. W., & Sundeen, S. J. (1995). *Pocket guide to psychiatric nursing* (3rd ed.). St. Louis: Mosby-Yearbook.

Sullivan, E. J. (1995). *Nursing care of clients with substance abuse.* St. Louis: Mosby-Yearbook.

Townsend, M. C. (1991). *Nursing diagnoses in psychiatric nursing: A pocket guide for care plan construction* (2nd ed.). Philadelphia: Davis.

U.S. Department of Health and Human Services, Public Health Service, Agency for Health Care Policy and Research. (1993).

Depression in primary care: Detection, diagnosis and treatment. *Journal of Psychosocial Nursing, 31,* 1—9-28.

Wells, K. B., Stewart, A., & Hays, R. D. (1989). The functioning and well being of depressed patients: Results from the Medical Outcomes Study. *Journal of the American Medical Association, 262,* 914–919.

Winter, A., & Winter R. (1993). *Consumer's guide to free medical information by phone and by mail.* Englewood Cliffs, NJ: Prentice Hall.

Wise, M. G. & Rundell, J. R. (1994). *Concise guide to consultation psychiatry* (2nd ed.). Washington, DC: American Psychiatric Press.

Yudofsky, S. C., Hales, R. E., & Ferguson, T. (1991). *What you need to know about psychiatric drugs.* New York: Ballantine Books.

Zauszniewski, J. A. (1994). Potential sequelae of family history of depression: Identifying family members at risk. *Journal of Psychosocial Nursing and Mental Health Services, 32*(9), 15–21.

Index

Will you know what to do if your in-home patient...

✔ **becomes depressed and refuses to eat?**
✔ **is mobile but incontinent?**
✔ **shows signs of chemical abuse?**

Prepare today for the home-care challenges you'll face tomorrow!

Lippincott's Guide to
Behavior Management in Home Care

By **Nina A. Klebanoff, PhD, RN, CS, LPCC**
and **Nina Maria Smith, RNC, MEd**

Here's your survival guide to the management of behavior problems in today's home-care environment. With this compact reference, you'll discover a wealth of easy-to-follow nursing interventions geared specifically to promote mental wellness, facilitate patient education, and provide holistic care while helping you to cope with the stress of in-home nursing practice!

You'll cover the basics and address all important aspects of behavior management to help you...

- *Improve communication skills*
- *Discover safety and crisis intervention techniques*
- *Examine basic defensive, protective, and coping mechanisms*

And find practical discussions of more than 70 behaviors — including 40 categories of behavior problems — which are listed alphabetically and cross-referenced for easy access. Don't face your next in-home patient unprepared...

Meet the demands of home behavioral health care with confidence!

ISBN 0-397-55432-X

90000

9 780397 554324